AF757010

THEORIES AND PRACTICES OF PSYCHOANALYSIS IN CENTRAL EUROPE

Theories and Practices of Psychoanalysis in Central Europe explores the close relationship between psychoanalysis, psycho-medical discourses, literature, and the visual arts of the late 1800s and early 1900s in Central Europe.

Agnieszka Sobolewska addresses the issue of theories and practices of psychoanalysis in Central Europe and the need to undertake interdisciplinary reflection on the specificity of psychoanalytic literary genres and fin-de-siècle psycho-medical discourses. With a focus on the circulation of Freudianism in the territories of present-day Austria, Hungary, the Czech Republic, Poland, and Germany, the book considers the creative transformations that psychoanalytic thought underwent in these countries and reflects on the specificity of psychoanalytic literary genres and the pivotal role of lifewriting genres in the psychoanalytic movement. Sobolewska's work both fills a visible gap in research on the history of psychoanalysis in Central Europe before the outbreak of World War II and offers the first insightful analysis of the role of life writing in the development of psychoanalytic thought.

Theories and Practices of Psychoanalysis in Central Europe will be of great interest to psychoanalysts in practice and in training as well as scholars of the history of psychoanalysis, the history of psychology, literature, cultural anthropology, and modernism.

Agnieszka Sobolewska, PhD, teaches at the Institute of Polish Culture, University of Warsaw. She specializes in the cultural history of psychoanalysis in Central and Eastern Europe. She is the author of articles and books devoted to life writing and psychoanalysis, the cultural history of psychology in Poland, and German colonial imagination.

HISTORY OF PSYCHOANALYSIS

Series Editor
Peter L. Rudnytsky

This series seeks to present outstanding new books that illuminate any aspect of the history of psychoanalysis from its earliest days to the present, and to reintroduce classic texts to contemporary readers.

Other titles in the series:

Karl Abraham
Life and Work, a Biography
Anna Bentinck van Schoonheten

The Freudian Orient
Early Psychoanalysis, Anti-Semitic Challenge, and the Vicissitudes of Orientalist Discourse
Frank F. Scherer

Occultism and the Origins of Psychoanalysis
Freud, Ferenczi and the Challenge of Thought Transference
Maria Pierri, Translated by Adam Elgar

Sigmund Freud and the Forsyth Case
Coincidences and Thought-Transmission in Psychoanalysis
Maria Pierri, Translated by Adam Elgar

A Brief Apocalyptic History of Psychoanalysis
Erasing Trauma
Carlo Bonomi

Theories and Practices of Psychoanalysis in Central Europe
Narrative Assemblages of Self Analysis, Life Writing, and Fiction
Agnieszka Sobolewska

For further information about this series please visit https://www.routledge.com/The-History-of-Psychoanalysis-Series/book-series/KARNHIPSY

THEORIES AND PRACTICES OF PSYCHOANALYSIS IN CENTRAL EUROPE

Narrative Assemblages of Self-Analysis, Life Writing, and Fiction

Agnieszka Sobolewska

Routledge
Taylor & Francis Group
LONDON AND NEW YORK

Designed cover image: Getty | Krimzoya

First published 2024
by Routledge
4 Park Square, Milton Park, Abingdon, Oxon OX14 4RN

and by Routledge
605 Third Avenue, New York, NY 10158

Routledge is an imprint of the Taylor & Francis Group, an informa business

British Library Cataloguing-in-Publication Data
A catalogue record for this book is available from the British Library

ISBN: 978-1-032-57976-4 (hbk)
ISBN: 978-1-032-57975-7 (pbk)
ISBN: 978-1-003-44189-2 (ebk)

DOI: 10.4324/9781003441892

Typeset in Times New Roman
by Taylor & Francis Books

For Kasia

CONTENTS

Acknowledgments ix

Introduction 1

1 Reading Sigmund Freud's correspondence with Wilhelm Fliess: Between a lover's discourse and self-analysis 34

2 The sexological discourse on non-normative sexuality: Sándor Ferenczi, Richard von Krafft-Ebing, and Magnus Hirschfeld 68

3 The interpretation of literary dreams: Psychoanalysis, trauma, and painful modernity – the case of Mihály Babits 92

4 The specters of psychoanalysis in interwar Prague: Bohuslav Brouk and Jindřich Štyrský 122

5 The queer case of Piotr Odmieniec Włast: (Psycho)biography, psychoanalysis, and the origins of anti-psychiatric discourse in Poland 150

6 Freud's queer fellow: Georg Groddeck between psychoanalytic theory and literary modernism 172

7 Practicing friendship – a new beginning for psychoanalytic theory and practice: Ferenczi between Georg Groddeck and Elizabeth Severn 206

8 Conclusion 236
9 Appendix 245

Index *251*

ACKNOWLEDGMENTS

This book would not have been possible without the intellectual collaboration, friendship, and support I have received from researchers specializing in different fields whom I was fortunate to meet over the past few years. I am deeply indebted to the scientific community of my home, the Institute of Polish Culture at the University of Warsaw. The intellectual ferment I found there has nurtured my interest in critical theory, anthropology of culture, anthropology of writing, and anthropology of literature. My studies at Sorbonne University, first in its master's program and then its doctoral school, have sensitized me to the philosophical aspects of translation, gradually leading me to an inexhaustible fascination with the polyphonic languages of Central European culture(s). The Eur'Orbem (Sorbonne University/CNRS) team in Paris and the Centre français de recherche en sciences sociales (USR 3138 CNRS-MAEDI) in Prague proved to be most helpful in expanding my knowledge of Central and Eastern Europe. I am certainly unable to mention all the scholars and academics to whom this book and myself are beholden. Nonetheless, I would like to express special gratitude to: Antal Bókay, Adam Bžoch, Maciej Duda, Josef Fulka, Daniela Finzi, Jean-François Laplénie, Adam Lipszyc, Marta Rakoczy, Paweł Rodak, Clara Royer, Peter L. Rudnytsky, Max Saunders, Małgorzata Smorąg-Goldberg, Sandra Sparber, and Mónika Takács.

Most of the chapters in this book were written in Prague and Vienna, where I lived from 2021 to 2023. The final title and subject matter owe much to an international series of seminars entitled "Rethinking Psychoanalysis in Central Europe: Interdisciplinary and Transnational Perspectives," which were held in 2022 at the Centre français de recherche en sciences sociales in Prague. I am very thankful to the wonderful scholars who took part in the event I organized and shared their knowledge. I would like to extend my special thanks to all the guest speakers and discussants at the event: Adam Bžoch, Judit

Mészáros, Peter L. Rudnytsky, Klara Naszkowska, Anna Borgos, Paweł Rodak, Jean-François Laplénie, Mónika Takács, Clara Royer, Mateusz Chmurski, and Mathieu Lericq. Moreover, this cycle of seminars would not have been possible without the institutional and organizational support of Jérôme Heurtaux and Claire Madl.

My book is the outcome of an individual grant project entitled "Between Self-Analysis and Autobiography. Everyday Writing Practices of Freud's Disciples and Their Impact on the Psychoanalytic Theory," no. DI2017 004647, awarded by the Ministry of Science and Higher Education of the Republic of Poland (2018–2022). Scholarships I received from the Centre français de recherche en sciences sociales (USR 3138 CNRS-MAEDI) for the academic year 2021/2022 and from the Institute for Human Sciences (Institut für die Wissenschaften vom Menschen, IWM) in Vienna, under the Józef Tischner Award and Fellowship (2022/2023), not only gave me unlimited access to libraries and archives in Central European cities (primarily in Prague, Vienna, and Budapest), but also ensured excellent working conditions in intellectually stimulating international scientific communities.

It sometimes happens that a book owes much to one person in particular. I would like to express my utmost gratitude to Peter L. Rudnytsky, who has provided me with remarkably caring and thoughtful scientific supervision in recent years. His critical comments on my papers, including extensive excerpts from this book, have become a veritable source of inspiration and a compass directing me into yet uncharted territories of the fascinating world of psychoanalytic thought. His excellent books, especially *Reading Psychoanalysis: Freud, Rank, Ferenczi, Groddeck* (2002) and *Mutual Analysis: Ferenczi, Severn, and the Origins of Trauma Theory* (2022), remain the greatest influence on my thinking *about* and thinking *with* psychoanalysis. I also want to thank Peter for the careful reading of the first version of this book's manuscript and for accepting it for publication in the History of Psychoanalysis book series.

Finally, Susannah Frearson, Saloni Singhania, and Alanna Donaldson have been a great help in the process of preparing the manuscript for publication. I thank them for their comments and their patience in improving its final version. I am also very grateful to Aleksandra Paszkowska for her excellent language guidance. Her valuable comments and revisions helped me to avoid potential stylistic awkwardness and language errors.

INTRODUCTION

In this book, I treat psychoanalysis as a heterogeneous amalgam of theories and practices immersed in specific social and cultural contexts not only of fin-de-siècle Vienna but – more broadly – of turn-of-the-century Central Europe. I will look at psychoanalysis as a polyphonic discourse formed at the intersection of psycho-medical science, literature, and life writing. In the following chapters, I write about psychoanalysis as a *narrative assemblage* – a set of cultural practices involving specific writing forms, narrative strategies, and analytical techniques rather than a purely theoretical system.

I define this "narrative assemblage" as a set of narrative strategies that were typical of the psycho-medical and literary discourses of the late 1800s and early 1900s that bred early psychoanalytic discourse. Freud's writings, like those of his closest associates, were based on diverse models of psychoanalytic knowledge expression and required the development of narrative strategies. The perspective I propose in this book will allow me to rediscover the heterogeneity of psychoanalytic literature as a fusion of scientific, literary, and lifewriting discourses developed under specific cultural, social, and political contexts. The development of such perspectives as intellectual and social history, cultural history, and then comparative cultural history made it possible to write about psychoanalysis not as an abstract theoretical system, but a component of the hybrid and polyethnic culture of turn-of-the-century Habsburg Empire.

As Carl E. Schorske has pointed out, psychoanalysis was a key component of the "modernist turn taken in Viennese high culture in the fin-de-siècle" (Schorske 1998: 15). As part of this turn, Freud's works brought a new understanding of the human psyche and of psycho-sexual development. As Schorske put it:

DOI: 10.4324/9781003441892-1

> The very word "modernism" has come to distinguish our lives and times from what had gone before, from history as a whole, as such. Modern architecture, modern music, modern science – all these have defined themselves not so much *out* of the past, indeed scarcely *against* the past, but detached from it in a new, autonomous cultural space. The modern mind grew indifferent to history, for history, conceived as a continuous nourishing tradition, became useless to its projects.
>
> *(Ibid.: 4)*

The new "autonomous cultural space" was marked by a rupture with the past and with well-established models of understanding the self. The modernist revolution that took place in economics and technology in the second half of the nineteenth century in Central Europe found a reflection in fin-de-siècle psycho-medical discourses, the visual arts, music, and literature. As Laura Marcus has noted in the context of the emergence of the so-called new modernist studies, "at the turn of the twentieth century literature, culture, and technology entered into a close relationship with each other, determining the ways of experiencing modernity" (Marcus 2014: 3; Berman 1983: 87–130; Figes 2019). To this triad, we should also add science, especially psycho-medical literature, which by the late 1800s had adopted the genres and narrative structures typical of personal writing (literary genres, lifewriting genres), rarely associated with scientific language.

The modernists' genuine desire to break the chains of tradition paradoxically resulted in their repeated efforts to redefine it. Ultimately, the rejection of tradition became a way of establishing a new relationship with it. The revolution of those who called themselves "The Young Ones" (*Die Jungen*) in the 1880s and 1890s was a rebellion against the Laws of the Fathers. As Schorske added in this context:

> Over time their initial search for community and for a reordering of society gave place to a preoccupation with the psychological. This concern found creative expression not only in psychoanalysis but also in a new intellectual cohort of visual and literary artists. For them social pessimism and existential anguish fueled the quest for a new art beyond generational or historical concerns. This psychological tendency gave its special stamp to Viennese modernism.
>
> *(Schorske 1998: 12)*

In the case of psychoanalysis, the modernist break with the "virtue of absorbing history and its elements eclectically" manifested itself in the pursuit of inventing a universal theory – a story about human nature that would work regardless of the place, time, and cultural context in which it was told.

As a man educated in the culture of the second half of the nineteenth century, Sigmund Freud invented psychoanalysis that was both a discourse critical of the past and one that transmitted certain aspects of the nineteenth-century order of thought (i.e. evolutionism, a linear view of the development of cultures) to twentieth-century sciences (Khanna 2003; Zaretsky 2005; Müller 2019; Mazurel 2021; Swartz 2022). Both Freud's early and late writings, in which he reflected on the origins of Judeo-Christian culture (*Totem and Taboo*) and the roots of monotheism (*The Man Moses and the Monotheist Religion*), established psychoanalysis as an innovative language that would prevail in intellectual thought throughout the twentieth century as well as a subjective tool for critically situating the self in relation to the past and present. This resulted in an "ambiguous mixture of self-conscious rupture and transmuted tradition" (Schorske 1998: 15; Le Rider 1993).

The cities of psychoanalysis

As a city woven of contrasts, Vienna 1900 was "the capital of both the high nobility and of liberal intellectuals, of the splendid Ringstrasse and endless slum areas, of anti-Semitism and Zionism, of a rigid conservatism and emerging Modernism" (Wipplinger 2019: 4). I argue that the "special stamp" of Viennese modernism was in fact impressed onto the broader fin-de-siècle culture in Central Europe in its polyphonic and hybrid nature (Magris 2013; Le Rider 1994). The dynamic dialogue between artists, writers, and representatives of psycho-medical sciences suggested that the boundaries between literature, the visual arts, music, and medicine were fluid. The effort holistically to rethink human nature did not take place in a single discipline but required the exploration of diverse media (the word, the image, the sound) and the fusion of many mutually interacting modes of expression (Janik & Toulmin 1973; Worbs 1983; Frankland 2000).

Painters such as Gustav Klimt, Egon Schiele, and Károly Kernstok, composers like Gustav Mahler, Anton Bruckner, Arnold Schoenberg, and Béla Bartók, and writers such as Hugo von Hofmannsthal, Artur Schnitzler, and Mihály Babits, among many others, exploited various media to challenge the prevailing trends of expressing the experiences of inner and outer worlds. By putting their audiences' senses to the test, the artists sought to transfigure and expand their perceptual capabilities. The worlds that they created, in which logical structures of thought confronted the dynamics of the unconscious, were built on thousands of pages of manuscripts, musical scores, and canvases: in Mahler's and Bruckner's monumental symphonies, Mann's novels, Musil's *Man Without Qualities* and small forms such as Schoenberg's *Sechs kleine Klavierstücke*, Bartók's *Mikrokosmos*, Hugo von Hofmannsthal's tragedies, Arthur Schnitzler's novellas, Babits's verses, and Franz Kafka's short stories. In this context, psychoanalysis – as an assemblage of theories and practices – can also be perceived as a monumental pursuit of reorganizing the image of humankind and the culture it has produced.

Scholars' initial interest in fin-de-siècle Vienna was quickly followed by an increased fascination with other Central and Eastern European capitals, particularly Budapest and Prague. In the last decades of the Austro-Hungarian Empire, Vienna and Budapest shared "a common destiny, tradition, and culture," and at the same time were "divided by their history, character, tradition, and culture" (Hanák 1998: xv). Significantly, Budapest proved to be a key city for the transmission and development of psychoanalysis before the outbreak of the First World War, second only to Vienna (Mészáros 2014).

In the first decades of the twentieth century, Freud's thought became rapidly internationalized. Psychoanalysis – the subject of lively discussion and reflection in medical, literary, and artistic circles in Central and Eastern Europe – was transmitted to Western European countries and the United States (Dybel 2019). Subsequently, by becoming an international language, psychoanalysis as a cultural practice gained its local iterations. Freud's thought reached the furthest corners of the Habsburg Empire, finding followers in Central and Eastern European cities now in the Czech Republic, Slovakia, Poland, Hungary, Romania, Ukraine, Croatia, and Serbia (Mészáros 2017: 91–103).

Local psychoanalytic societies and groups that formed before World War II strove for close alignment with the centers of psychoanalysis, which were represented pre-1938 by the Vienna Psychoanalytic Society and the International Psychoanalytic Association (established in 1910). At the same time, local groups also invented original theories and therapeutic methods, of which the Budapest Psychoanalytic School was the best example (Rachman 2016). The heterogeneity of psychoanalytic literature also resulted from translating works by Freud and his closest followers into national languages, in which categories fundamental to the psychoanalytic theory gained new meanings directly stemming from local cultural and linguistic contexts.

The plurality of modernisms

The decentralized perspective recently proposed by scholars of modernist cultures made it possible to look at psychoanalysis as an internally diversified cultural practice – one that was geographically dispersed and embedded in local temporalities. From such a belief came the seminal category of the "cultural parataxis," introduced by Susan Stanford Friedman (2007: 35–52). It allowed researchers to examine the specificity of local modernisms while at the same time shifting away from the "postcolonial paradigms of centers and peripheries" (Kornhauser & Siewior 2015: 12). Several years later, in opposition to Friedman's "cultural parataxis" – the transnational "development of a common program, the construction of theories and the creation of manifestos" – Polish researchers of Central European avant-garde movements proposed the category of "cultural paralaxis": one that concerned the development of local vanguard groups and their unique aesthetic propositions (Ibid.: 12–13). The categories of "parataxis" and "paralaxis" brilliantly capture not only the dynamics of the development of Central European vanguards, but can also be applied to Central and Eastern European modernist cultures evolving simultaneously locally and supra-locally.

At the outset, this book's perspective is that of a "comparative cultural history" as defined by Péter Hanák. Emerging from Carl Schorske's work on the social, political, and intellectual history of fin-de-siècle Vienna (Schorske 1980), this comparative cultural history asks about cultural practices developed in varied social and political contexts. As Hanák pointed out, "culture" cannot be seen purely as:

> the manifestation of an "absolute" spirit, but in a constant interaction with society. In this sense, cultural history is akin to social and intellectual history, but goes beyond it, by embracing also a society's principal conventions (*Gewohnheitskultur*). This in turn brings cultural history close to the field of research dealing with everyday life, and at the same time expand its horizons to encompass the mentality and traditions that govern everyday life.
>
> *(Hanák 1998: xviii)*

A focus on everyday life makes it possible to show the heterogeneity of local cultural practices. It also helps us to appreciate more deeply the determinants of people's everyday experiences in given cultural, social, and political contexts. In such a perspective, the cultural reality consists of everyday practices – reading books and newspapers, writing letters, visiting sanatoriums, and walking around urban metropolises. A comparative cultural history also allows the study of writing, reading, and research practices in their local (paralaxis) as well as supra-local dimensions (parataxis).

As I will demonstrate, the recognition of psychoanalysis as a cultural practice raises questions not only about the social and political context of its origins but also about its languages (plural form intended) and the specific genres they represented, in which the personal, the subjective and the autobiographical merged with the objective and impersonal. Once psychoanalytic literature is examined for its generic features, it can be treated as one of the experimental languages of Central European modernism(s). As Schorske wrote: "All autobiography is personal history, a narrative construction that involves both remembering and forgetting, evoking some parts of one's past and repressing others" (Schorske 1998: 5). The autobiographical text is considered here as the record of what is remembered and forgotten (repressed). Autobiography (and, more broadly, any lifewriting practices) is always a narrative construction and consists of diverse forms of written expression. In the case of psychoanalytic literature, the theoretical text and the case study never purported to be an impersonal discourse, but were rather a record of the subjective perception of the patient's story, in which the observation of another was confronted with the knowledge and self-awareness of the physician-author.

Psychoanalysis and life writing

In his monumental biography *Freud: A Life for Our Time*, Peter Gay observed that "the entanglement of autobiography with science has bedeviled psychoanalysis from its beginnings" (Gay 1988: 89). The languages of psychoanalysis emerged at the intersection of the subjective (personal) and the scientific (impersonal) – between self-analysis and autobiography on the one hand and between psycho-medical discourses and literary narratives on the other hand. To the early psychoanalysts, who later became Freud's biographers, the autobiographical dimension of his theoretical writings was evident.

In 1946, an article by Siegfried Bernfeld entitled "An Unknown Autobiographical Fragment by Freud" was published. The author drew attention to the autobiographical character of Freud's essay "Screen Memories" (1899), calling it "a dense mosaic of memory and fantasy" (Mautner 1994: 326). Freud himself suggested such an interpretive key to his followers and invited them to do an autobiographical reading of his works. In the preface to the second edition of *The Interpretation of Dreams*, he wrote:

> An equal durability and power to withstand any far-reaching alterations during the process of revision has been shown by the *material* of the book, consisting as it does of dreams of my own which have for the most part been overtaken or made valueless by the march of events and by which I illustrated the rules of dream-interpretation. For this book has a further subjective significance for me personally – a significance which I only grasped after I had completed it. It was, I found, a portion of my own self-analysis, my reaction to my father's death – that is to say, to the most important event, the most poignant loss, of a man's life. Having discovered that this was so, I felt unable to obliterate the traces of the experience.
>
> *(Freud [1899] 2010: xxvi)*

Although its author admitted that *The Interpretation of Dreams* was a sort of autobiography and "part of [his] own self-analysis," it became for that very reason the founding text of a new science.

It should be noted, though, that pointing to the autobiographical dimension of any text is not the same as considering it an autobiography (Saunders 2010: 165–207). *The Interpretation of Dreams* revealed only selected tropes from Freud's affective life. Rather than offer a linear account of how one "becomes what one is," to paraphrase Nietzsche (2007), it remained a distorted and flickering reflection of its author (Marcus 1999: 1–65). Similar to the dynamics of a dream, there were many overt and covert deformations. But while dreams are produced by the unconscious, the author deliberately covered his tracks and deceived his readers, including future biographers.

Freud wrote about his dislike for the biographical genre to his fiancée Martha Bernays as early as the mid-1880s: "As for the biographers, let them worry, we have no desire to make it easy for them. […] I am already looking forward to seeing them go astray" (Clark 1980: 63).[1] Therefore, to make things more difficult for potential biographers, Freud decided to destroy all personal notes and letters which in the future could expose "to the public gaze more of the intimacies of [his] mental life" (Freud 2010: xxiv). And yet, although distrustful of the biography, Freud (1914: 207–260) reached for this genre in 1914, when he was outlining the history of the psychoanalytic movement. Later, in 1925, he turned to the genre of autobiography, drafting his "Autobiographical Study" – a text that combined the psychoanalytic movements' collective autobiography and the subjective portrait of its creator (Freud 1959b: 7–74).

After World War I, autobiographies and biographies began to gain a more prominent position in psychoanalytic literature. Freud's first associates, such as Ernest Jones, Fritz Wittels, and Isidor Sadger, devoted themselves to writing biographies of the psychoanalytic movement, creating psychological portraits of Freud and composing their own memoirs. From the advent of the Vienna Psychoanalytic Society, psychoanalysts were also eager to create psychological studies of famous writers and artists. Early psychoanalytic literature, combining the idea of unmasking and deduction drawn from detective fiction with the classic case study, gave birth to a new lifewriting genre – the psychoanalytic psychography (German: Psychographie) (Sobolewska 2021b: 561–578).

Sadger had already written about psychography as a psychoanalytic genre in 1912. In his article "From Pathography to Psychography" ("Von der Pathographie zur Psychographie"), published in *Imago*, he argued:

> One of the new and most important tasks of any future biography will be to trace the intimate and constant interrelationships between [the subject's] love life and his work. […] Any future psychography, therefore, in order to be exhaustive, will have to include a pathographic chapter […]. The most important matter, however, remains always and at all times the explanation of the psychic connections evident in the life as well as in the work of every genius.
>
> *(Sadger 1912: 162, 164)*[2]

The gradual psychologization of the image of the creative genius led to the replacement of pathography – a popular writing genre among nineteenth-century physicians and psychiatrists which combined psychiatric diagnosis (usually indicating a hereditary burden on the artist or writer) with a biographical narrative – with psychography, in which psychoanalytic theory now functioned as the basic framework for understanding the life story of a great creator. Freud referred to the psychoanalytic psychography in his Goethe Prize speech:

> I am prepared for the reproach that we analysts have forfeited the right to place ourselves under the patronage of Goethe because we have offended against the respect due to him by trying to apply analysis to him himself: we have degraded the great man to the position of an object of analytic investigation. But I would dispute at once that any degradation is intended or implied by this.
>
> *(Freud [1930] 1961b: 210–211)*

The most important idea behind the psychoanalytic psychography was to abandon the pathologization of the writer or artist – which had been a distinctive element of the nineteenth-century pathography. Both Sadger's early theoretical article and Freud's remarks indicated the importance of the psychographic genre in early psychoanalytic literature. In the first decades of the twentieth century, psychographies and psychoanalytic interpretations of selected literary, musical, and visual works were written by Isidor Sadger, Karl Abraham, Theodor Reik, Ernest Jones, Fritz Wittels, Otto Rank, and Max Graf, among others.[3] The psychoanalytic psychography as a writing genre – an amalgam of the biography and the psychoanalytic case study – contributed to the birth of the so-called "new biography" after the Great War (Saunders 2010: 438–483).

In the following chapters, I will show that life writing became central to psychoanalytic literature in both overt and covert ways. Along with psychoanalytic psychographies, autobiographies, and biographies by Freud's followers, lifewriting genres laid the foundations for psychoanalytic theoretical writings. Autobiographies, alongside diaries and letters, very often served the first psychoanalysts as primary sources in their work on psychographies and psychoanalytic case studies. Moreover, occasionally, instead of working directly with the patient, the psychoanalyst used daily quasi-ethnographic records of the patient's behavior and condition made by a family member and later delivered to the psychoanalyst (Freud [1909] 1955b: 3–154). The psychoanalyst's narrative work consisted in transforming the patient's fragmented story into a linear discourse that also corresponded with the formal structure of psychography as a psychoanalytic biography of the patient's affective life.

In addition to being biographers (of their patients, of the psychoanalytic movement, of its creator) and autobiographers, psychoanalysts also stepped into the role of lifewriting genre theorists. They wrote about the psychoanalytic understanding of life writing (including the autobiography, the biography, and the diary) and the uses that psychoanalysis could make of lifewriting genres. In "Psycho-Analytic Notes on an Autobiographical Account of a Case of Paranoia," Freud stated that published memoirs provided sufficient material for analytical work:

> Since paranoics cannot be compelled to overcome their internal resistances, and since in any case they only say what they choose to say, it follows that this is precisely a disorder in which a written report or a printed

> case history can take the place of personal acquaintance with the patient. For this reason I think it is legitimate to base analytic interpretations upon the case history of a patient suffering from paranoia (or, more precisely, from dementia paranoides) *whom I have never seen, but who has written his own case history and brought it before the public in print* [italics mine].
>
> *(Freud [1911] 1958: 9)*

In the absence of any possibility of working directly with the patient, psychoanalysis would be transformed from a "talking cure" into a tool for interpreting the autobiographical text.

Later, in post-war psychoanalytic reflection, the autobiographical genre was very often considered a "contradiction in terms" (Rycroft 1985: 191–277). The emerging psychoanalytic understanding of "the self" and the emphasis on the crucial role played by the unconscious changed the image of the writing subject in the first half of the twentieth century. Subsequently, psychoanalysis came to consider the genre of formal autobiography as a kind of mask or narcissistic projection. Allegations of a lack of authenticity were also directed against the biographical genre. In this context, Freud stated:

> We all, who revere Goethe, put up, without too much protest, with the efforts of his biographers, who try to recreate his life from existing accounts and indications. But what can these biographers achieve for us? Even the best and fullest of them could not answer the two questions which alone seem worth knowing about.
>
> *(Freud [1930] 1961b: 211)*

Freud asked what the point of writing a biography was if it did not solve the "riddle of the miraculous gift" or capture the "value" of a great artist's work.

A different, positive attitude towards the biographical genre was expressed by Marie Bonaparte in her text titled "A Defense of Biography" (1939: 231–240). Shortly after Freud's death, Bonaparte reflected on the psychology of life preservation in life writing and personal documents. The desire to preserve a part of oneself collided with the desire for its complete destruction – the obliteration of any written traces that might posthumously reveal the most intimate details of one's emotional and erotic life. Biography – as a genre that relies on diaries and private correspondence – was, in Bonaparte's eyes, a written form of "the battle against oblivion" (Ibid.: 240). She also added:

> Biography indeed, has another and higher function than the mere satisfaction of an idle or unhealthy curiosity. [...] Biographies of men and women of the past bring to light the unity of human nature and are really like family portraits in which we recognize now one and now another of our own features.
>
> *(Ibid.: 239)*

In Bonaparte's view, the biographical genre was a kind of intimate "family portrait." In a similar way, Siegfried Bernfeld also saw lifewriting genres as a written "battle against oblivion." In his text entitled "Relics and Diaries" ("Reliquien und Tagebücher") (Bernfeld 1930: 370–381), Bernfeld wrote about diaries as "relics" – material pieces of their authors. In the eyes of the first psychoanalysts, the most personal records (maintained in the form of secret diaries, unpublished autobiographical sketches, memoirs or letters) functioned as a best way to reveal the emotional life of the patient.

From the perspective of its generic features, psychoanalytic literature can be treated as a set of heterogeneous discourses formed at the intersection of scientific expertise, self-analysis, life writing, and literature. While self-analysis became the *sine qua non* of psychoanalytic reflection, the narrative that stemmed from it required the insertion of one's story (or the patient's story) into the specific framework of a genre. In the first psychoanalysts' everyday writing practices, (self-)analytical material was transformed into both theoretical and autobiographical/biographical narratives. A close reading that is sensitive to the narrative polyphony and plasticity of psychoanalytic languages will allow me to examine it as a multilayered narrative assemblage combining elements of turn-of-the-century psycho-medical discourses, life writing, philosophy, and literature – rather than as a defined and stable discourse with a fixed system of meaning.

Psychoanalysis and fiction

The literary dimension of Freud's great case studies prompts deeper reflection not only on the relationship between psychoanalysis and literature but also on psychoanalytic writings as literary documents (Mahony 1987; Brooks 1992: 90–112). From the patient's dreams, childhood memories, and confessions, the psychoanalyst created a new story which – as an interpretation of the patients' words – transcended mere description, functioning instead as a narrative that was at once psychobiographical (a reconstruction of the patient's psycho-sexual development), psychoanalytic (interpretative), and literary (the patient as the protagonist of the case study).

The work of the psychoanalyst, requiring the development of specific narrative structures and skillful storytelling, approximated the work of the writer, although it was not identical to it. Freud wrote about this in his "Delusion and Dream in Jensen's *Gradiva*":

> An author, we hear them say, should keep out of the way of any contact with psychiatry and should leave the description of pathological mental states to the doctors. The truth is that no truly creative writer has ever obeyed this injunction. The description of the human mind is indeed the domain which is most his own; he has from time

> immemorial been the precursor of science, and so too of scientific psychology. But the frontier between states of mind described as normal and pathological is in part a conventional one and in part so fluctuating that each of us probably cross it many time in the course of a day. [...] Thus the creative writer cannot evade the psychiatrist nor the psychiatrist the creative writer, and the poetic treatment of a psychiatric theme can turn out to be correct without any sacrifice of its beauty.
>
> *(Freud [1907] 1959a: 43–44)*

Writing about the encounter between a psychiatrist and a writer, Freud pointed out their common working tool, which was the text. If a literary work can provide the treatment of a patient, then a psycho-medical study can also have aesthetic value. Freud stressed the universality of creative fantasy and the psychological mechanisms responsible for literary production. In "Creative Writers and Daydreaming," he stated:

> If we could at least discover in ourselves or in people like ourselves an activity which was in some way akin to create writing! An examination of it would then give us a hope of obtaining the beginnings of an explanation of the creative work of writers. And, indeed, there is some prospect of this being possible. After all, creative writers themselves like to lessen the distance between their kind and the common run of humanity; they so often assure us that every man is a poet at heart and that the last poet will not perish till the last man does.
>
> *(Freud [1908] 1959a: 143)*

The close relationship between psychoanalytic and literary textual production does not mean that a psychoanalytic text always has a literary dimension. Great case studies (especially that of Dora as a quasi-novel *à clef*), even when read as literary texts, do not qualify as novels *sensu stricto*.

Nevertheless, some of Freud's early associates devoted themselves to literature, combining analytical practice with literary creation. A perfect example of this was Fritz Wittels, who, as a psychoanalyst and writer, functioned in two circles: the Vienna Psychoanalytic Society and the literary milieu of Karl Kraus.[4] In the 1920s, Georg Groddeck demonstrated that the language of psychoanalysis could become literature and that the literary narrative could serve to develop psychoanalytic theory. As we will see, his literary work – especially his 1923 epistolary novel *The Book of the It* (*Das Buch vom Es. Psychoanalytische Briefe an eine Freundin*) – is a prime example of the entanglement of self-analysis, autobiography, and fiction. It also points to the letter as the primary written genre for communication between the patient and the analyst.

The letter as a psychoanalytic genre

Groddeck's intuition was confirmed in the daily writing practices of the first psychoanalysts, for whom correspondence – along with personal meetings – became a proper space for intellectual and affective exchange. Whereas the mosaic-like nature of psychoanalytic literature leads to inherent tensions between self-analysis, autobiography, (psycho)biography, and fiction, looking at the role of the epistolary genre provokes a better understanding of the very dynamics of psychoanalytic production at the level of the formation of its theory (textual production) and the establishment of its practices (analysis). Correspondence – as a written exchange of ideas – best illuminates the relational and interpersonal dimensions of knowledge formation and transmission (Espagne 1999). Throughout the history of psychoanalysis, the letter did not only facilitate the flow of ideas, but it also maintained the ties without which the diaspora of the psychoanalytic community in the first decade of the twentieth century could not have survived. Moreover, as a genre of writing, the letter also served as a tool for transmitting the most intimate details related to self-analysis and, in special cases, it enabled analyses to be carried out at all.

The genre of the letter has a special significance in the history of psychoanalytic literature. Correspondence, as the primary tool of long-distance communication of *le monde savant* of the nineteenth century, formed a network of personal ties based on mutual appreciation, trust, and friendship (Hoock-Demarle 2008). The letter, to a greater extent than other lifewriting genres such as the diary or journal, was rooted in the dynamics of an encounter, conversation, and mutual listening – the key elements in the psychoanalytic practice. After World War I, the letter (in the form of an epistolary novel) became a full-fledged part of psychoanalytic literature, alongside biography and autobiography.[5]

Psychoanalysis between the spoken and written word

A psychoanalytic text can be seen as the result of psycho-somatic activity based on (self-)reflection, writing, and reading practices. As a practice, writing is both a form of thinking and a medium through which one understands and defines reality. Daniel Chandler described writing as a record of the writer's psychosomatic activity that cannot be reduced to an abstract message (Chandler 1995: 3). As anthropologists of writing have shown, "the text" is not a transparent abstraction, but a specific medium that significantly influences the message.

The choice of genre (e.g. scientific treatise, case study, psychography, biography, autobiography) mediates the content and meaning of the text itself. In the case of psychoanalytic literature, if we look at how theory is mediated by the genre in which it is written, we can understand more fully the underlying tension between the spoken and the written word. Freud first mentioned the literary dimension of his case studies in *Studies on Hysteria*. In the case of Elisabeth von R., he wrote:

> I have not always been a psychotherapist. Like other neuropathologists, I was trained to employ local diagnoses and electro-prognosis, and it still strakes me myself as strange that the case histories I write should read like short stories and that, as one might say, they lack the serious stamp of science. I must console myself with the reflection that the nature of the subject is evidently responsible for this, rather than any preference of my own.
>
> *(Freud [1895] 1955a: 160)*

According to Freud, the dynamics of literature, contrary to the narrative typical of the psychiatric treatise, facilitated the "detailed depiction of mental processes" (160). Thus, the texts could be read "like short stories." Like a writer, the psychoanalyst had to use the narrative strategies available to him in order to transform his patients' fragmentary affective histories into coherent narratives.

Hysterical patients primarily suffered due to their memories that could be processed through speech. His patients' "stories of suffering" (Ibid.: 6) took the form of expressing a painful secret (Ibid.: 8). In this context, Freud and Breuer added:

> For we found, to our great surprise at first, that *each individual hysterical symptom immediately and permanently disappeared when we had succeeded in bringing clearly to light the memory of the event by which it was provoked and in arousing its accompanying affect, and when the patient had described that event in the greatest possible detail and had put the affect into words.*
>
> *(Ibid.: 6)*

The troubled memory is processed in speaking, which transforms affects into words. As August Ruhs summarized it:

> Turning away from the amphitheatrical showroom of Charcot's hysteria, moving from the visual to the auditive, and dispensing with the suggestive gaze of the hypnotist in favor of the patient ear of the analyst, Freud succeeded in detecting a previously unheard as well as unheard-of speech in hysterical behavior.
>
> *(Ruhs 2019: 51)*

The transition from the image (eye/seeing) to speech (ear/hearing) can be considered the real source of the emergence of early psychoanalytic practices.

The case of Katharina C. is a prime example of preserving in a written text the oral dynamics of a doctor-patient encounter. The structure of this case is dialogical and corresponds to a conversation between two people (who meet accidentally). In the opening paragraphs of this case study, Freud explained: "I report the conversation that followed between us just as it is impressed on my memory and I have not altered the patient's dialect" (Freud [1895] 1955a: 125). Through a relational reading of "the text," glimpses of the authors' actual everyday experiences can be revealed. Crucial is the role of the patient, who, as the case of Anna O. brilliantly demonstrates, guides the physician to the most effective method of therapy (Ibid.: 30). In the history of psychoanalysis, the problem of the patients' influence on therapeutic techniques returned in the 1930s with mutual analysis developed by Ferenczi with Elizabeth Severn.

The attempt at making the patient's fragmented story coherent resulted in a new narrative structure. But the patient had to make the first move. As Freud emphasized:

> Once a picture has emerged from the patients's memory, we may hear him say that it becomes fragmentary and obscure in proportion as he proceeds with his description of it. *The patient is, as it were, getting rid of it by turning it into words.*
>
> *(Ibid.: 280)*

The psychoanalyst was someone who followed his patients' initiating gestures when he transformed their affective stories into text. Moreover, the content of a psychoanalytic case study was not only determined by the analyst's subjective interpretation of a patient's case, but it was also shaped by the narrative models (oral and textual) and writing genres (e.g. story, tale, psychiatric case study) to which the case study adhered.

As Roy Harris noted, the text, especially a theoretical or scientific one, can be seen as the highest development of Western rationalism. The *Homo typographicus* learns about the inner and outer reality primarily through printed texts, which in the Western culture have long been identified with logical, rational reasoning (Harris 2009: 1–16). Harris stressed that the dominance of written forms can lead to "scriptism" (Godlewski 2018: 61–78) – "a belief in the superiority in various respects of written languages over spoken languages, and of the mastery of writing, as an *intellectual achievement*, over the mere command of fluent speech [italics mine]" (Harris 2009: 11). However, the blurring of the boundaries between the conscious and the unconscious, which was typical of fin-de-siècle modernist cultures, complicated the distinction between the rational (intellectual) and the irrational (emotional).

The Romantic appreciation for irrationality returned in the psycho-medical literature of the late 1800s and early 1900s as the unconscious was ascribed a special role in literary, poetic, and artistic production. For the early psychoanalysts, the spoken word was the raw material for constructing their own narrative. In this book, I stress that a psychoanalytic text is always created in relation *to* and in a relationship *with* someone: the patient and future readers.

A relational understanding of psychoanalytic theories and practices shows that they were primarily the result of dialogue and personal ties. The following chapters will demonstrate that the dialogical nature of psychoanalytic literature is evident in both its "private" (letters, daily notes, diaries) and "public" (case studies, articles, psychographies, biographies, autobiographies) circulation.

Psychoanalysis, literary modernism, and gender

Interdisciplinary reflection on turn-of-the-century modernism and modernity has accentuated two major themes: the departure from a rigid distinction between high and low culture, and the inseparability of the private and the public spheres. New modernist studies, which have been developing for more than two decades, have raised important questions about the everyday lives of modernist writers and artists, personal ties in creative circles, and the impact of experiencing modernization and technological shifts on literature, the visual arts, and music. Among the most important assumptions of new modernist studies were: the adoption of a broad chronological framework for literary and artistic modernism (1890–1945), a transnational and multilingual perspective, the valuation of mass media as important in the formation of modernist cultures and various approaches through categories such as identity, gender, race, and class.[6]

One fundamental source for investigating the everyday lives of modernist authors is their life writing: letters, diaries, memoirs, autobiographies, and biographies. Another central element in the contemporary reflection on literary modernism is the question of experiments with written forms, most importantly with the self-portraiture, autobiography, and the self-reflective narrative (Saunders 2010: 4). As Max Saunders (2009: 1041–1059) has demonstrated, literary criticism of the early 1900s in Britain developed theoretical tools to analyze the fluid boundaries between autobiography and fiction – between the discourse of "the truth" and the languages of the imagination. In this context, Saunders recalls the category of "autobiografiction," introduced in 1906 by English writer and literary critic Stephen Reynolds (1881–1919) (Reynolds 1906: 28, 30). In his essay, Reynolds had searched for a term that could best describe the phenomenon of texts that merged fiction with auto/biography. As he had written, autobiografiction was a "literary form more direct and intimate probably than any to be found outside poetry" (Ibid.: 28; Saunders 2009: 1047). Authors can talk about themselves both in an autobiography and in a fictional work in which they conceal elements of their personal stories.

Reynolds had understood the autobiographical dimension of a literary text as a form of spiritual experience and associated it with the process of consolation. Autobiografiction as an experimental literary genre, by combining autobiography with fiction, allowed authors to reveal details from their personal life and, at the same time, remain hidden. As Reynolds emphasized:

> And, after all, when a writer has revealed to the world more of his inner self than he would exhibit to his friends, it is only natural that he should wish to stay behind the scenes, at least until he finds out how the world will take his revelation – whether with inattention, ridicule, or with sympathy.
> *(Reynolds 1906: 28; cited in Saunders 2009: 1047)*

As a literary and lifewriting genre, autobiografiction appears to be a mask put on by writers in order to speak freely about themselves. If writers could hide behind the protagonists of their work, the psychoanalysts could also make the case study a space of self-expression. In this light, *The Interpretation of Dreams* can be seen as a perfect example of autobiografiction, in which personal reflection is fused with fantastic dream histories and analytical discourse. Freud's paper "Screen Memories," which I have mentioned above, can also be considered a form of autobiografiction, in which – following Reynolds's suggestions – the patient's story became a *porte parole* for the psychoanalyst's personal story.

In his interpretation of Reynolds's essay, Saunders pointed to another key element of autobiografiction. The tension between the private and the public manifested in a burning need to speak up about one's own experience. The desire to peel off the mask sometimes collided with the fear of exposure which could potentially be dangerous and destructive to the author. I am deliberately introducing this context because I find it particularly relevant to the early history of psychoanalysis. If many writers of the time, such as Oscar Wilde, E.M. Forster, Thomas Mann, Robert Musil, André Gide, as well as Gertrude Stein, Virginia Woolf, and Radclyffe Hall, addressed non-normative sexuality in their works, while being able to hide behind their protagonists, the psychoanalyst was also able to exploit the rapidly developing sexological discourses as a safe way of speaking about a culturally repressed topic to which he could personally relate. Reynolds's essay had presented autobiography as a literary genre that always relied on the authors' creative invention (i.e. autobiography as the creation of self-images) (Saunders 2009: 1051–1052). Therefore, readers of autobiographies could no longer be sure of their confessional nature, and at the same time, they were increasingly eager to find the autobiographical dimension in any literary fiction. As I will show in this book, psychoanalytic reflections on sexuality and the formation of gender identity functioned as a space for masked self-revelations. In this light, Freud's considerations on the etiology of neurosis, bisexuality and the sources of paranoia in repressing homosexual desire assume a personal dimension.

Diane Fuss writes about the place of psychoanalysis in reflection on gender and sexuality in the last decades of the twentieth century. Any subsequent attempts to rethink the established notion of gender and the dynamics of psycho-sexual development had to go back to their origins – to psychoanalysis. Fuss argues:

> in what presently goes under the name "queer theory," there is little or no consensus on the subject of psychoanalysis. Theorists of sexuality remain largely divided over the issue of the instrumental importance of psychoanalytic frames of thinking for an antihomophobic cultural politics. [...] On one side [...] psychoanalysis appears as simply the latest chapter in the history of a powerful cultural system of sexual classification, while on the other it emerges as one of the most important conceptual challenges to that system. Rather than cancel each other out, these two positions together register the internal contradiction that propel psychoanalysis, highlighting both this theory's enormous disruptive potential and its complicity with the very symbolization of power it seeks to subvert.
>
> *(Fuss 1995: 1)*

The topic of non-normative sexuality has been at the heart of psychoanalytic literature (Zaretsky 2005: 4–11). However, in feminist criticism, gender studies, and queer theory, psychoanalysis has very often been treated as a product of patriarchalism, rather than an attempt to rethink it (Mitchell 1974).

Similarly, considerations by Michel Foucault, Gilles Deleuze, and Félix Guattari played a role in propagating an image of psychoanalysis as the product of oppressive psychiatric practices formed in the 1700s and 1800s (Foucault 2006).[7] For example, Deleuze and Guattari wrote about the oppressive dynamics of psychoanalytic discourse in the following way:

> Oedipus restrained is the figure of the daddy-mommy-me triangle, the familial constellation in person. But when psychoanalysis makes of Oedipus its dogma, it is not unaware of the existence of relations said to be pre-oedipal in the child, exo-oedipal in the psychotic, para-oedipal in others. The function of Oedipus as dogma, or as the "nuclear complex," is inseparable from a forcing by which the psychoanalyst as theoretician elevates himself to the conception of a generalized Oedipus.
>
> *(Deleuze & Guattari 1983: 51)*

According to Deleuze and Guattari, the concept of a "generalized Oedipus" has become a major obstacle to the exploring of the inner dynamics of human desire. They argued that as a framework for understanding the structure of the human psyche, it rejected the unpredictability of imaginative production and sexual desire, weaving them into the rigid fabric of the patriarchal family. As the authors added:

> It is certain that the two preceding modes of generalization attain their full scope only in structural interpretation. Structural interpretation makes Oedipus into a kind of universal Catholic symbol, beyond all the imaginary modalities. It makes Oedipus into a referential axis not only

> for the pre-oedipal phases, but also for the pra-oedipal varieties, and the exo-oedipal phenomena.
>
> *(Ibid.: 52)*

In such a view, the Oedipal triangle became a crucial trope for psychoanalytic interpretations. Consequently, the number of possible readings prove to be limited:

> The productive unconscious makes way for an unconscious that knows only how to express itself – express itself in myth, in tragedy, in dream. But who says that dream, tragedy, and myth are adequate to the formations of the unconscious, even if the work of transformation is taken into account? Groddeck remained more faithful than Freud to an autoproduction of the unconscious in the coextension of men and Nature. It is as if Freud had drawn back from this world of wild production and explosive desire, wanting at all costs to restore a little order there, an order made classical owing to the ancient Greek theater.
>
> *(Ibid.: 54)*

Deleuze and Guattari argued that Freud shaped the human psyche following a theatrical model. Starting from his own self-analysis, he created a universal theory in which themes drawn from a particular ancient culture became the model for understanding oneself and the surrounding cultural, social, and political reality. As the authors added:

> For what does it mean to say that Freud discovered Oedipus in his own self-analysis? Was it in his self-analysis, or rather in his Goethian classical culture? In his self-analysis he discovers something about which he remarks: Well now, that looks like Oedipus! And at first he considers this something as a variant of the "familial romance," a paranoiac recording by which desire causes precisely the familial determinations to explode. It is only little by little that he makes the familial romance on the contrary, into a mere dependence on Oedipus, and that he neuroticizes everything in the unconscious at the same time as he oedipalizes, and closes the familial triangle over the entire unconscious. [...] Oedipus is the idealist turning point.
>
> *(Ibid.: 55)*

Although at its starting point, Oedipus was a response to Freud's malaise, the psychoanalytic theory quickly evolved into a universal model for understanding human psycho-sexual development. The authors emphasized that acknowledging the diversity and multidirectional dimension of human desire did not save psychoanalysis from reinforcing the boundary between what is normal (and desirable) and what is abnormal (undesirable). This conviction was later echoed by Deleuze and Guattari in their *Thousand Plateaus*. As they argued: "In truth, Freud seeks nothing and understands nothing. He has no idea what a libidinal assemblage is, with all the machineries it brings into play, all the multiple loves" (Deleuze & Guattari 1987: 37). In their eyes, Freud was a poor listener, while psychoanalysis was a language that understood very little about the dynamics of the unconscious.

The image of psychoanalytic theories and practices as inherently conservative (preserving the *status quo*) has overlooked the fundamental dimension of psychoanalysis as a set of therapeutic techniques. After all, in practical terms, psychoanalysis was supposed to help patients whose suffering most often stemmed from their specific social and cultural backgrounds. Nevertheless, the conviction expressed by Fuss about the ambivalent character of psychoanalytic theory, at once emancipatory and conservative, can also be applied to the broader context of modernism. At the turn of the twentieth century, two cultural currents flowed parallel to one another: emancipatory and identitarian movements by women, homosexuals, national, and religious minorities rose alongside nationalist and conservative sentiments, such as misogyny, racism, anti-Semitism, and homophobia (Fone 2001).[8] During this time, psycho-medical science, art, and literature became not only a tool for creating a new image of man and his sexuality but also a means of both upholding and breaking with the existing image of social reality.

In this book, I would like to show that previous reflections on Freud's understanding of gender and sexuality often failed to recognize the complex nature of psycho-medical literature in the late 1800s as a component of the modernist turn in Central Europe. One of my objectives has been to deepen the understanding of the role and meanings attached to non-normative sexuality in psychoanalysis and psycho-medical literature in Central Europe in the first half of the twentieth century.[9] In the following chapters, I will argue that by investigating the genres of early sexological literature, and especially looking at the role that lifewriting genres played in the formation of the modern *scientia sexualis*, I have discovered a complex dialogue between patients and physicians. Therefore, in opposition to Foucault, Deleuze, and Guattari, I propose a more relational method of examining early sexological discourses, seen as a polyphonic instrument for the exchange of ideas between authors and their patients. The autobiographic manifestos of non-normative people that appeared at the turn of the twentieth century – and were later used by physicians in their writings – should also be viewed as part of the psycho-medical literature of the time. The theme of non-normative sexuality recurs in each chapter of this book.

Methodological scope

The purpose of my book is not to present a total overview of the transmission of psychoanalytic theory and practice in Central Europe. Neither is my objective to exhaust the broad topic of the role of life writing in the history of psychoanalytic literature. Instead, in the following chapters, I trace the origins of the heterogeneity and polyphony of psychoanalysis emerging from the personal writing and everyday writing practices of the first psychoanalysts, modernist writers, and surrealists. My analysis can be placed at the intersection of literary studies, lifewriting studies, the history of psychoanalysis, cultural history, and the anthropology of writing. The cross-disciplinary dimension of my work makes it possible to cover a wide range of issues in the theory and practice of psychoanalysis. I also emphasize the Central European specificity of psychoanalytic discourses, which I consider a medium for international communication and local forms of expression shaped by varied linguistic cultures (Austrian, Hungarian, Czech, Polish, German). The following chapters are intended as a series of case studies based on the close reading of selected psychoanalytic, literary, life writing, and visual works. They treat psychoanalysis as a narrative assemblage – a set of theories and practices, and a hybrid mosaic of themes, languages, and forms of expression.

In recent years, the rise of modernism in Central and Eastern Europe has become the subject of numerous studies. The relationship between psychoanalysis, literature, and the visual arts has also now been substantially covered in literature. In addition, research on the history of Central and Eastern European psychoanalysis has been developing rapidly for the last three decades (Mészáros 1998: 202–214; 2010: 600–622; 2017: 91–103; Bžoch 2013; Kobylińska-Dehe & Prot-Klinger 2021; Borgos 2021; Sobolewska 2022b). In this book, I want to expand these perspectives by looking at the theories and practices of psychoanalysis as part of the modernist turn in Central Europe. I believe that a careful examination of the circulation of psychoanalytic knowledge in diverse linguistic contexts and the reflection on the heterogeneity of psychoanalytic literature will shed new light on the comparative cultural history of Freudianism in Central Europe.

It should be noted, however, that despite the popularity of psychoanalytic studies, the diversity of genres in psychoanalytic literature has not yet received a systematic description. Therefore, I argue that it is necessary to reflect on the importance of the writing forms developed by Freud's first associates in pre-war psychoanalytic literature. This book begins with the question of the role of personal writing in the formation and transformation of the theories and practices of psychoanalysis in Central Europe. In the following chapters, I propose to bring together two ways of thinking about psychoanalysis. On the one hand, I would like to inquire into psychoanalysis as a Central European cultural phenomenon and a part of the modernist turn. On the other hand, I will consider it as a form of oral and textual expression via a wide range of literary and lifewriting genres. By highlighting the oral/textual mediation of psychoanalytic literature, I stress the fact (often overlooked in literary studies and critical theory) that psychoanalysis was (and still is) both a theoretical practice and a therapeutic technique.

Reflection on experimentalism in literary modernism and the hybridity of its genres has had to rely on attentive interactions with the text that would lead to a better understanding and tuning into the particularities of authors' varied languages. Close reading is a form of listening. As such, it requires mindful attention from the person who interprets and writes. Sometimes it also demands empathy and open-mindedness to prevent hasty and universalizing judgments. Such a practice of deep comprehension engages the reader intellectually and emotionally. Therefore, modernist studies have absorbed close reading as an essential methodology. Because for many scholars "studying modernism has also meant studying close reading," David James called these two areas of research "convivial bedfellows" (James 2020: 1). However, if "close reading after all forms the baseline competence for the infinite number of topics one might engage or the infinite number of arguments one might make" (Kramnick 2021: 220), how does it inform reflection on psychoanalysis in particular? "What exactly is close reading and how does it work as an explanatory practice?" (Ibid.: 220), Kramnick asks, and answers as follows:

> The expression "close reading" would seem to imply a particularly intense version of the ordinary practice of reading, an especially hard concentration on or attention to the written word. As an explanatory method, however, close reading is not exactly reading in that sense. […] Rather, the interpretive work we call close reading is a form of writing. It is "a genre of commentary," in Andrew Goldstone's words, in which a critic writes about writing in order to pursue an idea or make a point or shed light on a topic. Close reading as method thus involves the confrontation and commingling of one's own words and words out there in the world. Such writing about writing is reading only in the metaphorical sense.
>
> *(Ibid.: 221–222)*

Literary studies cannot be conducted without close reading – which, as a practice, goes beyond understanding and interpreting into the territory of performativity. In my view, such close, everyday encounters with texts result in new constellations of meanings, created through the interpreter's writing. An intimate encounter with the object of our study involves both listening (to the author's voice) and storytelling (interpretation). In this context, David James stressed:

> looking closer at close reading means looking at matters of expression as well as exegesis. Revealing this about close reading shouldn't be surprising, for it's a practice that remains inescapably affective, as I've hinted, and therefore temperamentally idiosyncratic, notwithstanding its pretensions to systematicity or its reputation for stringency.
>
> *(James 2020: 15)*

This way, close reading becomes a practice of mediation between listening and recognizing the meanings of a given text (or work). Moreover, our daily emotions and beliefs mature as a result of interacting with the interpreted work. All of these considerations urge the reader to answer the crucial questions: how to read? How to look? How to listen?

From a psychoanalytic perspective, the method of close reading can be compared to a meeting between the analyst and the analysand. The patient speaks, and the analyst listens. However, according to the relational approach inspired by Sándor Ferenczi and Elizabeth Severn's mutual analysis and applied in this book, the therapeutic encounter of close reading is based on reciprocity rather than unidirectional hierarchy (from the patient's story to the psychoanalyst's narrative). Like the psychoanalyst accompanying their patient in the process of analysis, the scholar can experience an intellectual and affective exchange in intimate contact with a text or a work of art. The French psychoanalyst Nicolas Abraham proposed a similar way of interacting with a literary text in his interpretation of Mihály Babits's famous work *The Book of Jonah* (*Jonas könyve)* (1938). The title of Abraham's text, *The Case Jonas. Translation and Psychoanalytic Comment on the Book of Jonah by Michael Babits* (*Le cas Jonas. Traduction et commentaire psychanalytique du Livre de Jonas de Michael Babits*) (1973), was a reference to the psychoanalytic genre of case study (Abraham 1981). The story of the titular Jonas became the object of reflection for the psychoanalyst-listener. In his introduction, Abraham wrote:

> I propose, this evening, to recount to you the complete sequence of a case of analysis. [...] You will therefore have to arm yourself with patience to follow, for two hours, the meanders of an evolution, which – it is true – usually spreads over several years. If I have decided to present a case to you, ignoring all the rules of discretion, it is because I have a patient who will not be shocked by the revelation of his intimate life. [...] This privileged patient is none other than a poem.
>
> *(Ibid.: 63)*

The practice of listening and translating transforms into an exegesis that is based on maintaining a close personal bond between the text (the storyteller) and the interpreter (the psychoanalyst). In my book, I will attempt to show that studying psychoanalytic literature and the dynamics of its circulation is both a work of listening and translation.

As we will see, engaging with works created in diverse cultural contexts requires not only noticing the varied forms of expression they employ but also developing a sensitivity to their linguistic heterogeneity. Therefore, in this case, understanding the other (the writer, the psychoanalyst, the artist) through the kind of listening that is close reading requires immersion in the linguistic wealth of Central Europe. This is only possible by developing something that I would call a *multilingual ear*. This problem turns out to be particularly important if one investigates output in languages as different from one another as German, Polish, and Hungarian. Consequently, listening to the voice of Central European authors also becomes a method of better comprehending the diversity and linguistic polyphony of Central European modernisms.

When I write about the theories and practices of psychoanalysis, I am referring both to theories by Freud and his closest associates, and to the therapeutic techniques they developed. My deliberate juxtaposition of these two words – "theory" and "practice" – underscores the practical dimension of any theory as well as the theoretical foundation of any practice. In this book, I will look at theory as the result of research, reflection, reading, and writing practices and at practice as a form of a creative application of theories that specified ways of working with patients. By the term "psychoanalytic literature," I understand the entirety of psychoanalytic writings, which combined different genres such as analytic notes, case studies, reviews, psychographies, biographies, autobiographies, letters, diaries, and novels.

I discuss "psychoanalytic literature" rather than simply "psychoanalysis" or "psychoanalytic discourse(s)" in order to highlight the dynamic fluctuation of any boundaries between psycho-medical, literary, and lifewriting genres. As a result, I suggest the possibility of rereading the early psychoanalytic literature in terms of its content and various genres. In the following chapters, devoted to the theories and practices of psychoanalysis in Central Europe, I focus on the circulation of Freudianism in the territories of present-day Austria, Hungary, the Czech Republic, Poland, and Germany, and discuss the creative transformations that psychoanalytic thought underwent in these countries.

Chapter 1 ("Reading Sigmund Freud's Correspondence with Wilhelm Fliess: Between A Lover's Discourse and Self-Analysis") pursues the history of early psychoanalytic discourse as originating in the intellectual and emotional bond between Freud and Wilhelm Fliess. A close reading of their correspondence will allow me to demonstrate that the source of Freud's scientific creativity lay not only in intellectual stimulation, but also in love that prompted him to undertake self-analysis. I read Freud's letters to Fliess as an example of "a lover's discourse" as proposed by Roland Barthes. I show that they contain expressions of affection which were socially repressed as non-normative to Western culture. I also use Freud's love discourse addressed to his friend to re-examine the meanings of cultural concepts such as "friendship."

At a time of rapidly developing psycho-medical discourses on non-normative sexuality, writing about homosexual love required skillful masking, sometimes even against the beloved addressee. The fear of exposure affected not only published writings but also private discourses (e.g. letters). Thus, I read Freud's reluctance to publish his letters to Fliess, his emotions associated with the rupture of their relationship, and the publication of excerpts from their private correspondence by Fliess in 1906 in the perspective of his fear of being exposed – an emotion deeply inscribed in LGBTQA+ history. Chapter 1 has two purposes: first, to rethink the origins of psychoanalytic theory as taking shape in an epistolary exchange between self-analysis and lover's discourse; second, to reveal the personal dimension of Freud's reflections on non-normative sexuality, especially bisexuality.

Chapter 2 ("The Sexological Discourse on Non-Normative Sexuality: Sándor Ferenczi, Richard von Krafft-Ebing, and Magnus Hirschfeld") offers insights into the formation of early sexological literature on non-normative sexuality. A close reading of selected psycho-medical texts by Sándor Ferenczi, Richard von Krafft-Ebing, and Magnus Hirschfeld sheds light on the polyphonic nature of early sexological discourses, which at the turn of the twentieth century were based on patients' autobiographical notes. In the late 1800s, descriptive case studies entered into a close dialogue with lifewriting genres, allowing the creation of complex narratives about the patients' experiences. In this chapter, I search for the roots of a new image of human sexuality. The modernist turn in literature, the visual arts, music, and architecture did not omit psycho-medical sciences. Therefore, the pluralization of views on human sexuality was reflected in early sexological writings. I argue that the shift from the descriptive model, beginning in the 1890s, resulted in the psychological deepening of the patient's image and the abandonment of the physician's dispassionate and objective gaze.

My aim in this chapter is to take a closer look at the polyphonic nature of psycho-medical literature. At the turn of the twentieth century, drawing inspiration from German-, English-, and French-speaking authors, early sexological discourses developed rapidly in Hungary. I argue that Ferenczi's early text "Homosexualitas Feminina" (1902) can be seen as part of the "empathetic turn" – a shift that occurred in psycho-medical literature in the 1890s. In this chapter, I suggest that Ferenczi's empathetic turn was due to two main factors: the growing psychologization of patients as autobiographical writings began to occupy an increasingly central position in psycho-medical literature and his own critical reaction to the overproduction of early sexological discourses on homosexuality. Chapter 2 also demonstrates how significant this turn was in literary and artistic modernism, which transformed the image of the human body and its desires.

Chapter 3 ("The Interpretation of Literary Dreams: Psychoanalysis, Trauma, and Painful Modernity – The Case of Mihály Babits") continues the focus on the case study genre and its complicated relationship with autobiographical and biographical discourses. This time, however, the object of my analysis is not a psycho-medical text, but a work of literature. I describe the intertwining of literary modernism and psycho-medical literature before the outbreak of the First World War as a dynamic, mutual exchange of ideas rather than as an example of the passive reception of psychiatric knowledge in literary circles. I argue that this dialogue enabled writers to create complex psychological portraits of modernity.

In this chapter, I focus on the first novel by Hungarian writer and a leading representative of modernism, Mihály Babits, titled *The Caliph Stork* (*A gólyakalifa*). I argue that this work constitutes an outstanding example of a literary description of dissociation in Central European modernist literature. Drawing on the research of Pierre Janet, Morton Prince, and Sigmund Freud, Babits created his distinctive psychological portrait of a split personality. In the fictional case study of his protagonist, Elemér Tábory, stylized as an autobiography, Babits reflected on the mechanism of dissociation as a response to rapid modernization and the birth of modernity in Hungary. The literary description of mental illness allowed him to create an insightful psychographic portrait of a man experiencing urban transformation, the mechanization of daily life, growing social inequalities, the painful feeling of backwardness, and the increasing demands of mass education.

I also take a deeper look at the experiments with autobiography and psycho-medical discourses in *The Caliph Stork*. At the turn of the twentieth century, many German, Austrian, and Hungarian authors, such as Thomas Mann, Arthur Schnitzler, Robert Musil, and Géza Csáth, were using psycho-medical literature as suitable material for their literary work. By integrating elements of his contemporaries' psycho-medical discourses (Prince's dissociation theory, Janet's trauma theory, Freud's dream theory) into the literary text, Babits created a psychological diagnosis of the modernist turn in Hungary. A close reading of *The Caliph Stork* will also allow me to point out the parallel between Babits' psychological diagnoses and theories by Freud, Ferenczi, Sabina Spielrein, and Otto Gross, as well as Elizabeth Severn's reflections on nightmares.

Chapter 4 ("The Specters of Psychoanalysis in Interwar Prague: Bohuslav Brouk and Jindřich Štyrský") further notes the importance of how life writing, modernist literature, the visual arts and psycho-medical sciences converged in Central Europe. Using the example of Jindřich Štyrský's dream diaries and his erotic works from the interwar period, this chapter traces the complicated paths of the transfer of psychoanalysis into Czech culture before the outbreak of World War II. A careful examination of Štyrský's Surrealist work will demonstrate that in their reception of psychoanalytic theory, Czech artists were attracted to Freud's *The Interpretation of Dreams* as well as the psychoanalytic appreciation for the various forms in which human sexuality could express itself.

Analyzing Štyrský's erotic and oneiric work in the context of the influence of psychoanalytic knowledge on the medical milieu of interwar Prague provides a better view of how theories by Freud, Otto Rank, and Marxist psychoanalysts such as Otto Gross and Wilhelm Reich impacted the Czech Surrealist milieu. For them, psychoanalysis was not a stable system of meanings or determined therapeutic practices but a flexible material for both the free expression of their own intimate experiences (self-analysis) and the diagnosis of a society suspended between the trauma of the Great War and the specter of another destructive event – World War II.

This chapter orbits around the category of utopia, closely related to the irrational dynamics of daydreaming and to liberated sexuality. The idea of a sexual utopia was later developed by the "wild psychoanalyst" and Surrealist Bohuslav Brouk. A close reading of his reflections on the pornophilic work of Czech Surrealists published by Štyrský in his *Edice 69* series (Edition 69) will allow me to trace the unexplored circulation paths of psychoanalytic knowledge in Czech artistic circles. I demonstrate how Brouk's interpretations of erotic Surrealist art as breaking with the order of reproduction (involving the patriarchal system and war-as-legitimized-violence) anticipated Herbert Marcuse's later reflections on civilization and Eros as well as José Esteban Muñoz's thoughts on queer utopias.

Chapter 5 ("The Queer Case of Piotr Odmieniec Włast: Psychography, Psychoanalysis, and the Origins of Anti-Psychiatric Discourse in Poland") further pursues reflections on the shadowed paths of circulation of psychoanalytic knowledge in the intellectual and artistic circles of Central Europe. In this chapter, I propose a close reading of the psychographic essay by the Polish physician Aleksander Oszacki dedicated to the renowned modernist poet Piotr Włast (Maria Komornicka). A careful examination of Oszacki's remarks about Włast's psyche will offer a closer look at the dynamics of the transmission of psychoanalytic knowledge to Polish culture and science as the internalization of the entire structures of thinking about non-normative sexuality. My reading of Oszacki's essay, which was popular in Polish critical and literary circles in the second half of the twentieth century and greatly influenced the reception of Włast's work and biography, allows me yet again to accentuate the close relationship between lifewriting genres (the biography, the letter) and psychomedical discourses (the case study). I argue that his psychography can be viewed as a negative of the case study of Daniel Paul Schreber. While in "Psycho-Analytic Notes on an Autobiographical Account of a Case of Paranoia (Dementia Paranoides)" Freud focused on the dynamics of paranoia leading from masculinity to effeminacy, Oszacki, writing about Włast, pointed to the opposite dynamics that lead from renouncing femininity to embracing masculine identification.

This chapter also demonstrates that an essay that has been forgotten by contemporary literary criticism can act as an essential contribution to a better understanding of the shadow dynamics of knowledge transmission. I argue that this issue is particularly important in the Polish context, where psychoanalysis did not have an easy reception, and no formal psychoanalytic society or group was established before the outbreak of World War II. With the psychography of Piotr Włast as its starting point, this chapter also outlines the areas of Polish literary history where an emancipatory, anti-psychiatric discourse began to evolve. Włast's letters to his family are treated as an intimate testimony to his spiritual transition and a unique manifesto of transgender identity in Polish literature.

The shift away from the gender binary and the tangle of self-analysis, autobiography, and fiction in psychoanalytic literature are the central themes of Chapter 6 ("Freud's Queer Fellow: Georg Groddeck, Between Psychoanalytic Theory and Literary Modernism"). In this chapter, I offer a detailed analysis of the literary works of Georg Groddeck, one of the most extravagant figures in the psychoanalytic movement. I read his two psychoanalytic novels, *Der Seelensucher. Ein psychoanalytischer Roman* and *The Book of the It*, from the perspective of modernist literary experimentalism. In his novels, Groddeck fused psychoanalytic theory with reflection on the psychology of the creative process and with autobiographical discourse. In his second novel, *The Book of the It*, he offered a combination of autobiography, psychoanalytic lectures, and an epistolary novel, which allowed him to create an (auto)psychographic study of the psycho-sexual life of Patrik Troll, his alter ego. Playing with the tension between self-analysis and the oral dynamics of the analytic session, Groddeck showed how epistolary exchanges, self-analysis, autobiography, biography, and fiction intertwined in the history of theories and practices of psychoanalysis.

The chapter opens with a reconstruction of Groddeck's position in the psychoanalytic movement and his relationship with Freud and his closest associates. Emphasizing the innovative nature of Groddeck's concept of the unconscious and his category of the It (das Es) will allow me to rethink the influence of Friedrich Nietzsche's thought on Groddeck and Freud as well as to re-examine the long tradition of criticism directed against scientific conservatism in German-language philosophy and literature. Following Nietzsche, Groddeck expressed a strong aversion to all authority and stressed the creative dimension of research practices, which, according to him, were based on the dynamics of imagination – like literature or art. The belief in theoretical practice as a form of creativity led Groddeck to develop his vision of literature and artistic creation. In this chapter, I trace the most important tropes in Groddeck's thought related to sex theory. I demonstrate that his epistolary novel represented a unique combination of literary experimentalism typical for modernist literature with an innovative psychoanalytic text. I also stress that Groddeck's reflections on gender and sexuality revealed queer intuitions present in interwar psychoanalytic thought.

Chapter 7 ("Practicing Friendship – A New Beginning for Psychoanalytic Theory and Practice: Ferenczi Between Georg Groddeck and Elizabeth Severn") examines the centrality of the psychology of creation in Groddeck's and Ferenczi's reflections. Reading their correspondence for discussions on scientific work as a form of creative fertility will enable me to rethink boundaries between literary, artistic, and scientific creation. The chapter begins with a close reading of Groddeck and Ferenczi's letters. Again, they show how crucial personal ties were in the formation of psychoanalytic theory and how letter-writing fueled the history of psychoanalysis.

In this final chapter, I raise questions about the hybridity of genres in psychoanalysis, both in terms of the tension between life writing, literature, and psycho-medical discourses, and between the spoken and written word. I pay particular attention to Ferenczi's late lifewriting practices. I read his *Clinical Diary* as an example of valuing speech (the oral situation) over writing (writing practices), which sheds new light on the crucial relationship between listening and writing in psychoanalytic practice. I argue that the oral dimension of the *Clinical Diary* (a great part of which was dictated by Ferenczi and typed by his secretary) makes it possible to expand the research on the diversity of life-writing genres in psychoanalytic literature. I interpret Ferenczi's diary as a written-oral form, which, thanks to his appreciation of the medium of the spoken word, enabled him to extend the situation of the encounter between patient and analyst. In this final chapter, I will show how Ferenczi's sensitivity to his patients' words and the shift away from the case study genre to small, fragmentary forms were linked to his mutual analysis seen as a technique of empathizing with the patient. As I will demonstrate, focusing on listening instead of constructing narratives can contribute greatly to the conceptualization of the history of theories and practices of psychoanalysis as a shift from the interpretative to the relational model of analytic practice.

In the Conclusion, I return to my initial question on the future methodologies of writing the history of psychoanalysis in Central Europe. My focus is on the importance of the relational understanding of research and writing practices. I also emphasize the need to undertake interdisciplinary reflection on the specificity of psychoanalytic literary genres and fin-de-siècle psycho-medical discourses. The final remarks concern the comparative cultural and relational history of psychoanalysis in Central Europe, which I have developed in this book. As the following chapters will show, such a vantage point permits the free combination of diverse disciplines and perspectives. The cross-disciplinary dimension of the adopted research methods proves to be crucial for any attempt to describe the inherent hybridity of psychoanalytic languages and practices.

Notes

1 Cf. Freud, M. Bernays, *Die Brautbriefe 1882–1886*. Ungekürzte Ausgabe in fünf Bänden, Gerhard Fichtner, Ilse Grubrich-Simitis & Albrecht Hirschmüller (Eds.) (Frankfurt am Main: S. Fischer Verlag, 2011–2019); Dale M. Moyer, *The Flash and Outbreak of a Fiery Mind: The Love Letters of Martha Bernays Freud, 1882–1886* (Bloomington: Author House, 2010).
2 All translations mine unless noted otherwise.
3 Early psychographic literature by the first Freudians is very substantial. See, for example: Sadger, *Konrad Ferdinand Meyer. Eine pathographisch-psychologische Studie*. Grenzfragen des Nerven- und Seelenlebens vol. 59 (Wiesbaden: Bergmann, 1908); *Heinrich von Kleist. Eine pathographisch-psychologische Studie*, Grenzfragen des Nerven- und Seelenlebens vol. 70 (Wiesbaden: Bergmann, 1910); Ernest Jones, *Das Problem des Hamlet und Ödipus-Komplex* (Leipzig-Wien: Deuticke, 1911); Karl Abraham, *Giovanni Segantini: ein psychoanalytischer Versuch* (Leipzig-Wien:

Deuticke, 1911); Theodor Reik, *Flaubert und seine Versuchung des heiligen Antonius. Ein Beitrag zur Künstlerpsychologie* (J.C.C. Bruns, Minden, 1912); *Arthur Schnitzler als Psycholog* (Frankfurt am Main: Fischer Taschenbuch Verlag, 1993); Fritz Wittels, *Tragische Motive: das Unbewußte von Held und Heldin* (Berlin: Fleischel, 1911); Otto Rank, *Das Inzest-Motiv in Dichtung und Sage: Grundzüge einer Psychologie des dichterischen Schaffens* (Leipzig: Deuticke, 1912); Max Graf, *Richard Wagner im "Fliegenden Holländer": ein Beitrag zur Psychologie künstlerischen Schaffens* (Leipzig-Wien: Deuticke, 1911). The most known psychographic case studies by Freud are his works on Leonardo (1910) and Schreber (1911), see: Freud, "Leonardo da Vinci and a Memory of his Childhood," in *The Standard Edition of the Complete Psychological Works of Sigmund Freud.* Vol. 11, ed. James Strachey (London: The Hogarth Press, 1957), 59–137; "Psycho-Analytic Notes on an Autobiographical Account of a Case of Paranoia," in *The Standard Edition of the Complete Psychological Works of Sigmund Freud.* Vol. 12, ed. James Strachey (London: The Hogarth Press, 1958), 3–82.

4 On Fritz Wittels, see: Elke Mühlleitner, *Biographisches Lexikon der Psychoanalyse* (Tübingen: Edition Diskord, 1992), 369–372; cf. Le Rider, *Karl Kraus. Phare et brûlot de la modernité viennoise* (Paris: Seuil, 2018). On Kraus's criticism of psychoanalysis, see the classical work by Thomas Szasz, *Anti-Freud: Karl Kraus's Criticism of Psychoanalysis and Psychiatry* (Syracuse-New York: Syracuse University Press, 1990).

5 In the psychoanalytic movement, diaries were seen as a perfect source for researching the psycho-sexual development of children and young adults, see: Siegfried Bernfeld, "Reliquien und Tagebücher," *Zeitschrift für psychoanalytische Pädagogik* vol. 4, no. 10 (1930): 370–381; "Ein Mißglücktes Tagebuch," *Almanach der Psychoanalyse* 6 (1931): 249–257; Hermine Hug-Hellmuth, "Aus dem Tagebuch eines halbwüchsigen Mädchens," *Almanach der Psychoanalyse* 1 (1926): 145–160; cf. *Tagebuch eines halbwüchsigen Mädchens*, ed. H. Hug-Hellmuth (Wien-Leipzig: Internationale Psychoanalytische Verlag, 1919). After the publication of the *Tagebuch eines halbwüchsigen Mädchens*, Hug-Hellmuth was accused of writing this diary in a pseudo-childlike style to illustrate Freud's theories on infantile sexuality, see: Marie Lenormand, "Hug-Hellmuth or the Impasses of an Objectifying Conception of the Infantile," *Recherches en Psychanalyse* vol. 13, no. 1 (2012): 74–86.

6 "New modernist studies" are related to the founding of the Modernist Studies Association in 1999. Over the past two decades, the Society's annual international conferences as well as its two scholarly journals, *Modernism/Modernity* and *Modernist Cultures*, have provided a platform for a transnational discussion on the future of modernist studies. A good overview of the most important objectives of this perspective was proposed by Douglas Mao and Rebecca L. Walkowitz, "The New Modernist Studies," *PMLA* vol. 123, no. 3 (2008): 737–748. One of the leading research centers for new modernist studies is the Oxford Centre for Life-Writing. For the most important works in this area, see: Marcus, *Auto/biographical Discourses: Theory, Criticism, Practice* (Manchester: Manchester University Press, 1994); *Moving Modernisms: Motion, Technology, and Modernity*, ed. David Bradshaw, L. Marcus, and Rebecca Roach (Oxford: Oxford University Press, 2016); Max Saunders, *Imagined Futures: Writing, Science, and Modernity in the To-Day and To-Morrow Book Series, 1923–31* (Oxford: Oxford University Press, 2019).

7 See especially the lecture from December 12, 1973, 123–142, and the lecture from January 9, 1974, 173–199.

8 On the recent history of homophobia (the second half of the twentieth century), see: Peter Hegarty, *A Recent History of Lesbian and Gay Psychology: From Homophobia to LGBT* (London-New York: Routledge, 2018), especially chapters "Normative Creativity" and "Revolutionary Science"; cf. *The Dictionary of Homophobia: A Global History of Gay & Lesbian Experience*, ed. Louis-Georges Tin, trans. Marek Redburn et al. (Vancouver: Arsenal Pulp Press, 2008). On the

intersection of antisemitism and homophobia in the times of Freud's life and work, see: Sander L. Gilman, *Freud, Race, and Gender* (Princeton: Princeton University Press, 1993).

9 By the term "queer sexuality," I understand all forms of sexual expressions that do not fit into the heteronormative model.

References

Abraham, K. (1911). *Giovanni Segantini: ein psychoanalytischer Versuch*, Leipzig/Wien: Deuticke.

Abraham, N. (1981). *Jonas. Anasémies* III, Paris: Aubier Flammarion.

Bernfeld, S. (1930). Reliquien und Tagebücher, in *Zeitschrift für psychoanalytische Pädagogik* 4 (10), 370–381.

Bernfeld, S. (1931). Ein Mißglücktes Tagebuch, in *Almanach der Psychoanalyse* 6, 249–257.

Bernfeld, S. (1946). An Unknown Autobiographical Fragment by Freud, in *American Imago* 4, 3–19.

Berman, M. (1983). *All That Is Solid Melts Into Air: The Experience of Modernity*, New York/London: Verso.

Bonaparte, M. (1939). A Defence of Biography, in *The International Journal of Psychoanalysis* 20, 231–240.

Borgos, A. (2021). *Women in the Budapest School of Psychoanalysis: Girls of Tomorrow*, New York/London: Routledge.

Brooks, P. (1992). *Reading for the Plot: Design and Intention in Narrative*, Cambridge Massachusetts/London: Harvard University Press.

Bžoch, A. (2013). *Psychoanalyse in der Slowakei. Eine Geschichte zwischen Enthusiasmus und Widerstand*, Gießen: Psychosozial Verlag.

Chandler, D. (1995). *The Act of Writing: A Media Theory Approach*, Aberystwyth: University of Wales.

Clark, R. W. (1980). *Freud: The Man and the Cause*, New York: Random House.

Deleuze, G. & Guattari, F. (1983). *Anti-Oedipus: Capitalism and Schizophrenia*. Translated by Robert Hurley, Mark Seem, & Helen R. Lane. Minneapolis: University of Minnesota Press.

Deleuze, G. & Guattari, F. (1987). *A Thousand Plateaus: Capitalism and Schizophrenia*. Translated by Brian Massumi. Minneapolis/London: University of Minnesota Press.

Dybel, P. (2019). *Psychoanalysis – the Promised Land? The History of Psychoanalysis in Poland 1900–1989, Part I. The Sturm und Drang Period. Beginnings of Psychoanalysis in the Polish Lands during the Partitions 1900–1918*, Bern: Peter Lang.

Espagne, M. (1999). *Les transferts culturels franco-allemands*, Paris: Presses Universitaires de France.

Figes, O. (2019). *The Europeans: Three Lives and the Making of a Cosmopolitan Culture*, New York: Metropolitan Book.

Fone, B. R. S. (2001). *Homophobia: A History*, New York: Metropolitan Books.

Foucault, M. (2006). *Psychiatric Power: Lectures at the Collège de France 1973–1974*. Translated by Graham Burchell. New York: Palgrave Macmillan.

Frankland, G. (2000). *Freud's Literary Culture*, Cambridge: Cambridge University Press.

Freud, S. (1914). Zur Geschichte der psycho-analytischen Bewegung, in *Jahrbuch für psychoanalytische und psychopathologische Forschung* 6, 207–260.

Freud, S. ([1895] 1955). Studies on Hysteria, in J. Strachey (Ed.), *The Standard Edition of the Complete Psychological Works of Sigmund Freud*. Vol. 2, London: The Hogarth Press.

Freud, S. ([1909] 1955). Analysis of a Phobia in a Five-Year-Old Boy, in J. Strachey (Ed.), *The Standard Edition of the Complete Psychological Works of Sigmund Freud.* Vol. 10, London: Hogarth Press, 3–154.
Freud, S. ([1910] 1957). Leonardo da Vinci and a Memory of his Childhood, in J. Strachey (Ed.), *The Standard Edition of the Complete Psychological Works of Sigmund Freud.* Vol. 11, London: The Hogarth Press, 59–137.
Freud, S. ([1911] 1958). Psycho-Analytic Notes on an Autobiographical Account of a Case of Paranoia, in J. Strachey (Ed.), *The Standard Edition of the Complete Psychological Works of Sigmund Freud.* Vol. 12, London: The Hogarth Press, 1–82.
Freud, S. ([1907] 1959a). Delusions and Dreams, in Jensen's *Gradiva*, in J. Strachey (Ed.), *The Standard Edition of the Complete Psychological Works of Sigmund Freud.* Vol. 9, London: The Hogarth Press, 43–44.
Freud, S. ([1908] 1959a). Creative Writers and Day-Dreaming, in J. Strachey (Ed.), *The Standard Edition of the Complete Psychological Works of Sigmund Freud.* Vol. 9, London: The Hogarth Press, 141–154.
Freud, S. ([1925] 1959b). An Autobiographical Study, in J. Strachey (Ed.), *The Standard Edition of the Complete Psychological Works of Sigmund Freud.* Vol. 20, London: The Hogarth Press, 7–74.
Freud, S. ([1930] 1961b). The Goethe Prize, in J. Strachey (Ed.), *The Standard Edition of the Complete Psychological Works of Sigmund Freud.* Vol. 21, London: The Hogarth Press, 205–214.
Freud, S. ([1899] 2010). *The Interpretation of Dreams.* Translated by James Strachey. New York: Basic Books.
Freud, S. & Bernays, M. (2011–2019). *Die Brautbriefe 1882–1886.* Ungekürzte Ausgabe in fünf Bänden, Gerhard Fichtner, Ilse Grubrich-Simitis & Albrecht Hirschmüller (Eds.). Frankfurt am Main: S. Fischer Verlag.
Friedman, S. S. (2007). Cultural Parataxis and Transnational Landscapes of Reading. Toward a Locational Modernist Studies, in A. Eysteinsson & V. Liska (Eds), *Modernism*, Amsterdam-Philadelphia: John Benjamins Publishing Company, 35–52.
Fuss, D. (1995). Pink Freud, in *GLQ* 2 (1–2),1–9.
Gay, P. (1988). *Freud: A Life for Our Time*, New York: Norton.
Gilman, S. L. (1993). *Freud, Race, and Gender*, Princeton: Princeton University Press.
Godlewski, G. (2018). Poza nachylenie tekstowe, w stronę doświadczenia przedtekstowego. Wskazówki terapeutyczne, in *Teksty Drugie* 1, 61–78.
Graf, M. (1911). *Richard Wagner im "Fliegenden Holländer": ein Beitrag zur Psychologie künstlerischen Schaffens.* Leipzig-Wien: Deuticke.
Hanák, P. (1998). *The Garden and the Workshop: Essays on the Cultural History of Vienna and Budapest*, Princeton: Princeton University Press.
Harris, R. (2009). *Rationality and the Literate Mind*, New York/London: Routledge.
Hegarty, P. (2018). *A Recent History of Lesbian and Gay Psychology: From Homophobia to LGBT*, London/New York: Routledge.
Hoock-Demarle, M.-C. (2008). *L'Europe des lettres: Réseaux épistolaires et construction de l'espace européen*, Paris: Albin Michel.
Hug-Hellmuth, H. (1926). Aus dem Tagebuch eines halbwüchsigen Mädchens, in *Almanach der Psychoanalyse* 1, 145–160.
Hug-Hellmuth, H. (Ed.) (1919). *Tagebuch eines halbwüchsigen Mädchens*, Wien/Leipzig: Internationaler Psychoanalytischer Verlag.
James, D. (2020). Introduction, in D. James (Ed.), *Modernism and Close Reading*, Oxford: Oxford University Press, 1–16.
Janik, A. & Toulmin, S. E. (1973). *Wittgenstein's Vienna*, New York: Simon and Schuster.

Jones, E. (1911). *Das Problem des Hamlet und Ödipus-Komplex*, Leipzig/Wien: Deuticke.
Khanna, R. (2003). *Dark Continents. Psychoanalysis and Colonialism*, Durham/London: Duke University Press.
Kobylińska-Dehe, E. & Prot-Klinger, K. (Eds.) (2021). *Jak feniks z popiołów? O odradzaniu się psychoanalizy w powojennej i dzisiejszej Polsce*, Kraków: Universitas.
Kornhauser, J. & Siewior, K. (Eds.) (2015). *Głuchy brudnopis. Antologia manifestów awangard Europy Środkowej*, Kraków: Wydawnictwo Uniwersytetu Jagiellońskiego.
Kramnick, J. (2021). Criticism and Truth, in *Critical Inquiry* 47 (4), 218–240.
Le Rider, J. (1993). *Modernity and Crises of Identity: Culture and Society in Fin-de-siècle Vienna*, New York: Continuum.
Le Rider, J. (1994). *Modernité viennoise et crises de l'identité*, Paris: Presses Universitaires de France.
Le Rider, J. (2018). *Karl Kraus. Phare et brûlot de la modernité viennoise*, Paris: Seuil, 2018.
Lenormand, M. (2012). Hug-Hellmuth or the Impasses of an Objectifying Conception of the Infantile, in *Recherches en Psychanalyse* 13 (1), 74–86.
Magris, C. (2013). *Der habsburgische Mythos in der modernen österreichischen Literatur*. Translated by Madeleine von Pásztory. Wien: Paul Zsolnay Verlag.
Mahony, P. J. (1987). *Freud as a Writer*, New Haven: Yale University Press.
Mao, D. & Walkowitz, R. L. (2008). The New Modernist Studies, in *PMLA* 123 (3), 737–748.
Marcus, L. (1994). *Auto/biographical Discourses: Theory, Criticism, Practice*, Manchester: Manchester University Press.
Marcus, L. (Ed.) (1999) *Sigmund Freud's The Interpretation of Dreams: New Interdisciplinary Essays*, Manchester/New York: Manchester University Press.
Marcus, L. (2014). *The Dreams of Modernity*, Cambridge: Cambridge University Press.
Marcus, L., Bradshaw, D. & Roach, R. (Eds.) (2016). *Moving Modernisms: Motion, Technology, and Modernity*, Oxford: Oxford University Press.
Mautner, B. (1994). Freud's Lost Dream and the Schism with Wilhelm Fliess, in *International Journal of Psycho-Analysis* 75, 321–333.
Mazurel, H. (2021). *L'inconscient ou l'oubli de l'histoire*, Paris: La Découverte.
Mészáros, J. (1998). The Tragic Success of European Psychoanalysis: The Budapest School, in *International Forum of Psychoanalysis* 7, 202–214.
Mészáros, J. (2010). Progress and Persecution in the Psychoanalytic Heartland: Antisemitism, Communism and the Fate of Hungarian Psychoanalysis, in *Psychoanalytic Dialogues* 20, 600–622.
Mészáros, J. (2014). *Ferenczi and Beyond: Exile of the Budapest School and Solidarity in the Psychoanalytic Movement during the Nazi Years*, London: Karnac.
Mészáros, J. (2017). The Saga of Psychoanalysis in Eastern Europe: Repression and Rebirth in Hungary, and in Former Czechoslovakia and Yugoslavia, in *História Ciências Saúde-Manguinhos* 24, 91–103.
Mitchell, J. (1974). *Psychoanalysis and Feminism: Freud, Reich, Laing, and Women*, New York: Pantheon Books.
Moyer, D. M. (2010). *The Flash and Outbreak of a Fiery Mind: The Love Letters of Martha Bernays Freud, 1882–1886*, Bloomington: Author House.
Mühlleitner, E. (1992). *Biographisches Lexikon der Psychoanalyse*, Tübingen: Edition Diskord.
Müller, L. (2019). *Freuds Dinge: der Diwan, die Apollokerzen und die Seele im technischen Zeitalter*, Berlin: Die Andere Bibliotek.
Nietzsche, F. (2007). *Ecce Homo: How to Become What You Are.* Translated by Duncan Large. Oxford: Oxford University Press.

Rachman, A. W. (Ed.) (2016). *The Budapest School of Psychoanalysis: The Origin of a Two-Person Psychology and Emphatic Perspective*, London/New York: Routledge.
Rank, O. (1912). *Das Inzest-Motiv in Dichtung und Sage: Grundzüge einer Psychologie des dichterischen Schaffens.* Leipzig: Deuticke.
Reik, T. (1912). *Flaubert und seine Versuchung des heiligen Antonius. Ein Beitrag zur Künstlerpsychologie*, Minden: J.C.C. Bruns.
Reik, T. (1993). *Arthur Schnitzler als Psycholog*, Frankfurt am Main: Fischer Taschenbuch Verlag.
Reynolds, S. (1906). Autobiografiction, in *Speaker* 15 (366), 28, 30.
Ruhs, A. (2019). Nervous Times: Something of What Preceded the Culture of the Fin-de-Siècle and Viennese Modernism, in *Vienna 1900: Birth of Modernism*, ed. Hans-Peter Wipplinger, Vienna: Leopold Museum.
Rycroft, C. (1985). On Autobiography, in *Psychoanalysis and Beyond*, London: Chatto & Windus, 191–277.
Sadger, I. (1908). *Konrad Ferdinand Meyer. Eine pathographisch-psychologische Studie.* Grenzfragen des Nerven- und Seelenlebens vol. 59. Wiesbaden: Bergmann.
Sadger, I. (1910). *Heinrich von Kleist. Eine pathographisch-psychologische Studie*, Grenzfragen des Nerven- und Seelenlebens vol. 70. Wiesbaden: Bergmann.
Sadger, I. (1912). Von der Pathographie zur Psychographie, in *Imago* 1, 158–175.
Saunders, M. (2009). Autobiografiction: Experimental Life-Writing from the Turn of the Century to Modernism, in *Literature Compass* 6 (5), 1041–1059.
Saunders, M. (2010). *Self Impression: Life-Writing, Autobiografiction, and the Forms of Modern Literature*, Oxford: Oxford University Press.
Saunders, M. (2019). *Imagined Futures: Writing, Science, and Modernity in the To-Day and To-Morrow Book Series, 1923–31*, Oxford: Oxford University Press.
Schorske, C. E. (1980). *Fin-de-siècle Vienna. Politics and Culture*, New York: Vintage.
Schorske, C. E. (1998). *Thinking with History: Explorations in the Passage to Modernism*, Princeton: Princeton University Press.
Sobolewska, A. (2021b). Isidor Sadger's Images as the Other: Psychoanalysis Between Life Writing and Literary Experimentalism, in *Biography: An Interdisciplinary Quarterly* 44 (4), 561–578.
Sobolewska, A. (2022b). Theories and Practices of Psychoanalysis in Central Europe Immediately After World War II, in *The International Journal of Psychoanalysis* 103 (5), 828–850.
Swartz, S. (2022). *Psychoanalysis and Colonialism: A Contemporary Introduction*, London-New York: Routledge.
Szasz, T. (1990). *Anti-Freud: Karl Kraus's Criticism of Psychoanalysis and Psychiatry*, Syracuse/New York: Syracuse University Press.
Tin, L.-G. (Ed.) (2008). *The Dictionary of Homophobia: A Global History of Gay & Lesbian Experience.* Translated by Marek Redburn. Vancouver: Arsenal Pulp Press.
Wipplinger, H.-P. (Ed.) (2019). *Vienna 1900: Birth of Modernism*, Vienna: Leopold Museum.
Wittels, F. (1911). *Tragische Motive: das Unbewußte von Held und Heldin.* Berlin: Fleischel.
Worbs, M. (1983). *Nervenkunst. Literatur und Psychoanalyse im Wien der Jahrhundertwende*, Frankfurt am Main: Europäische Verlagsanstalt.
Zaretsky, E. (2005). *Secrets of the Soul: A Social and Cultural History of Psychoanalysis*, New York: Vintage.

1

READING SIGMUND FREUD'S CORRESPONDENCE WITH WILHELM FLIESS

Between a lover's discourse and self-analysis

In this chapter, I take a closer look at the emotional dimension of Freud's letters to Wilhelm Fliess. By doing so, I wish to rethink the problem of the emotional nature of their relationship as well as its influence on the formation of early psychoanalytic thought (Anzieu 1998; 2000: 1201–1216). As we will see, in the space of these letters, early psychoanalytic discourse became closely intertwined with personal, self-analytic, and a lover's discourse.

The second half of the twentieth century saw the publication of written correspondence between early psychoanalysts. First, Freud's selected letters to Wilhelm Fliess (1950) were published, followed by a selection of Freud's correspondence with various addressees (1960), then letters to Oskar Pfister (1963), Karl Abraham (1965), Lou Andreas-Salomé (1966), Arnold Zweig (1968), Edoardo Weiss (1970), Georg Groddeck (1974), Carl Gustav Jung (1974), and Stefan Zweig (1989). These, however, were incomplete editions in which many letters – including those with content deemed too confidential by the editors – were omitted. As Ernst Falzeder aptly wrote:

> None of these was a complete, unabridged edition: whole letters were left out, and passages that were considered unimportant, repetitive, indiscreet, offensive, or not fit for print for whatever other reason were deleted. Sometimes the place where something had been omitted was marked, sometimes not; in no case was it indicated how many words, phrases, or paragraphs had been omitted. [...] *As a result, until the mid-1970s, what the reader – the English-speaking reader in particular – took to be Freud's letters was not Freud but a censored and distorted version of what he had actually written* [italics mine].
>
> *(Falzeder 2002: 13–15)*

DOI: 10.4324/9781003441892-2

The price to pay for editorial interference was the formation of a particular image of the history of psychoanalysis, which could not fully reflect the affective nature of the personal ties between the first analysts.

By that time, though, autobiographies and memoirs by Freud's closest collaborators had begun to appear. These autobiographical texts contributed greatly to the pluralization of the image of the psychoanalytic movement, revealing its collective and intellectual-affective dynamics. Theodor Reik (1949), Wilhelm Stekel (1950), Ludwig Binswanger (1956), Ernest Jones (1959), Bruno Goetz (1969), Edoardo Weiss (1970), Max Schur (1973), Helena Deutsch (1973), and (posthumously) Fritz Wittels (1996) published their memoirs during this period. Psychoanalysts were also fond of the biographical genre. The monumental biography of Freud by Jones (1953–1957) was preceded by earlier works by Wittels (1924), Sadger ([1930] 2006), and Helena Deutsch (1940: 184–194).[1] These texts should be considered the earliest attempts to create subjective (micro)histories of the psychoanalytic movement. Since the 1980s, full editions of Freud's correspondence with his most important associates have also been published: with Fliess (1985), Sándor Ferenczi (1992, 1996, 2000), Jones (1993), and Abraham (2009). That way, in the second half of the twentieth century, life writing – and letter-writing specifically – found itself at the heart of psychoanalytic literature.

Like many postmodern thinkers, Roland Barthes was preoccupied with the complex relationship between the spoken word and the text.[2] As he argued:

> Only writing can accommodate extreme subjectivity, because in writing there is an agreement between the indirectness of the expression and the truth of the subject – an agreement that is impossible at the level of the word (and therefore of the lecture), which is always [...] both direct and theatrical. The book on the *Lover's Discourse* is perhaps poorer than the seminar, but I maintain that it is truer.
>
> *(Barthes 2007: 19)*[3]

The cited fragment refers to the seemingly simple fact that an oral situation (such as a meeting or lecture) is governed by different laws than an event in which a written text remains the basis of intellectual or emotional exchange.[4] Barthes confronted this problem not only in theory, but also in practice, as he was preparing the publication in print of his two-year cycle of lectures at the École pratique des hautes études (1974–1976) on "a lover's discourse" (*le discours amoureaux*).[5] According to Barthes, the book as a selection of structured and cohesive notes cannot fully capture the dynamics of a face-to-face encounter. At the same time, it was the published text of the lectures that appeared to him as more truthful and directly communicative. In this view, writing would be a means of "the expression and the truth of the subject" (*l'expression et la vérité du sujet*).

The tension between the spoken word and the written text also becomes an essential element of epistolography. Correspondence is a series of encounters – from the exchange of customary courtesies to intellectual and emotional discussions – that maintain professional and personal ties (Hoock-Demarle 2008; Saint-Gille 2010: 387–391; Całek 2019). However, letters have their own dynamics which are unlike direct conversation: they require time (waiting for a reply, factoring in the risk of a letter being lost), activate certain writing conventions (courtesy expressions resulting from linguistic customs), and are characterized by reduced confidentiality (a letter may fall into the wrong hands) compared to an intimate conversation. Despite the inconvenience, the impossibility of a face-to-face meeting would frequently force senders to confess their feelings in epistolary exchange, even if their love was forbidden.[6]

In Barthes's eyes, the feelings that are expressed in the letters, although they remain the subjective and unique voice of the sender, become part of the supra-individual structure of "a lover's discourse" – a linguistic system of meanings that has its own tradition. Lovers' voices are shaped by their specific historical and cultural contexts (dependent on the time, language, and geographical location). The same can be said of theoretical discourse, whether scientific, philosophical, or psychoanalytic, seen as the result of daily reflective reading and writing practices (Anzieu 1981; Sobolewska 2021a).[7] In this light, any theory should be regarded as processual work – it takes time to form and is based on writing and reading (Hébrard 1995: 473–523; 2005: 105–140; Rodak 2009; Darnton 1992: 237–270). As anthropologists of literacy have well demonstrated, writing – as a practice that is both reflective and self-reflective – mediates text and influences its meaning.[8] These considerations provide a good introduction to the study of the history of psychoanalytic literature with its specificity as a genre. In addition to individual daily writing practices, letters – understood as private and yet collective practices of the regular exchange of thoughts – proved crucial for the early development of psychoanalytic theory (Grubrich-Simitis 1993a; May 2015).[9]

In the nineteenth century, epistolography was a basic form of communication, both between close friends and business partners. Correspondence constituted a specific cultural practice that filled a good part of the letter-writers' everyday lives. As Sigmund's Freud son, Ernst L. Freud, wrote:

> As a Letter Writer, my father was unusually prolific and conscientious. He dealt with his voluminous correspondence unassisted and in longhand. He answered every letter he received, no matter from whom, and as a rule this answer was in the post within twenty-four hours. His evenings he devoted to scientific writing, but every spare minute between analyses was dedicated to his correspondence. In the course of his long life, strict observance of this routine resulted in the composition of many thousands of letters.
>
> *(Freud 1961: vii–viii)*

Epistolary practices were a key part of Freud's daily routine – a private ritual. Freud used his letters to his closest associates to discuss current issues related to the psychoanalytic movement and psychoanalytic societies.

During the time of the movement's internationalization, letters primarily functioned as a means of consolidating the psychoanalytic community. Moreover, they became a site for practicing (self-)analysis.[10] Freud's correspondence with his closest collaborators constitutes an unparalleled source of knowledge about psychoanalytic theories and practices. It also gives insight into the nature and emotional dimension of the personal ties linking psychoanalysts, which significantly influenced the inner dynamics of the Freudian movement. The letters exchanged between the first analysts facilitated both the expression and the suppression of emotions, the clashing of views, discussions, and the eruption of conflicts.

In this light, Freud's body of letters to Wilhelm Fliess constitutes an exceptional document. That is because it reveals the origins of certain specific psychoanalytic theories and, at the same time, establishes a model for an affective-intellectual partnership subsequently reproduced by Freud in his later relationships with his closest associates. Freud's correspondence with Fliess also provides a material record of Freud's self-analysis, thus bringing to light a crucial moment in his personal biography.

As Barthes pointed out, a lover's discourse expresses a variety of emotional states, such as "amour-passion, amour-total, amour-limite, mal d'amour (passionate love, total love, limited love, lovesickness)."[11] Moreover, this discourse speaks not so much to the feeling itself, but to who is confessing love. Read through this prism, Freud's letters to Fliess become a material trace of Freud's "moi amoureux" – "myself in love." Finding a language of expression for his feelings, he – like many people in love before him – actively contributed to love literature.

As a form of expression, a lover's discourse is not dialectical, but rather "it turns like a perpetual calendar, an encyclopedia of affective culture" (Barthes 1990: 7). In Western culture's foundational texts from Plato and Ovid,[12] through Abelard, Shakespeare,[13] Montaigne,[14] to Rimbaud and Verlaine,[15] forbidden love (in its different forms) has found a place for itself.[16] Sometimes, however – because it was socially stigmatized and repudiated – it had to adopt a mask, thus becoming a form of linguistic sublimation referred to as "friendship," "companionship" or intellectual "partnership."[17] As Barthes accurately pointed out: "La grammaire du discours opprime deux classes de sujet: les femmes et les homosexuels (The grammar of discourse oppresses two groups of subjects: women and homosexuals)" (Barthes 2007: 701). At the same time, he added:

> L'amoureux ne peut se définir ni par son objet, ni par sa tendance, mais par son discours. L'amoureux est tout discours (The lover can be defined neither by his object, nor by his tendency, but by his discourse. The lover is all discourse).
>
> *(Ibid.: 675)*

One gets to know a lover through his words, through the language of his letters. The lover, who has to use masks for the expression of his affection, readily resorts to other discursive genres, not only those customarily associated with love discourse (e.g. life writing, literature, poetry). Similarly – and perhaps counter-intuitively – a scientific theory could also become a space for describing and examining one's emotional life. As we will see, at the origin of psychoanalytic theories and practices, these two spheres – the romantic/affective and intellectual/professional – intersected constantly.

1.1 The personal dimension of knowledge transmission in the psychoanalytic movement

A closer look at the emotional dimension of personal ties in the psychoanalytic movement enables one to reflect more on the impact of positive feelings (such as respect or admiration) on the formation of close relationships between the first analysts. At the same time, it also allows one to rethink the importance of negative affects (such as jealousy or feelings of hurt and rejection) on the dissolution of intellectual communities (in this case, the psychoanalytic circles). Recall Randall Collins's reflections on the importance of personal ties for the production and transmission of knowledge (Collins 1998). The American sociologist wrote:

> I suggest three processes, overlapping but analytically distinct, that operate through personal contacts. One is thc passing of cultural capital, of ideas and the sense of what to do with them; another is the transfer of emotional energy, both from the exemplars of previous successes and from contemporaneous buildup in the cauldron of a group; the third involves the structural sense of intellectual possibilities, especially rivalrous ones.
>
> *(Ibid.: 71)*

The problems of the transmission of cultural capital, the entanglement of everyday research practices in scholars' emotional life, and the affective dimension of the relationships that bind researchers together led Collins to distinguish two basic types of personal ties in scientific communities: the vertical and the horizontal. While vertical ties defined the collaboration between teacher and student, horizontal ties involved independent researchers, often of similar age and professional status (Ibid.: 71–72).

In the case of Freud's closest circle, many of the conflicts between analysts arose, I believe, from the disruption of the boundaries between vertical and horizontal ties: the student wanted to be equal to the master, while the master did not want to see an equal in his colleague. The contradictory desires of Freud and his younger colleagues most often led to the exclusion of the "unruly" thinker from the community, also serving to suppress theories that did not suit the teacher. This problem was brilliantly diagnosed by Ferenczi. In his letter from September 27, 1932, to Freud, Ferenczi wrote:

> You can be assured that I remember all the beautiful earlier visits, even though I also have to concede that more courage and *more open talk on my part about practical and theoretical things would have been advantageous to me. But, unfortunately, there is usually a lack of such courage in those who are younger and weaker* [italics mine].
>
> *(Freud & Ferenczi 2000: 444)*

Ferenczi addressed the problem of an authoritarian attitude affecting the student-master relationship. Relative to the teacher, the younger and less experienced colleague had to assume the position of a child who, as the "younger and weaker," needed support both intellectually and emotionally. This dynamic, however, inevitably led to the suppression of the student's potential as well as to emotional exploitation on the part of the teacher. Freud's response on October 2, 1932, illustrates this mechanism perfectly:

> For three years you have been systematically turning away from me, probably developed a personal hostility that goes further than it could express itself. Each of those who were once near to me and then fell away was able to find more to reproach me with than you, of all people.
>
> *(Freud & Ferenczi 2000: 444–445)*

Freud held Ferenczi responsible for the rupture of their friendship ("The traumatic effect dissipates in me, I am prepared, and used to it"), thus avoiding confrontation with his authoritarian attitude toward his associates. At the same time, as the history of the development of the psychoanalytic movement from the 1910s onward demonstrates, Freud owed the success of his theory to his colleagues. In the context of knowledge transmission, Collins commented:

> what we consider intellectual greatness is having produced ideas which affect later generations, who either repeat them, develop them further, or react against them. [...] I would add that it is possible to assess whether some individuals received more retrospective eminence than they deserve, *in the sense that they did not really produce the ideas which are later attributed to them* [italics mine].
>
> *(Collins 1998: 69)*

Recognition very often occurs retrospectively and is determined by the involvement of followers who continue, transform, and challenge the teacher's thoughts. In other words, those who come later largely account for the reputation of the "master." Thus, they are also able to freely reshape the memory of their "teacher," allowing some stories to come to the fore, while keeping others silenced.

1.2 Psychoanalysis as one man's invention?

Beginning in 1902, Freud surrounded himself with disciples, gradually moving out of something he considered scientific alienation. Psychoanalysis, developed by a group of physicians and intellectuals, quickly became an interdisciplinary and intergenerational language, appealing to the representatives of a great variety of fields, from psychiatrists and neurologists to philosophers and musicologists. For many of the young intellectuals joining the Freudian movement, such as Karl Abraham, Sándor Ferenczi, Otto Rank, Isidor Sadger, Fritz Wittels, Max Graf, Georg Groddeck, Lou Andreas-Salomé, and Siegfried Bernfeld, psychoanalysis was a new paradigm of thinking. In the memoirs of his students, the conviction that Freud was an extraordinary person, a genius, and the master and discoverer of the unconscious came to the fore very often. Max Graf (1942) wrote his memoir in this spirit:

> I met Freud in the same year in which he published the *Interpretation of Dreams* [1900, sic!] – in other words, in the most important and decisive year of his life. Freud had at the time been treating a lady whom I knew. […] I was invited to visit him in his office. Freud was then forty-four years old. The very black hair on his head and beard had begun to show traces of gray. The most striking thing about the man was his expression. *His beautiful eyes were serious and seemed to look at man from the depths.* There was then something distrustful in this look; later, there was to appear bitterness as well. *Freud's head had something artistic about it; it was the head of a man of imagination* [italics mine].
>
> *(Graf 1942: 467)*

For some, Freud was a miracle worker, while for others (like Isidor Sadger or Erich Fromm) he seemed to be a tyrant, exercising quasi-authoritarian rule (Sadger 2006; Fromm 1972; 2017).

Freud also attempted to create a portrait of the birth and development of psychoanalysis. In the very first sentences of "On the History of the Psycho-Analytic Movement" (1914), he wrote that psychoanalysis was his invention ("die Psychoanalyse ist meine Schöpfung"), and recalled that for a decade he had been striving alone to develop his own theory ("ich war durch zehn Jahre der einzige, der sich mit ihr beschäftigte") (Freud 1914: 207). Thus, he transformed the beginnings of psychoanalysis into a quasi-mythical story about the birth of the new science, which perfectly coincided with the personal history of its creator. Of those earliest and lonely years, Freud wrote: "Meanwhile, like Robinson Crusoe, I settled down as comfortably as possible on my desert island. When I look back to those lonely years, away from the pressures and confusions of to-day, it seems like a glorious heroic age" (Freud [1914] 1957: 22). Evidently, Freud constructed his intellectual biography along the lines of the literary hero and protagonist of Daniel Defoe's famous novel. Freud repeated this founding gesture in his "An Autobiographical Study" (Freud [1925] 1959b: 7–74). However, in both of his auto/biographies, he omitted the fact that at the origin of psychoanalysis lay an intellectual and emotional relationship with Wilhelm Fliess. As we will see, their correspondence significantly contributes to the study of the emotional history of psychoanalysis as originating from Freud's amorous discourse with his companion.

Freud's letters to Fliess introduced a new language – the psychoanalytic discourse understood as the assemble of self-analytic, autobiographical, love, and scientific discourses. The first edition of this correspondence, published under the title *Aus den Anfängen der Psychoanalyse. Briefe an Wilhelm Fließ, Abhandlungen und Notizen aus den Jahren 1887–1902* in 1950, included a selection of 153 out of his 284 letters to Fliess and was edited by Marie Bonaparte, Anna Freud, and Ernst Kris (Freud 1950). Based on the German edition, an English translation was published four years later, and a French version appeared in 1956 (titled *La naissance de la psychanalyse*). Another edition, prepared by Jeffrey Moussaieff Masson and published only in 1985, titled *The Complete Letters of Sigmund Freud to Wilhelm Fließ, 1887–1904*, included all the letters preserved by Marie Bonaparte and unpublished until then, including Freud's letter to Ida Fliess and several letters from Fliess (Freud 1985). The correspondence from the early years, compared to post-1890, was short and sent sporadically. After 1892, however, the frequency and personal nature of Freud's letters were increasing. By 1897, he had acquired the habit of sending lengthy epistles two or three times a month. The frequency of correspondence would only diminish again after 1900 and the letters would become progressively shorter. The 1904 letters around the "plagiarism affair" – which I will discuss below – show the breakdown of the friendship between Freud and Fliess.

1.3 "Auto-genesis" in self-analytical letters to Fliess

In the history of psychoanalysis, the letter, more than the formal autobiography or the journal, has been a space of *auto-genesis* – an attempt to understand oneself through self-analysis. In the introduction to the second volume of *Les Brouillons de soi*, Philippe Lejeune defined autobiography as follows: "Here, we will understand autobiography as all texts (stories, diaries, letters) in which one speaks about oneself" (Lejeune 2013: 13). Any lifewriting genre in which the element of "writing the self" appears thus takes on an autobiographical dimension. In this view, a letter understood as a form of self-writing is a space of auto-genesis *par excellence.*

The correspondence between Freud and Fliess began in 1887 and lasted seventeen years. In his letters, Freud more than once expressed his feelings for Fliess. On May 21, 1894, worried about his friend's silence, he wrote:

> Dearest friend, Dearest in truth, because I find it touching that you should so thoroughly go into my condition at a time when you are either very busy or not well or possibly both. There was a gap in your letters which had begun to look uncanny to me, and which almost induced me to write for information to a young lady in Berlin [...]. I promise you a detailed report on my illness next time; I feel better, but far from well; at least I am working again. Today I shall allow myself a good hour and chat only about science with you. It is obviously no special favor of fate that I have approximately five hours a year to exchange ideas with you, when I can barely do without the other – and you are the only other, the *alter* [German: wo ich den Anderen kaum entbehren kann und Du der einzige Andere, der alter, bist].
>
> *(Freud 1985: 73)*

Freud's impatience exposed his emotional involvement, which only intensified over time. In a letter dated August 26, 1898, Freud was already writing about love: "I already realized that it was necessary for me *to love you* [German: Dich zu lieben] in order to enrich my life [italics mine]" (Ibid.: 323). In December 1987, both men met in Breslau. Freud recalled their trip in the following manner:

> Back home and in harness again, with the *delicious aftertaste* [German: mit dem köstlichen Nachgeschmack] of our days in Breslau. Bi-bi [bisexuality-bilaterality] is ringing in my ears, but I am still *feeling too well* for serious work [italics mine].
>
> *(Ibid.: 290)*

The phrase "delicious [köstlich] aftertaste" used by Freud indicates that the trip was not only intellectual but also romantic in nature. Therefore, the evocation of the concept of bisexuality in the following sentence is not unexpected. For Freud, who was discovering his feelings, the idea of universal human bisexuality was the perfect opportunity to reveal the truth of his desires. He then began to write about the "feminine" side of his psyche. In a letter from May 7, 1900, referring to friendship between men, he emphasized: "no one can replace for me the relationship with the friend which a special – *possibly feminine* [German: etwa feminine] – side demands [italics mine]" (Ibid.: 291–293). This letter, too, can be read as a love confession. No one, says Freud, can replace a man as his companion. In his love letters, Fliess was the one Freud longed to see, whose portrait he had created in his mind, whom he wanted to trust, and whose opinion he placed above everything else. In another letter, Freud stated:

> Last night your dear wife, radiant as always, visited us, bringing *the short-lived illusion of all of us being happily together* [German: die kurze Illusion eines erfreulichen *Zusammenlebens* gebracht] and taking it away

> again with her departure. Such interruptions of loneliness have a salutary effect by reminding us how difficult renunciation actually is and how wrong one is to get used to it [italics mine].
>
> *(Ibid.: 284)*

Although physically absent, Fliess accompanied Freud in his imagination, becoming the object of his fascination and love.[18]

How significant the relationship with Fliess was for Freud is evidenced by his subsequent letters to his younger associates. To Sándor Ferenczi, Freud wrote:

> You not only noticed, but also understood, that *I no longer have any need to uncover my personality completely*, and you correctly traced this back *to the traumatic reason* for it. *Since Fliess, with the overcoming of which you recently saw me occupied*, that need has been extinguished. A part of *homosexual cathexis has been withdrawn and made use of to enlarge my own ego.* I have succeeded where the paranoiac fails [italics mine].
>
> *(Garner 1989: 86)*

The split with Fliess is described here as a traumatic experience. Freud diagnosed his overcoming of the love for his former friend as a struggle with his own homosexuality. This theme reappears in a famous letter to Ferenczi dated October 17, 1910, in which Freud wrote: "I feel capable of handling everything and am *pleased with the greater independence that results from having overcome my homosexuality* [italics mine]" (Ibid.: 87). What is particularly significant here is not necessarily the question of "overcoming" his non-normative desire, but the fact that Freud merges the two psychological struggles: with his homosexuality and with the memories of Fliess. Paradoxically, the return to the traumatic experience was an opportunity for Freud to revisit the lost love that later he was so eager to reduce to the "homosexual component" of his character.

While the discourse of friendship between men in modern Western culture permitted affection, tenderness, and sensitivity, the sphere of sexuality remained an unbridgeable boundary (Kosofsky Sedgwick 1990). In the early years of the psychoanalytic movement, Freud surrounded himself almost exclusively with men. The situation changed after World War I, when the first female psychoanalysts formally joined the movement. Still, his closest circle of collaborators (the so-called Geheimes Komitee) was formed exclusively by men. Writing about homosocial relationships, Eve Kosofsky Sedgwick noted:

> "Homosocial desire," to begin with, is a kind of oxymoron. "Homosocial" is a word occasionally used in history and the social sciences, where it describes social bonds between persons of the same sex; it is a neologism, obviously formed by analogy with "homosexual," and just as obviously meant to be distinguished from "homosexual." In fact, it is applied to such

> activities as "male bonding," which may, as in our society, be characterized by intense homophobia, fear and hatred of homosexuality. To draw the "homosocial" back into the orbit of "desire," of the potentially erotic, then, is to hypothesize the potential unbrokenness of a continuum between homosocial and homosexual – a continuum whose visibility, for men, in our society, is radically disrupted.
>
> *(Ibid.: 1)*

In Sedgwick's eyes, "male bonding" was based on the exclusion of women and the suppression of homosexual desire. While women were not equal partners to men, homosexuals were seen as the ones who (like Daniel Paul Schreber) had lost the battle against themselves, ending up as the subjects of psycho-medical case studies.

In *Between Men*, Sedgwick introduced the distinction between love and desire, which she related to the social phenomenon of male bonding:

> I have chosen the word "desire" rather than "love" to mark the erotic emphasis because, in literary critical and related discourse, "love" is more easily used to name a particular emotion, and "desire" to name a structure; in this study, a series of arguments about the structural permutations of social impulses fuels the critical dialectic. For the most part, I will be using "desire" in a way analogous to the psychoanalytic use of "libido" – not for a particular affective state or emotion, but for the affective or social force, the glue, even when its manifestation is hostility or hatred or something less emotively charged, that shapes an important relationship.
>
> *(Ibid.: 2)*

While Sedgwick's notion of love refers to a feeling that ties people together, desire is a category derived from a particular social structure – in this case based on homophobia and the patriarchal preservation of strong (asexual) relations between men. Although Freud and Fliess's partnership could easily be considered a form of homosocial desire, a careful reading of their correspondence shows that this bond could simultaneously transcend the patriarchal structure (as love) and realize itself discursively as homosocial male bonding (in the only acceptable way at the time).

Freud's relationship with Fliess was so intense that it soon began to arouse interest and jealousy in their closest circle and thus rapidly went beyond the socially acceptable model of male-male bonding. Freud's feelings for Fliess must have been so overt that at some point they were considered a threat to Fliess's marriage (Freud 1985: 447).[19]

Freud – who was raised in the bourgeois culture of Vienna in the second half of the nineteenth century in an assimilated Jewish community – was well aware of the cultural taboo against homosexuality. At the same time, even if it seemed impossible in the given socio-cultural conditions, love still demanded expression. Correspondence, with its culturally and traditionally defined norms and rules, became the perfect space for Freud to disclose his feelings. Shirley Nelson Garner, writing about the emotional dimension of Freud's letters to Fliess, aptly pointed out the similarities between Freud's epistolary love discourse and Shakespeare's poetic discourse. As she wrote:

> for both Freud and Shakespeare, male friendships were extremely important. Both evidently felt the pulls of bisexual attraction [...]. Shakespeare's homoerotic attraction may have been stronger than Freud's, or they may only appear to be so because the poetic mode in which the artist worked allowed him more freedom to express them. But as the two men reveal themselves in their writing; both have bisexual temperaments.
> *(Garner 1989: 87)*

The boundary between male platonic friendship and homoerotic desire turns out to be artificial. It operates not so much as a social fact, but as a linguistic construct – the result of the interactions of norms and rules that create the discursive space in which both sender and receiver of the letter function.

Following Garner's analysis, one must keep in mind that Freud and Shakespeare were writing in different social circumstances that viewed human sexuality in a completely opposite way. While the law severely punished "sodomy" in Shakespeare's time, the "question" of homosexuality as a psychological fact did not exist (Laqueur 1990). At the time when Freud was exchanging letters with Fliess and working on *The Interpretation of Dreams*, homosexuality was distinguished in psycho-medical science as a type of perversion, which was of particular interest to psychiatrists and sexologists (Foucault 2003). In the second half of the nineteenth century, homosexual desire started to be seen as a deviation from the "normal" path – one that demanded psychiatric intervention. While Garner seems to overlook this important aspect, she nevertheless accurately observes:

> Freud and Shakespeare, therefore, suspended their friendships with men between a crucial desire for intimacy and union and a need to keep those feelings at bay. It was within this space that Freud's friendship with Fliess unfolded. On the one hand, his love for Fliess served him as inspiration and gave him creative energy. On the other, his homophobia, his fear of homosexuality, was destructive. [...] *It was his relentless homophobia rather than his homosexual feelings that led Freud astray* [italics mine].
> *(Garner 1989: 88)*

The fear of social stigmatization due to sexual non-normativity in Freud's case was multiplied by his experience of anti-Semitic violence, which he openly mentioned both in *The Interpretation of Dreams* and in *An Autobiographical Study*. The fear of double exclusion – because of his ethnicity and (potential) homosexuality – can easily be understood in the context of the rising anti-Semitism and homophobia at the turn of the twentieth century. If Freud (1925) did not renounce his origins ("My parents were Jews, and I have remained a Jew myself" [1959b: 9]), he had to reject his love for men, reducing it to the kind of desire that can be "overcome."

The specter of Fliess reappeared in subsequent relationships with younger colleagues that reminded Freud of his lost beloved.[20] In one of his last letters to Jung, he wrote:

> I propose that we abandon our personal relations entirely. I shall lose nothing by it, for my only emotional tie with you has long been a thin thread – *the lingering effect of past disappointments* – and you have everything to gain, in view of the remark you recently made in Munich, to the effect that *an intimate relationship with a man inhibited your scientific freedom* [italics mine].
>
> *(Freud & Jung 1974: 539)*

Freud did not hide a sense of disappointment and betrayal by his colleague. The same tone – like a mantra – resurfaced in his last letters to Ferenczi. In a letter from January 11, 1933, Freud described their disintegrating relationship as follows:

> You write about our being on good terms, which has lasted for many years. I think it was more than that, rather an intimate community of life, feeling, and interest [German: es war mehr als das, eher eine innige Lebens-, Gefühls- und Interessengemeinschaft].
>
> *(Freud & Ferenczi 2000: 446)*

For Freud, the relationship with Ferenczi went beyond the professional: it was a kind of emotional and spiritual partnership.

It is no coincidence that the sense of loss occupied such an important place in the mechanism of the consolidation of the "ego" (das Ich) in Freud's thought. While the forbidden feeling itself could be overcome, the image of the lost object became part of the personality. This mechanism was brilliantly analyzed by Judith Butler. As she argued: "The ego ideal thus serves as an interior agency of sanction and taboo which, according to Freud, works to consolidate gender identity through the appropriate *rechanneling and sublimation of desire* [italics mine]" (Butler 1999: 85). In Freud's case, this "appropriate rechanneling" became the repudiation of homosexual desire and the consent to forced heterosexuality. Butler argues that at the level of the consolidation of one's identity, the taboo against homosexuality precedes the taboo against incest, making the repudiation of homosexuality a central point in human psycho-sexual development. It is worth recalling the following important passage from her argument:

> But clearly not all gender identification is based on the successful implementation of the taboo against homosexuality. [...] Further, this identity is constructed and maintained by the consistent application of this taboo, not only in the stylization of the body in compliance with discrete categories of sex, but in the production and "disposition" of sexual desire. *The language of disposition moves from a verb formation (to be disposed) into a noun formation, whereupon it becomes congealed (to have dispositions); the language of "dispositions" thus arrives as a false foundationalism, the results of affectivity being formed or "fixed" through the effects of the prohibition* [italics mine].
>
> *(Ibid.: 86)*

In this sense, the loss of a loved one (of the same sex) is necessary and inevitable in any individual biography. Significantly, the dynamics of identity formation described by Freud do not say much about "the primary sexual facts of the psyche"; rather, they represent "a law imposed by culture." Similarly, Freud's assertions about "overcoming" homosexual desire for Fliess provide no insight into his feelings, but evidence an apparently successful process of internalizing the homophobic law. The effect of suppression, Butler writes, is melancholy:

> The melancholia of gender identification which "answers" the Oedipal dilemma must be understood, then, as the internalization of an interior moral directive which gains its structure and energy from an externally enforced taboo. Although Freud does not explicitly argue in its favor, *it would appear that the taboo against homosexuality must precede the heterosexual incest taboo*; the taboo against homosexuality in effect creates the heterosexual "dispositions" by which the Oedipal conflict becomes possible. The young boy and young girl who enter into the Oedipal drama with incestuous heterosexual aims have already been subjected to prohibitions which "dispose" them in distinct sexual directions. *Hence, the dispositions that Freud assumes to be primary or constitutive facts of sexual life are effects of a law which, internalized, produces and regulates discrete gender identity and heterosexuality* [italics mine].
>
> *(Ibid.: 87)*

The repudiation of homosexual desire is seen here as equal to the suppression of affection and the loss of the loved object. In other words, the "heterosexual disposition" as the culmination of the process of psycho-sexual development is inevitably associated with loss. A close reading of the correspondence with Fliess can serve as a glimpse into the sources of psychoanalytic theory, which took shape in the face of the loss of the love object – at the intersection of the scientific and the personal.

1.4 The fragments of Freud's love discourse

Epistolary practices include both static/narrative and dynamic/performative genres. In the former case, the letter serves to transmit a specific piece of information. In the latter, it becomes a space for creating dialogue and maintaining a relationship. It is in this sense that letter-writing is a cultural practice (with its own tradition) and a performative act – a form of constructing and performing romantic love in correspondence – as well as a sort of action that affects the lives of the sender and the addressee. In this light, Freud's letters to Fliess can be read as the material trace of a kind of affection that, although it escaped social norms, could not overcome the homophobic culture in which the two physicians functioned.[21] Freud embraced culturally defined rules of genre and expression, seeking the best discursive formula for expressing his feelings. As Barthes has emphasized, the analysis of love discourse – rather than providing a psychological portrait of the lover himself – gives a view of the entire structure that "offers the reader a discursive site: the site of someone speaking within himself, *amorously*, confronting the other (the loved object), who does not speak" (Barthes 1990: 3).

In one of the already mentioned letters, Freud wrote: "I can barely do without the other – and you are *the only other, the alter* [italics mine]" (Freud 1985: 73). I believe this passage to be one of the most beautiful confessions of love in the history of Western literature. What catches the reader's attention is the tender ending of the sentence: "you are the only other, the alter" (German: der einzige Andere, der alter).

In Freud's eyes, Fliess was someone with whom he shared a unique spiritual connection. His words echo Michel de Montaigne's love confession to his late friend (Étienne de La Boétie) in *Essays* (1580).[22] In a chapter entitled "Of Friendship," Montaigne wrote:

> If a man should importune me to give a reason why I loved him, I find it could no otherwise be expressed, than by making answer: *because it was he, because it was I* (French: Parce que c'était lui, parce que c'était moi) [italics mine].
>
> *(Montaigne 1877: no pagination)*

Montaigne dedicated this chapter on friendship entirely to La Boétie, incorporating his friend's sonnets into the first editions of his *Essays.* These passages are not merely philosophical reflections on "male bonding," but a public declaration of love for a friend – a tribute to the companionship they once shared.

Montaigne understood friendship as an ideal union of souls. This contrasted with his idea of marriage, which appeared to him as a contract regulating the continuity of the species. Love for women, Montaigne argued, was the result of lust, not the impulse of the heart. Love that engaged both the heart and the spirit remained reserved for the man – because only he could become, in Freud's words, "der einzige Andere." Montaigne translated the distinction between love (for women) and friendship (between men) into the physical (erotic) as well as the spiritual realm. A careful reading of "Of Friendship" reveals that, according to the French essayist, the division between (the sexual) love and the spiritual (asexual) bond was fluid, because only friendship could develop into love and the rest belonged exclusively to "lust." Significantly, Montaigne referred to famous ancient lovers as examples of perfect friendships: Achilles and Patroclus as well as Harmodius and Aristogeiton. Although the philosopher criticized the "sexual practices" accepted in ancient Greece, what outraged him was not the amorous-erotic bond between men, but the hierarchy culturally inscribed in homosexual relationships. Friendship, which in Montaigne was synonymous with love, could only happen between equals. Therefore, the philosopher argued:

> And doubtless, if without this, there could be such a free and voluntary familiarity contracted, where not only the souls might have this entire fruition, but the bodies also might share in the alliance, and a man be engaged throughout, the friendship would certainly be more full and perfect.
>
> *(Montaigne 1877: no pagination)*

Montaigne postulated here a kind of male-male community in which friendship did not exclude homoerotic relationships. The amorous dimension of his vision of friendship is hard to miss:

> We sought one another long before we met, and by the characters we heard of one another, which wrought upon our affections more than, in reason, mere reports should do; I think 'twas by some secret appointment of heaven. *We embraced in our names; and at our first meeting, which was accidentally at a great city entertainment, we found ourselves so mutually taken with one another, so acquainted, and so endeared betwixt ourselves, that from thenceforward nothing was so near to us as one another* [italics mine].
>
> *(Montaigne 1877: no pagination)*

The effort to separate love (a community of bodies) from friendship (a community of souls) is a purely discursive operation. Montaigne's words, such as "We sought one another long before we met," "We embraced in our names" constitute the voice of a man deeply in love. The phrase "der einzige Andere" used by Freud manifested that the friendship he desired was exactly the sentiment lyrically described by Montaigne:

> This [friendship] has no other idea than that of itself, and can only refer to itself: this is no one special consideration, nor two, nor three, nor four, nor a thousand; 'tis I know not what quintessence of all this mixture,

> which, seizing my whole will, carried it to plunge and lose itself in his, and that having seized his whole will, brought it back with equal concurrence and appetite to plunge and lose itself in mine. *I may truly say lose, reserving nothing to ourselves that was either his or mine* [italics mine].
>
> *(Montaigne 1877: no pagination)*

The letters to Fliess show that Freud was dreaming of the kind of connection that found its description in the words of the French philosopher. Nevertheless, in order not to raise suspicion, homoerotic discourse had to be transformed into a discourse of friendship. A great example of the interplay between writing to a friend and writing to a lover is Freud's letter of July 14, 1894. In it, Freud wrote: "Dearest friend, Your praise *is nectar and ambrosia for me* [German: Liebster Freund! Nektar und Ambrosia ist mir Dein Lob] [italics mine]" (Freud 1985: 87). Less than a year later, in the same spirit, he added:

> My dear Wilhelm, *Your kindheartedness is one of the reasons I love you.* [German: Unter anderem liebe ich Dich auch wegen Deiner Gutmütigkeit]. Initially, it seemed to me that you had broken off contact with me because of my remarks about the mechanism of the symptoms distant from the nose, and I did not deem this improbable. Now you surprise me with a discussion that takes those fantasies seriously [italics mine]!
>
> *(Ibid.: 131)*

Freud's affection grew as he discovered in his friend a partner to discuss the most intimate facts of his own emotional life. The beginnings of his fascination with Fliess, however, were already clear in his earlier correspondence. Freud began a letter dated June 28, 1892 with the following words:

> I have had no opportunity other than in memory to refer back to *the beautiful evening on which I saw you among yours next to your bride.* […] *the comforting thought welled up in me: he is now well taken care of* [German: besorgt] *and in good hands* [German: gut aufgehoben]. This certainty also set the tone for my correspondence with you. *You will not misunderstand it* [italics mine].
>
> *(Ibid.: 31)*

In these words, Freud symbolically gave his companion away to the bride, which only confirmed the superior nature of their bond. A few years earlier Freud also wrote: "*I still do not know how I won you* [German: Ich weiß noch immer nicht, wodurch ich Sie gewonnen habe]. The bit of speculative anatomy of the brain cannot have impressed your rigorous judgment for long" (Ibid.: 16). Freud made no effort to hide his love, and in his letters – despite the hostile cultural context – his affection found its name.[23]

1.5 Self-analysis as a writing practice

In "textually biased"[24] Western culture, writing is treated as a practice that is both rationalizing and alienating (Lyons 1988; Brock 2013). In particular, self-reflective and introspective practices, which have a long tradition in the history of Western thought, have been accused of intensifying the isolation of the writer. Self-reflection, introspection, and self-analysis, as techniques of self-knowledge, served to subject lived experience (by evoking certain affects, impressions) to intellectual processing, based on the practice of writing. For their author, Montaigne's *Essays* became both a life project and a way to gain self-knowledge – and so did *The Interpretation of Dreams* for Freud. Montaigne treated his work as open, constantly adding new passages and rewriting old ones over the years (Calhoun 2014). The same was true of *The Interpretation of Dreams.* With subsequent editions, Freud transformed and extended his opus magnum. Both Freud and Montaigne placed themselves and the "other" (the friend, the beloved) at the center of their self-reflective and writing practices. The two works cited here are thus perfect examples of *relational writings* – texts developed in the light of the authors' relationships to their friend (as a source of inspiration).

When Freud discovered that he could freely confide in Fliess, his self-analytic practices intensified. The companion embraced the role of the confidant and a mirror in which Freud could truly see himself. On October 3, 1897, Freud wrote:

> There is still very little happening to me externally, but internally something very interesting. For the last four days my self-analysis, which I consider indispensable for the clarification of the whole problem, has continued in dreams and has presented me with the most valuable elucidations and clues.
>
> *(Freud 1985: 268)*

As the cited passage demonstrates, self-analysis – as a means of revealing the earliest details of one's personal history – was grounded in the work of memory. The materials examined by Freud were both explicit and implicit memories, with the latter only being accessible through the interpretation of one's dreams. On October 15, Freud again wrote about his progress in self-analysis:

> My self-analysis is in fact *the most essential thing I have at present and promises to become of the greatest value to me* [German: verspricht von höchstem Wert für mich zu werden] if it reaches its end. In the middle of it, it suddenly ceased for three days, during which I had the feeling of being tied up inside (which patients complain of so much) [italics mine].
>
> *(Ibid.: 270)*

Several days later, he added:

> As for myself, I have nothing to tell you about *except analysis, which I think will be the most interesting thing about me* for you as well. [...] I am beginning to perceive in the determining factors large, general, framing motives, as I should like to call them, and other motives, fill-ins, which vary according to the individual's experiences [italics mine].
>
> *(Ibid.: 274)*

Freud spent the entire month of October 1897 practicing self-analysis. During this time, the frequency of his letters also intensified. On the last day of the month, he wrote:

> *My analysis continues and remains my chief interest* [German: Hauptinteresse]. Everything is still obscure, even the problems, but there is a comfortable feeling in it that one has only to reach into one's storerooms to take out what is needed at a particular time. *The most disagreeable part of it is the moods, which often completely hide reality. Sexual excitement* [German: die sexuelle Erregung], *too, is no longer of use* [German: zu brauchen] *for someone like me* [italics mine].
>
> *(Ibid.: 276)*

Self-analysis practiced in written correspondence can be defined as a reflective practice that intensifies one's emotional state, thus becoming both physically and affectively exhausting. Freud's letters of the following months attest to his emotional burnout. Freud was increasingly bored and tired; his self-analysis was progressing too slowly, failing to produce the desired results.

To be successful, self-analysis as a practice carried out in epistolary form requires the presence of another person – a companion for whom it is worthwhile writing down the details of one's emotional life. In Freud's eyes, without a beloved, his own self-analysis would lose its meaning. For example, he wrote in this spirit on November 14, 1897:

> *My self-analysis remains interrupted. I have realized why I can analyze myself only with the help of knowledge obtained objectively (like an outsider). True self-analysis is impossible* [German: unmöglich]; otherwise there would be no [neurotic] illness. Since I am still contending with some kind of puzzle in my patients, this is bound to hold me up in my self-analysis as well [italics mine].
>
> *(Ibid.: 281)*

In the words "true self-analysis is impossible" one can hear an echo of the heated discussions on introspection as a method of self-examination that took place in philosophical and psychological circles in the second half of the nineteenth century. This is why Freud introduces the distinction between self-analysis and psychoanalysis as a meeting of two people. The long-held distinction between self-analysis (the one-person model) and analysis (the two-person model) was based on the conflation of self-analysis with introspection. In this view, Freudian self-analysis was no different from self-observation, which in the 1870s and 1880s attracted the interest of leading psychologists such as Franz Brentano and Wilhelm Wundt, and earlier of philosophers such as Auguste Comte and John Stuart Mill. The letters to Fliess, however, significantly complicate the idea of treating introspection and self-analysis synonymously. That is because, in these letters, expressions of feelings are intertwined with the language of self-analysis, which makes the two discourses – a lover's discourse and self-analysis – inseparable.

By placing Fliess as the object of love at the center of Freud's self-analytic practices, it is possible to see them as a complex technique of self-examination, which from the very beginning constituted a form of communication with a loved one. In this context, Freud asserted:

> *I still do not know what has been happening in me. Something from the deepest depths of my own neurosis set itself against any advance* in the understanding of the neuroses, and you have somehow been involved in it. *For my writing paralysis seems to me designed to inhibit our communication.* I have no guarantees of this, just feelings of a highly obscure nature. Has nothing of the kind happened to you [italics mine]?
>
> *(Ibid.: 255)*

It was writing as a daily practice that made it possible to rationalize the accumulated self-analytic material, which ceased to be obscure and vague. By subjecting himself to self-observation, Freud was able to distance himself from his past and stepped into the role of his own autobiographer. The next phase was to send the written self-reflections to his friend. At the climax of the self-analysis, however, Freud "discovered" the Oedipus complex and transformed his own story into a quasi-mythical tale. On October 15, 1897, he was already stating:

> the Greek legend seizes upon a compulsion which everyone recognizes because he senses its existence within himself. Everyone in the audience was once a budding Oedipus in fantasy and each recoils in horror from the dream fulfillment here transplanted into reality, with the full quantity of repression which separates his infantile state from his present one.
>
> *(Ibid.: 272)*

From this point on, self-analysis begins to develop primarily in the *imaginary* realm.

Significantly, during his intense correspondence with Fliess, Freud adopted many of his friend's theories. In a letter dated February 8, 1897, he wrote: "That I am the 'nobody' in Vienna who believes in your series you undoubtedly know" (Ibid.: 229). During this time, Freud was also experimenting with the theory of periodicity. He drew tables and carefully divided days into periods: female and male. The extent of his fascination with Fliess's theories is evidenced by a letter dated December 6, 1896, in which Freud admitted:

> One must also trace the derivation of the different epochs, psychological and sexual. *You have taught me to recognize the latter as special multiples of the 28-day female period.* [...] If I assume that all observed periods are such multiples, then on the one hand the 23-day period remains unutilized, and on the other hand, it remains unexplained why psychic and sexual phases do not coincide (4 years), and why sometimes perversion and at other times neurosis develops [italics mine].
>
> *(Ibid.: 210)*

Periodicity also became important to Freud in his practices of self-analysis. On October 15, 1897, he noted that he felt powerless during the "female period," and that self-analysis did not produce the anticipated results. As he stated: "From this one should draw the conclusion that the female period is not conducive to work" (Ibid.: 270). In fact, he had already argued: "It is to be supposed that the element essentially responsible for repression is always what is feminine" (Ibid.: 246). The next sentence of the letter is even more remarkable: "This is confirmed by the fact that women as well as men admit more readily to experiences with women than with men. What men essentially repress is the *pederastic element* [German: das päderastische Element] [italics mine]" (Ibid.: 246).[25] Although Freud abandoned the theory of periodicity in the years that followed, certain elements of Fliess's idea of bisexuality remained present in his future thought. On December 29, 1897, he wrote to Fliess: "I have not yet found the time to have a word with my female side" (Ibid.: 291). As can be deduced from his next letter (January 4, 1898), Freud devoted the last days of 1897 to this very task. In a letter dated January 22, 1898, he added: "The button business, which has received my fullest recognition, stands out like an oasis in the desert. In the carriage I already convinced myself, by unbuttoning my clothes, that you were right" (Ibid.: 295). According to Fliess, left-handedness was thought to indicate the predominance of a female element in a person, and thus latent homosexuality (Ibid.: 291).[26] However, he only made his ideas public later, in the work titled *The Course of Life: Basis for Exact Biology* (*Der Ablauf des Lebens. Grundlegung zur exakten Biologie*), where he interchangeably used two terms – "*die Zweigeschlechtlichkeit*" and "*die Doppelgeschlechtigkeit*" – to describe the man-woman nature of every human being (Fliess 1906a).

In his letters to Fliess, Freud would replace the term "*die Zweigeschlechtlichkeit*" employed by his friend with the term "*die Bisexualität*." The latter connotes a slightly different meaning. While "*die Zweigeschlechtlichkeit*" or "*die Doppelgeschlechtigkeit*" indicate a bisexual condition that is universal to man internally (psychically), "*die Bisexualität*" – due to the presence of the root word "*sexualität*" – tends to treat man's bisexual nature not as inherent (as in Weininger's view), but rather in the sense of a desire directed toward people of both sexes. Freud's substitution of terms is not accidental and reveals one of the most important results of his self-analysis. In fact, what Freud did was that he took over Fliess's theoretical discourse to write about something he was concerned with on a deeply personal level. In other words, his theoretical practice became a disguised manifestation of his own bisexuality.

The rupture of their relationship forced Freud both to renounce his unfulfilled love and to suppress the truth about its importance to the foundations of his theory. In his later writings, Freud maintained his belief that bisexuality was inherent to humans, while distancing himself from Fliess and his "plagiarism affair." In *Three Essays on the Theory of Sexuality*, he wrote:

> Every individual on the contrary displays a mixture of the character-traits belonging to his own and to the opposite sex; and he shows a combination of activity and passivity whether or not these last character-traits tally with his biological ones.
>
> *(Freud [1905] 1953: 220)*

The masculine (active) and the feminine (passive) were supposed to merge in every human being. That this intuition was conveyed to him by Fliess is mentioned by Freud only in the first edition of this work. In all subsequent editions, he omitted his friend's name. The appearance and disappearance of Fliess's name may also suggest that the affective entanglement lasted many years after the breakup of their relationship. The specter of the loss, which haunted him, turned Freud into a disappointed and abandoned lover. The price of coming to terms with his grief after losing Fliess was the transformation of the memory of a *vibrant feeling* into a surmountable *wishful projection*.

1.6 The plagiarism affair, with love correspondence in the background

In his letters to his younger colleagues, Freud returned more than once to his friendship with Fliess. At the same time, he reduced that relationship to an established psychological pattern, thus depriving it of its uniqueness – unlike Montaigne's descriptions. The emotional ties that Freud established with several of his closest colleagues in the following years acted as a recollection of

Fliess and a reenactment of the lost love object. As Ann Pellegrini has aptly written about the mechanism of substitute formation in the context of trauma: "The 'original' is displaced; when we return, we return elsewhere: to a re-place, not the same place we began" (Pellegrini 2009: 244). Exactly the same mechanism is at work with the loss of the love object ("the real thing"), which is later recalled from the "re-place," thereby marking all subsequent emotional-intellectual relationships.

Toward the end of Freud's life, the ghost of Fliess returned – not as an emotional disappointment, but as the dread of the public disclosure of the material traces of their relationship. In 1928, Freud received a request from Ida Fliess: she asked to be given the letters from her late husband.[27] Freud, however, destroyed most of this correspondence in 1904 – unlike Fliess, who preserved his letters. After the correspondence was acquired by Marie Bonaparte in the 1930s, Freud repeatedly wrote to her about his fear of making them public. In one letter, he claimed: "Our correspondence was *the most intimate* you can imagine. It would be highly embarrassing to have it fall into the hands of strangers. […] *I do not want any of them to become known to so-called posterity* [italics mine]" (Freud 1985: 7). Although Freud acknowledged that his correspondence with Fliess had a "most intimate" character, his feelings were not necessarily decipherable to outsiders. Bonaparte's reply illustrates this well:

> Can you *really remember after such a long time what is in these letters*? After all, you *even forgot whether you destroyed the letters* from Fliess or hid them. […] The breakup of this friendship must have been *so painful* [italics mine].
>
> *(Ibid.: 8)*

Aware of the longtime close friendship between Freud and Fliess as well as the importance of their correspondence for the entire history of psychoanalysis, Bonaparte wondered if the fear and trauma of the rupture with his companion had not provoked in Freud an emotional projection which had distorted the memory of the actual content of the letters. The fear of the publication of his intimate correspondence not only painfully reminded Freud of his lost love, but also forced him to confront anew the experience of revealing what was most intimate to him – fragments of love letters to his friend.

Since 1904, Fliess had publicly claimed the theories of bisexuality and periodization as his discoveries.[28] In 1906, in a text titled *On My Own Account* (*In eigener Sache*), Fliess (1906b) made use of Freud's correspondence as an argument in his quarrel with Herman Swoboda and Otto Weininger, thereby involving Freud in it (Schröter 1988: 141–183; 1999: 49–64; 2003: 147–171; Porge 1994). The publication featured extensive excerpts from Freud's correspondence (Freud's letters of July 20, July 23, July 26 as well as his letter of July 27, 1904). In the conclusion, Fliess pointed to Freud as the primary person responsible ("*spiritus rector*") for "stealing" his theory of bisexuality.[29] Referring (publicly) to their private correspondence, he wrote:

> These letters show Freud as the spiritus rector who not only knew about the illegitimate use of other people's [intellectual] property by Weininger but had made it possible. And yet he did not object and warned neither Weininger nor me!
>
> *(Fliess 1906b: 23)*

In his letters to Swoboda, Freud tried to show indifference to Fliess's actions. It is hard to believe, though, that for Freud the publication of *In eigener Sache* with excerpts from his own letters was not painful (Tögel & Schröter 2002: 313–337).[30] After all, Fliess did not only accuse him of scientific dishonesty, but also revealed what for Freud was a memory of a past intimate relationship.

The plagiarism affair cast a shadow over Freud's entire life story and became the subject of investigation by his biographers. Ernest Jones (1953), Vincent Brome (1968), as well as Paul Roazen (1975) wrote extensively about it. Works specifically dedicated to the affair, on the other hand, either inquired into the psychological condition of Fliess himself or emphasized the value and pioneering nature of his research. In 2003, Schröter took another look at the Fliess affair. Drawing on his published works as well as Freud's unpublished notes (kept at the Library of Congress), Schröter revisited the relationship between Freud and Fliess culminating in the scandal over the theory of bisexuality. However, Schröter completely ignored the emotional character of the two men's friendship, focusing exclusively on its professional dimension. As he wrote:

> The friendship between Freud and Fliess – in its intense phase, starting in 1893 – was based on sharing phantasies about a joint project: the development of a new theory of sexuality, spelt out in its relevance for biology, psychology and the etiology of the neuroses, with Fliess elaborating the organological and Freud the clinical/psychological aspects.
>
> *(Schröter 2003: 161)*[31]

Although Schröter reduced Freud's and Fliess's relationship to "a symbiotic intellectual relationship" (Ibid.: 161), a thorough reading of the letters to Fliess shows that their friendship was an intellectual and an emotional partnership.[32] As I have also tried to demonstrate in this chapter, for Freud the scientific discourse on sexuality expounded in the letters to his companion became an extension of his self-analysis.[33]

For Schröter, the main reason for the rupture of Freud and Fliess's friendship was the fact that "they were not working on the same subject [...], actually neither of them had much use for, or even comprehended, the findings of the other" (Ibid.: 162). Disagreements at the professional level, however, deepened the affective dimension of their relationship, with which certain expectations (at the professional and affective level) were connected: an expectation of full understanding, affectionate reciprocity, a desire to create new theories together, and full trust. Schröter accurately points out that the "fruit Freud gathered from his efforts to overcome the break-up with Fliess" was his theory of paranoia (Ibid.: 163). Its sources, however, were hidden in the personal reworking of the experience of the lost love object. Freud's consideration of Fliess's paranoia can thus be seen not only as an attempt to understand his friend's behavior, but also as a strategy for looking away from his own feelings – hurt and rejection.[34] Freud's struggle with his love for Fliess turns out to be not only an "overcoming" of homoerotic desire, but also a struggle with the experience of rejection, betrayal, and the fear of being publicly exposed by a once-loved person.

1.7 Conclusion

Freud's letters to Fliess are the most important source for exploring the emotional and relational roots of psychoanalysis. Joy, hope, uncertainty, ambition, jealousy, hurt, and anger mark the affective layer of these letters which provided the space for both Freud's self-analysis and the emergence of the early psychoanalytic discourse. If infatuation accompanied and propelled Freud's practices of self-analysis, then feelings of betrayal and disappointed love cast a shadow over his theory, and thus over the entire history of psychoanalysis. This chapter has sought to show that Freud's letters to Fliess – read as fragments of a lover's discourse – were a means of self-discovery and at the same time a vehicle for expressing non-normative love. In this light, the letters to Fliess provide insight into the psychology of relationships based on intellectual inspiration, friendship, erotic fascination, desire, and love. Today, they also can be read as one of the finest examples of homoerotic love discourse in Western literature.

Over time, Freud and Fliess's intimate relationship that initially provided the impetus for the practice of self-analysis and scientific creativity – in the form of the theory of sexuality – became a tool for the diagnosis and description of non-normative desire. It should not be forgotten that Freud's letters to Fliess were written at a time when modern sexological knowledge – and, with it, modern homophobic discourses – were being consolidated. As a material trace of non-normative love, these documents were therefore inevitably associated with the fear of social exclusion and stigmatization. To better understand the complex and even conflicting affects surrounding Freud and his fear of the disclosure of his correspondence with Fliess, it is necessary to take a closer look at the poetics of the psycho-medical discourses on non-normative sexuality that were emerging at the turn of the century.

Notes

1 Here, it is worth mentioning a collection of unpublished biographical essays by Siegfried Bernfeld, who had been working on Freud's biography since the 1940s. The manuscript is kept at the Library of Congress, see *Siegfried Bernfeld Papers*

1892–1953: Series 5: Sigmund Freud Biographical Material, 1854–1958, Library of Congress Manuscript Division Washington, DC 20540.

2 The problem of the relationship between the spoken and the written word is at the center of the anthropology of literacy and the anthropology of writing. The most important works in this field include: Daniel Chandler, *The Act of Writing: A Media Theory Approach* (Aberystwyth: University of Wales, 1995); Jack Goody, *La Logique de l'écriture. Aux origines des sociétés humaines*, trans. Anne-Marie Roussel (Paris: Armand Colin, 2018); David R. Olson, *The World on Paper: The Conceptual and Cognitive Implications of Reading and Writing* (Cambridge-New York: Cambridge University Press, 1994); Roy Harris, *The Semantics of Science* (London-New York: Continuum, 2005). Tim Ingold, *Lines: A Brief History* (New York-London: Routledge, 2007). The anthropology of writing is developing particularly rapidly in Polish anthropology, see for example: *Antropologia pisma. Od teorii do praktyki*, ed. Philippe Artières and Paweł Rodak (Warszawa: Wydawnictwa Uniwersytetu Warszawskiego, 2010); Grzegorz Godlewski, *Słowo, pismo, sztuka słowa. Perspektywy antropologiczne* (Warszawa: Wydawnictwa Uniwersytetu Warszawskiego, 2008); *Luneta i radar. Szkice z antropologicznej teorii kultury* (Warszawa: Wydawnictwa Uniwersytetu Warszawskiego, 2016).

3 In French: *Seule l'écriture peut recueillir l'extrême subjectivité, car dans l'écriture il y a accord entre l'indirect de l'expression et la vérité du sujet – accord impossible au plan de la parole (donc du cours), qui est toujours, quoi qu'on veuille, à la fois directe et théâtrale. Le livre sur le Discours amoureux est peut-être plus pauvre que le séminaire, mais je le tiens pour plus vrai.*

4 Structuralism as a result of the dominance of a text-centered view of reality is more extensively discussed by the Polish anthropologist Paweł Majewski in his book titled *Mantykora. Wczesna historia encyklopedii* (Warszawa: Wydawnictwa Uniwersytetu Warszawskiego, 2022); see especially the chapter "*Hommes des lettres* między słowami a rzeczami," 28–85, cf. François Dosse, *Histoire du structuralisme, vol. 1, Le champ du signe* (Paris: La Découverte, 1991), *vol. 2, Le chant du cygne* (Paris: La Découverte, 1992).

5 The book *Fragments d'un discours amoureux* (A Lover's Discourse: Fragments) was published in the spring of 1977 and was an immediate success, see: Barthes, *Le discours amoureux*, 19–23.

6 The twelfth-century letters between Abelard and Heloise are a key body of correspondence for the development of the love letter genre, see: Constant J. Mews, ed., *The Lost Love Letters of Heloise and Abelard. Perceptions of Dialogue in Twelfth-Century France*, trans. C. J. Mews and Neville Chiavaroli (New York: Palgrave Macmillan, 2008). The history of the discovery of the manuscript (a collection of anonymous love letters) and their attribution to Heloise and Abelard is traced by Mews in the first part of the book (see Chapters 1 and 5: "The Discovery of a Manuscript," 3–27; "The Language of the Love Letters," 115–144).

7 For more on writing practices in the context of Polish experimental psychology, see my book entitled *Autoekonomie zapisu Juliana Ochorowicza. Codzienne praktyki piśmienne i badawcze psychologa*/Julian Ochorowicz's Self-Economies of Writing. Everyday Writing and Research Practices of the Psychologist (Warszawa: Wydawnictwa Uniwersytetu Warszawskiego, 2021). On the psychology of the creative process in the context of everyday writing practices, see: Didier Anzieu, *Le corps de l'œuvre. Essais psychanalytiques sur le travail créateur* (Gallimard, Paris 1981).

8 In the context of psychology, I have written about it in the chapter "Psychoarcheologia bezwiednego. Introspekcja i autoanaliza: eksperyment – automatyzm – dialog," in Sobolewska, *Autoekonomie Juliana Ochorowicza*, 172–260. Here, it is worth mentioning three pioneering works in the field of the Polish anthropology of literacy which directly raised the problem of the interrelationship between the experience of writing (and the various difficulties associated with it) and what is written (the content of the work), see: Marta Rakoczy, *Słowo – działanie –*

kontekst. O etnograficznej koncepcji języka Bronisława Malinowskiego (Warszawa: Wydawnictwa Uniwersytetu Warszawskiego, 2012); P. Majewski, *Pismo, tekst, literatura. Praktyki piśmienne starożytnych Greków i matryca pamięci kulturowej Europejczyków* (Warszawa: Wydawnictwa Uniwersytetu Warszawskiego, 2013); *Tekstualizacja doświadczenia. Studia o piśmiennictwie greckim* (Toruń: Wydawnictwo Naukowe Uniwersytetu Mikołaja Kopernika, 2015).

9 For English translation, see: U. May, *Freud at Work: On the History of Psychoanalytic Theory and Practice, with an Analysis of Freud's Patient Record Books* (London-New York: Routledge, 2018).

10 Complete editions and selections of Freud's letters to family, friends, and colleagues have been published, including exchanges with Martha Freud, Eugene Bleuler, Wilhelm Fliess, Minna Bernays, Eduard Silberstein, Anna Freud, Ludwig Binswanger, Arnold Zweig, Carl Gustav Jung, Sándor Ferenczi, Ernest Jones, Karl Abraham, Lou Andreas-Salomé, Otto Rank, Nikolai Y. Ossipow, Georg Groddeck, Oskar Pfister, and Max Eitingon. Numerous letters exchanged with collaborators, including Groddeck and Ferenczi, Ferenczi and Jones, Anna Freud and Lou Andreas-Salomé, Abraham with Fliess, and Jones, are also available in print. A selection of Freud's early letters to miscellaneous addressees has been published under the title *Sigmund Freud. Briefe 1873–1939*, ed. Ernst and Lucy Freud (Frankfurt am Main: S. Fischer Verlag, 1960). Freud's letters to his children were also published as *Sigmund Freud. Unterdess halten Wir zusammen. Briefe an die Kinder*, ed. Michael Schröter (Berlin: Aufbau Verlag 2010), Freud's travel letters as *Sigmund Freud. Unsere Herz zeigt nach dem Süden. Reisebriefe 1895–1923*, ed. Christfried Tögel and Michael Molnar (Berlin: Aufbau Verlag 2002), and a selection of Freud's letters with Havelock Ellis, Ivan Pavlov, George Bernard Shaw, Romain Rolland as *Freudiana*, ed. A. A. Roback (Cambridge, Massachusetts: Sci-Art Publishing, 1957).

11 I am referring here to the previously unpublished notes on a lover's discourse by Barthes, see Barthes, *Le discours amoureux*, 673. Cf. Denis De Rougemont, *Love in the Western World*, trans. Montgomery Belgian (Princeton: Princeton University Press, 1983), 5–7.

12 I refer here to a particularly significant case for the formation of the love letter genre in the history of European literature: Ovid's "Epistle from Sappho to Phaon" from the Heroides cycle. For a discussion of this short work attributed to Ovid, see Albert R. Baca, "Ovid's Epistle from Sappho to Phaon (Heroides 15)," *Transactions and Proceedings of the American Philological Association* 102 (1971): 29–38. Within queer readings of Western literature, Sappho is treated as a poet of lesbian and queer love as well as a non-normative figure (as a woman-author, a queer woman, and the first poetess in the canon of European literature). For more on this, see Harriette Andreadis, "The Sappho Tradition," in *The Cambridge History of Gay and Lesbian Literature*, ed. E. L. Mccallum and Mikko Tuhkanen (Cambridge: Cambridge University Press, 2014), 15–33; Melissa Mueller, "Sappho and Sexuality," in *The Cambridge Companion to Sappho*, ed. P. J. Finglass and Adrian Kelly (Cambridge: Cambridge University Press, 2021), 36–52. In this chapter, Mueller, after Eve Kosofsky Sedgwick, writes about the "queer affect" as a conceptual tool for reading and interpreting Sappho's poems and a remedy for the error of interpreting her writings (and life) through binary oppositions (heterosexuality/homosexuality and lesbian/straight), 50.

13 For the most recent queer readings of Shakespeare's works, see: *Shakesqueer: A Queer Companion to the Complete Works of Shakespeare*, ed. Madhavi Menon (Durham-London: Durham University Press, 2011); *Queer Shakespeare: Desire & Sexuality*, ed. Goran Stanivukovic (London-New York: Bloomsbury Publishing, 2017); Melissa E. Sanchez, *Shakespeare and Queer Theory* (London-New York: Bloomsbury Publishing, 2019).

14 For a queer reading of Montaigne's writings, see Gary Ferguson, *Queer (Re) readings in the French Renaissance: Homosexuality, Gender, Culture* (New York:

Routledge, 2016), especially the chapter "Montaigne's Itchy Ears. Friendship, Marriage, Homosexuality, and Scepticism," 191–244.

15 On Verlaine's queerness, see *The Cambridge History of Gay and Lesbian Literature*, 326, 327, 379–80, 381–82; cf. Louise Alison Brown, "Rethinking Queer Poetry: Queerness in the French Lyric Tradition from 1819 to 1918" (PhD diss., University of California, 2020); the manuscript of this doctoral dissertation is available online: https://escholarship.org/content/qt68s5453d/qt68s5453d_noSplash_81acdb29a87113874d01e9d6b564aa25.pdf (accessed 07.07.2022), 122–142.

16 For nineteenth-century authors, especially queer ones, Plato's *Symposium* was particularly important, as was his *Phaedrus*. In the nineteenth century, the *Symposium* was also used by representatives of the psycho-medical sciences of the time (along with a particular vision of Greek ancient culture) as an argument for the depenalization of homosexuality. See, for example, David Decosta Leitao, "Plato and the Philosophical Dialogue," in *The Cambridge History of Gay and Lesbian Literature*, 34–50.

17 On companionship, lesbianism, and female husbands in the first half of the nineteenth century, see Jack Halberstam, *Female Masculinity*, 65–73. Cf. *I Know My Own Heart: The Diaries of Ann Lister*, ed. Helena Whitbread (New York: New York University Press, 1992).

18 It is worth mentioning that Freud's affective life at the time was also occupied by his sister-in-law Minna Bernays, with whom he probably began an affair in the summer of 1900. His love for Fliess did not necessarily preclude affectionate involvements with other people. On the contrary, an affair with Minna could only strengthen the indication that Freud was in fact bisexual. Referring to the importance of Freud's love relationship with Minna, Peter L. Rudnytsky writes: "If Freud did engage in a sexual affair with Minna, four years younger than his wife, Martha, and his own junior by nine years, the effects of this primordial boundary violation would not have been confined to Freud's 'private' life, but would, rather, have extended to the professional sphere in manifold ways, and would, indeed, haunt the entire history of psychoanalysis," P. L. Rudnytsky, *Rescuing Psychoanalysis from Freud and Other Essays in Re-Vision* (London: Karnac, 2011), 13–14.

19 Ida Fliess was jealous of Freud's intimate relationship with Fliess. She was also warned against Freud by Josef Breuer. Freud mentioned this on August 7, 1901: "he [Breuer] told her [Ida] how lucky she was that *I did not live in Berlin and could not interfere with her marriage* [italics mine]."

20 Freud will recognize this pattern in his emotional life in a letter dated 3.10.1897 to Fliess.

21 As linguistic anthropologist Laura M. Ahearn has accurately stated, love is not an abstract category or an ahistorical feeling: "love, like all other emotions, accrues meanings (note the plural here – meanings) only in specific sociocultural interactions, in particular places and at given moments in history," L. M. Ahearn, *Invitations to Love: Literacy, Love Letters, and Social Change in Nepal* (Ann Arbor: The University of Michigan Press, 2001), 48.

22 Michel de Montaigne, *Essays of Michel de Montaigne*, ed. William Carew Hazlitt, trans. Charles Cotton (London: Reeves and Turner, 1877). This book is available online: www.gutenberg.org/files/3600/3600-h/3600-h.htm#link2HCH0027, accessed December 1, 2021.

23 See letter dated January 22, 1898, where Freud mentions his left-handedness in the context of Fliess's bilateral theory.

24 On "the textual bias" in Western culture, see David R. Olson, *The World on Paper*; G. Godlewski, "Poza nachylenie tekstowe, w stronę doświadczenia przedtekstowego. Wskazówki terapeutyczne," *Teksty Drugie* 1 (2018): 61–78. Godlewski states that "the textual bias" dominates Western science and culture, and explains that this tendency "results from advanced literacy" and "leads to the textualization of reality": 78. However, in the context of psychoanalysis and analytic practices,

the question of "the textual bias" is more complicated. Indeed, the spoken word plays a key role in the therapeutic process. At the same time, the method and technique of interpretation are immersed in written (theoretical) texts which define the framework of analytic work in a given therapeutic approach. I will return to this problem in the final chapter of this book.

25 Cf. his letter on November 14, 1897: "This is where I have got to so far – with all the inherent obscurities. I have resolved, then, henceforth to regard as separate factors what causes libido and what causes anxiety. I have also given up the idea of explaining libido as the masculine factor and repression as the feminine one," 281.

26 See footnote number 5: "The reference is to a test to see if a person is left-handed. Fliess believed that people who were left-handed showed the psychological (and physical) characteristics of the opposite sex," ibid.: 291.

27 The two letters from Ida Fliess to Freud and two from Freud to Ida Fliess are in the Jewish National and University Library in Jerusalem, see Deborah Margolis, "Freud, Fliess, and the Lost Dream," *Modern Psychoanalysis* 15 (1990): 131–148.

28 During this time, Fliess published several texts accusing Otto Weininger and Herman Swoboda of plagiarism, see Wilhelm Fliess, *Der Ablauf des Lebens. Grundlegung zur exakten Biologie* (Leipzig-Wien: Deuticke, 1906); *In eigener Sache*; Richard Pfennig, *Wilhelm Fliess und seine Nachentdecker: O. Weininger und H. Swoboda* (Berlin: E. Goldschmidt, 1906).

29 In his *In eigener Sache*, Fliess wrote: "Otto Weininger, now deceased, claimed permanent bisexuality, Hermann Swoboda periodicity. Both authors were intimate friends and had access to one and the same source: Prof. Sigmund Freud in Vienna," 5.

30 Excerpts from their private correspondence also appeared in Pfenning's pamphlet, to whom Fliess must have passed this confidential material before 1906.

31 See also Schröter, "Freud und Fließ im wissenschaftlichen Gespräch. Das Neurasthenie projekt von 1893," in *Jahrbuch der Psychoanalyse* 22 (1988), 175–178.

32 Schröter, "Fliess versus Weininger," 161. I do not think Schröter is right when he writes: "Beginning in the summer of 1897, Freud set it [the friendship with Fliess] aside in favour of writing his *Interpretation of Dreams* which was almost exclusively restricted to the field of psychology," 161. 1897 was a pivotal year for Freud's self-analytical practices, which he reported to Fliess. In his biography of Freud, Peter Gay notes an important detail about the relationship between Freud and Fliess. As he writes: "Freud's friendship with Fliess ripened with fair speed, rather uncharacteristic for an age in which intimacy was usually slow to develop and sometimes resisted decades of close association," P. Gay, *Freud: A Life for Our Time*, 61. On Fliess, 55–63.

33 Schröter mentions that Freud even planned to write a book on human bisexuality together with Fliess, 161. At the same time, bisexuality recurred as a theme and a source of conflict during Freud's last meeting with Fliess in Achensee in 1900, and also later during the plagiarism affair; cf. Barbara Mautner, "Freud's 'Lost' Dream and the Schism with Wilhelm Fliess," *International Journal of Psychoanalysis* 75 (1994), 321–333.

34 Schröter refers to Freud's unpublished notes in which he diagnosed paranoia in Fliess, 163.

References

Ahearn, L. M. (2001). *Invitations to Love: Literacy, Love Letters, and Social Change in Nepal*, Ann Arbor: The University of Michigan Press.

Anzieu, D. (1981). *Le corps de l'œuvre. Essais psychanalytiques sur le travail créateur*, Paris: Gallimard.

Anzieu, D. (1998). *L'auto-analyse de Freud et la découverte de la psychanalyse*, Paris: Presses Universitaires de France.
Anzieu, D. (2000). Vues nouvelles sur l'auto-analyse de Freud et la découverte de la psychanalyse, in *Revue française de psychanalyse* 64, 1201–1216.
Artières, P. & Rodak, P. (Eds.) (2010). *Antropologia pisma. Od teorii do praktyki*, Warszawa: Wydawnictwa Uniwersytetu Warszawskiego.
Baca, A. R. (1971). Ovid's Epistle from Sappho to Phaon (Heroides 15), in *Transactions and Proceedings of the American Philological Association* 102, 29–38.
Barthes, R. (1990). *A Lover's Discourse: Fragments*. Translated by Richard Howard. London/New York: Penguin Books.
Barthes, R. (2007). *Le discours amoureux. Séminaire à l'École pratique des hautes études 1974–1976 suivi de Fragments d'un discours amoureux: inédits*, Paris: Seuil.
Binswanger, L. (1956). *Erinnerungen an Sigmund Freud*, Bern: Francke.
Brock, A. C. (2013). *The History of Introspection Revisited*, New York/London: Routledge.
Brome, V. (1968). *Freud and His Early Circle*, New York: W. Morrow & Co.
Brown, L. A. (2020). *Rethinking Queer Poetry: Queerness in the French Lyric Tradition from 1819 to 1918*, non-published PhD-thesis: University of California.
Butler, J. (1999). *Gender Trouble*, New York/London: Routledge.
Całek, A. (2019). *Nowa teoria listu*, Kraków: Księgarnia Akademicka.
Calhoun, A. (2014). *Montaigne and the Life of Philosophers: Life Writing and Transversality in the Essais*, Newark: University of Delaware Press.
Chandler, D. (1995). *The Act of Writing: A Media Theory Approach*, Aberystwyth: University of Wales.
Collins, R. (1998). *The Sociology of Philosophies: A Global Theory of Intellectual Change*, Cambridge, Massachusetts: Harvard University Press.
Darnton, R. (1992). *Gens de lettres, gens du livre*. Translated by Marie-Alyx Revellat, Paris: Éditions Odile Jacob.
De Rougemont, D. (1983). *Love in the Western World*. Translated by Montgomery Belgian, Princeton: Princeton University Press.
Decosta Leitao, D. (2014). Plato and the Philosophical Dialogue, in L. Marcus & P. Nicholls, *The Cambridge History of Twentieth-Century English Literature*, Cambridge: Cambridge University Press, 34–50.
Deutsch, H. (1940). Freud and his Pupils: A Footnote to the History of the Psychoanalytic Movement, in *Psychoanalytic Quarterly* 9, 184–194.
Deutsch, H. (1973). *Confrontations with Myself: An Epilogue*, New York: W. W. Norton.
Dosse, F. (1991). *Histoire du structuralisme: vol. 1, Le champ du signe*, Paris: La Découverte.
Dosse, F. (1992). *Histoire du structuralisme: vol. 2, Le chant du cygne*, Paris: La Découverte.
Falzeder, E. (Ed.) (2002). *The Complete Correspondence of Sigmund Freud and Karl Abraham: 1907–1925: Completed Edition*. Translated by Caroline Schwarzacher. London/New York: Karnac.
Ferguson, G. (2016). *Queer (Re)readings in the French Renaissance: Homosexuality, Gender, Culture*, New York: Routledge.
Finglass, P. J. & Kelly, A. (2021). *The Cambridge Companion to Sappho*, Cambridge: Cambridge University Press.
Fliess, W. (1906a). *Der Ablauf des Lebens. Grundlegung zur exakten Biologie*, Leipzig/Wien: Deuticke.

Fliess, W. (1906b). *In eigener Sache. Gegen Otto Weininger und Hermann Swoboda*, Berlin: E. Goldschmidt.

Foucault, M. (2003). *Le pouvoir psychiatrique*, Paris: Seuil.

Freud, E. L. (Ed.) (1960). *Sigmund Freud. Briefe 1873–1939*, Frankfurt am Main: S. Fischer Verlag.

Freud, E. L. (1961). Preface to Letters of Sigmund Freud 1873–1939, in *Classic Books* 51: vii–viii.

Freud, S. (1950). *Aus den Anfängen der Psychoanalyse: Briefe an Wilhelm Fliess, Abhandlungen und Notizen aus den Jahren 1887–1902*, London: Imago.

Freud, S. ([1905] 1953). Three Essays on the Theory of Sexuality, in J. Strachey (Ed.), *The Standard Edition of the Complete Psychological Works of Sigmund Freud.* Vol. 7, London: The Hogarth Press, 125–245.

Freud, S. ([1914] 1957). On the History of Psycho-Analytic Movement, in J. Strachey (Ed.), *The Standard Edition of the Complete Psychological Works of Sigmund Freud*, Vol. 14, London: The Hogarth Press, 1–66.

Freud, S. ([1925] 1959b). An Autobiographical Study, in J. Strachey (Ed.), *The Standard Edition of the Complete Psychological Works of Sigmund Freud.* Vol. 20, London: The Hogarth Press, 7–74.

Freud, S. & Pfister, O. (1963). *Briefe 1909–1939*, Frankfurt am Main: S. Fischer Verlag.

Freud, S. & Abraham, K. (1965). *Briefe 1907–1926*, Frankfurt am Main: S. Fischer Verlag.

Freud, S. & Andreas-Salomé, L. (1966). *Briefwechsel*, Frankfurt am Main: S. Fischer Verlag.

Freud, S. & Zweig, A. (1968). *Briefwechsel*, Frankfurt am Main: S. Fischer Verlag.

Freud, S. & Weiss, E. (1973). *Briefe zur psychoanalytischen Praxis. Mit den Erinnerungen eines Pioniers der Psychoanalyse*, Frankfurt am Main: S. Fischer Verlag.

Freud, S. & Groddeck, G. (1974). *Briefe über das Es*, Frankfurt am Main: S. Fischer Verlag.

Freud, S. & Jung, C. G. (1974). *Briefwechsel*, Frankfurt am Main: S. Fischer Verlag.

Freud, S. & Zweig, A. (1968). *Briefwechsel*, Frankfurt am Main: S. Fischer Verlag.

Freud, S. (1985). *The Complete Letters of Sigmund Freud to Wilhelm Fliess*, 1887–1904, Cambridge, Massachusetts: Harvard University Press.

Freud, S. (1988). *Brautbriefe. Briefe an Martha Bernays aus den Jahren 1882 bis 1886*, Frankfurt am Main: S. Fischer Verlag.

Freud, S. & Ferenczi, S. (1993). *The Correspondence of Sigmund Freud and Sándor Ferenczi. Vol. 1: 1908–1914*, Cambridge, Massachusetts: Harvard University Press.

Freud, S. & Ferenczi, S. (1996). *The Correspondence of Sigmund Freud and Sándor Ferenczi. Vol. 2: 1914–1919*, Cambridge, Massachusetts: Harvard University Press.

Freud, S. & Ferenczi, S. (2000). *The Correspondence of Sigmund Freud and Sándor Ferenczi. Vol. 3: 1920–1933*, Cambridge, Massachusetts: Harvard University Press.

Freud, S. & Jones, E. (1993). *The Complete correspondence of Sigmund Freud and Ernest Jones: 1908–1939*, Cambridge, Massachusetts: Harvard University Press.

Freud, S. & Jones, E. (1993). *Briefwechsel Sigmund Freud - Ernest Jones: 1908–1939*, Frankfurt am Main: S. Fischer Verlag.

Freud, S. & Abraham, K. (2009). *Briefwechsel 1907–1925. Band I: 1907–1914*, Wien: Verlag Turia plus Kant.

Freud, S. & Abraham, K. (2009). *Briefwechsel 1907–1925. Band II: 1915–1925*, Wien: Verlag Turia plus Kant.

Fromm, E. (1972). *Sigmund Freud's Mission: An Analysis of his Personality and Mission*, New York: Harper Colophon Books.

Fromm, E. (2017). *Beyond the Chains of Illusion: My Encounter with Marx and Freud*, London: Bloomsbury Academic.
Garner, S. N. (1989). Freud and Fliess: Homophobia and Seduction, in D. Hunter (Ed.), *Seduction and Theory. Readings of Gender, Representation, and Rhetoric*, Chicago: University of Illinois Press.
Gay, P. (1988). *Freud: A Life for Our Time*, New York: Norton.
Godlewski, G. (2008). *Słowo, pismo, sztuka słowa. Perspektywy antropologiczne*, Warszawa: Wydawnictwa Uniwersytetu Warszawskiego.
Godlewski, G. (2016). *Luneta i radar. Szkice z antropologicznej teorii kultury*, Warszawa: Wydawnictwa Uniwersytetu Warszawskiego.
Godlewski, G. (2018). Poza nachylenie tekstowe, w stronę doświadczenia przedtekstowego. Wskazówki terapeutyczne, in *Teksty Drugie* 1, 61–78.
Goetz, B. (1969). *Das ist alles, was ich über Freud zu erzählen habe: Erinnerung an Sigmund Freud*, Berlin: Friedenauer Presse.
Goody, J. (2018). *La Logique de l'écriture. Aux origines des sociétés humaines*. Translated by Anne-Marie Roussel. Paris: Armand Colin.
Graf, M. (1942). Reminiscences of Professor Sigmund Freud, in *Psychoanalytic Quarterly* 1, 465–476.
Grubrich-Simitis, I. (1993a). *Zurück zu Freuds Texten: Stumme Dokumente sprechen machen*, Frankfurt am Main: S. Fischer Verlag.
Grubrich-Simitis, I. (1993b). *Back to Freud's Texts: Making Silent Documents Speak*. Translated by Philip Slotkin. New Haven: Yale University Press.
Halberstam, J. (1998). *Female Masculinity*, New York/London: Duke University Press.
Harris, R. (2005). *The Semantics of Science*, London/New York: Continuum.
Hébrard, J. (1995). Des écritures exemplaires: l'art du maître écrivain en France entre XVIe et XVIIIe siècle, in *Mélanges de l'École française de Rome, Italie et Méditerranée* 107 (2), 473–523.
Hébrard, J. (2005). Peut-on faire une histoire des pratiques populaires de lecture à l'époque moderne? Les 'nouveaux lecteurs revisités' / Histoires de lecture, XIXe-XXe siècles présentées par Jean-Yves Mollier, in *Matériaux pour une histoire de la lecture et de ses institutions* 17, 105–140.
Hoock-Demarle, M.-C. (2008). *L'Europe des lettres: Réseaux épistolaires et construction de l'espace européen*, Paris: Albin Michel.
Ingold, T. (2007). *Lines: A Brief History*, New York/London: Routledge.
Jones, E. (1953). *The Life and Work of Sigmund Freud*. Vol. I, New York: Basic Books.
Jones, E. (1955). *The Life and Work of Sigmund Freud*. Vol. II, New York: Basic Books.
Jones, E. (1957). *The Life and Work of Sigmund Freud*. Vol. III, New York: Basic Books.
Jones, E. (1959). *Free Associations: Memories of a Psychoanalyst*, London: The Hogarth Press.
Kosofsky Sedgwick, E. (1990). *The Epistemology of the Closet*, Berkeley, Los Angeles: University of California Press.
Laqueur, T. (1990). *Making Sex: Body and Gender from the Greeks to Freud*, Cambridge Massachusetts: Harvard University Press.
Lejeune, P. (2013). *Autogenèses. Les Brouillons de soi*, vol. 2, Paris: Seuil.
Lyons, W. (1988). *The Disappearance of Introspection*, Branford: The MIT Press.
Mccallum, E. L. & Tuhkanen, M. (Eds.) (2014). *The Cambridge History of Gay and Lesbian Literature*, Cambridge: Cambridge University Press.
Majewski, P. (2013). *Pismo, tekst, literatura. Praktyki piśmienne starożytnych Greków i matryca pamięci kulturowej Europejczyków*, Warszawa: Wydawnictwa Uniwersytetu Warszawskiego.

Majewski, P. (2015). *Tekstualizacja doświadczenia. Studia o piśmiennictwie greckim*, Toruń: Wydawnictwo Naukowe Uniwersytetu Mikołaja Kopernika.
Majewski, P. (2022). *Mantykora. Wczesna historia encyklopedii*, Warszawa: Wydawnictwa Uniwersytetu Warszawskiego.
Margolis, D. (1990). Freud, Fliess, and the Lost Dream, in *Modern Psychoanalysis* 15, 131–148.
Mautner, B. (1994). Freud's Lost Dream and the Schism with Wilhelm Fliess, in *International Journal of Psycho-Analysis* 75, 321–333.
May, U. (2015). *Freud bei der Arbeit. Zur Entstehungsgeschichte der psychoanalytischen Theorie und Praxis, mit einer Auswertung von Freuds Patientenkalender*, Gießen: Psychosozial-Verlag.
May, U. (2018). *Freud at Work: On the History of Psychoanalytic Theory and Practice, with an Analysis of Freud's Patient Record Books*, London/New York: Routledge.
Menon, M. (Ed.) (2011). *Shakesqueer: A Queer Companion to the Complete Works of Shakespeare*, Durham/London: Durham University Press.
Mews, C. J. (Ed.) (2008). *The Lost Love Letters of Heloise and Abelard. Perceptions of Dialogue in Twelfth-Century France*. Translated by C. J. Mews & Neville Chiavaroli. New York: Palgrave Macmillan.
Montaigne, M. de (1877). *Essays of Michel de Montaigne*. Translated by Charles Cotton. London: Reeves and Turner.
Olson, D. R. (1994). *The World on Paper: The Conceptual and Cognitive Implications of Reading and Writing*, Cambridge/New York: Cambridge University Press.
Pellegrini, A. (2009). The Dogs of War and the Dogs of Home, in *American Imago* 66 (2), 231–251.
Pfennig, R. (1906). *Wilhelm Fliess und seine Nachentdecker: O. Weininger und H. Swoboda*, Berlin: E. Goldschmidt.
Porge, E. (1994). *Vol d'idées? Wilhelm Fliess, son plagiat et Freud*, Paris: Denoel.
Rakoczy, M. (2012). *Słowo – działanie – kontekst. O etnograficznej koncepcji języka Bronisława Malinowskiego*, Warszawa: Wydawnictwa Uniwersytetu Warszawskiego.
Reik T. (1949). *Fragment of a Great Confession: A Psychoanalytic Autobiography*, New York: Farrar, Straus, and Company.
Roazen, P. (1975). *Freud and his Followers*, Harmondsworth: Penguin.
Roback, A. A. (Ed.) (1957). *Freudiana*, Cambridge, Massachusetts: Sci-Art Publishing.
Rodak, P. (2009). *Pismo,* książka, *lektura. Rozmowy: Le Goff, Chartier, Hébrard, Fabre, Lejeune*, Warszawa: Wydawnictwa Uniwersytetu Warszawskiego.
Rudnytsky, P. L. (2011). *Rescuing Psychoanalysis from Freud and Other Essays in Re-Vision*, London: Karnac.
Sadger, I. (2006). *Recollecting Freud*. Translated by Johanna Micaela Jacobsen. Madison: University of Wisconsin Press.
Saint-Gille, A.-M. (2010). L'Europe des lettres, in *Études Germaniques 2*, 387–391.
Sanchez, M. E. (2019). *Shakespeare and Queer Theory*, London/New York: Bloomsbury Publishing.
Schröter, M. (1988). Freud und Fliess im wissenschaftlichen Gespräch. Das Neurasthenie projekt von 1893, in *Jahrbuch der Psychoanalyse* 22, 141–183.
Schröter, M. (1999). Hermann Swoboda (1873–1963): Früher Freud-Schüler und Kritiker der Traumdeutung, in *Luzifer-Amor. Zeitschrift zur Geschichte der Psychoanalyse* 12 (24), 49–64.
Schröter, M. (2003). Fliess vs. Weininger, Swoboda und Freud: Der Plagiatsstreit von 1906 im Licht der Dokumente, in *Psyche* 56, 147–173.

Schröter, M. (Ed.) (2010). *Sigmund Freud. Unterdess halten Wir zusammen. Briefe an die Kinder*, Berlin: Aufbau Verlag.
Schur, M. (1973). *Sigmund Freud: Leben und Sterben*, Frankfurt am Main: Suhrkamp.
Siegfried Bernfeld Papers 1892–1953: Series 5: Sigmund Freud Biographical Material, 1854–1958, Library of Congress Manuscript Division, Washington, DC 20540.
Sobolewska, A. (2021a). *Autoekonomie zapisu Juliana Ochorowicza. Codzienne praktyki piśmienne i badawcze psychologa*, Warszawa: Wydawnictwa Uniwersytetu Warszawskiego.
Stanivukovic, G. (Ed.) (2017). *Queer Shakespeare: Desire & Sexuality*, London/New York: Bloomsbury Publishing.
Stekel, W. (1950). *The Autobiography of Wilhelm Stekel: The Life Story of a Pioneer Psychoanalyst*, New York: Liveright.
Tögel, C. & Molnar, M. (Eds.) (2002). *Sigmund Freud. Unsere Herz zeigt nach dem Süden. Reisebriefe 1895–1923*, Berlin: Aufbau Verlag.
Tögel, C. & Schröter, M. (2002). Sigmund Freud und Hermann Swoboda. Ihr Briefwechsel (1901–1906), in *Psyche* 56, 313–337.
Weiss, E. (1970). *Sigmund Freud as a Consultant: Recollections of a Pioneer in Psychoanalysis*, New York: Intercontinental Medical Book Corporation.
Wittels, F. (1924). *Sigmund Freud. Der Mann, die Lehre, die Schule*, Leipzig: E. P. Tal.
Wittels, F. (1996). *Freud and the Child Women: The Memoirs of Fritz Wittels*, New Haven: Yale University Press.

2

THE SEXOLOGICAL DISCOURSE ON NON-NORMATIVE SEXUALITY

Sándor Ferenczi, Richard von Krafft-Ebing, and Magnus Hirschfeld

At the turn of the twentieth century, psycho-medical literature was transformed into a space for negotiating and redefining what was normal or abnormal, healthy or unhealthy (Oosterhuis 2012: 133–155). In German-language medical literature of the late 1800s, the publication of theses by such authors as Richard von Krafft-Ebing, Albert Moll, Albert von Schrenck-Notzing, and Magnus Hirschfeld shaped new ways of describing and perceiving human sexuality. At that time, medical case studies were both the representative genre of psycho-medical literature and "modernity's vital narrative forms and means of explanation" (Lang & Damousi 2017: 1).

The classic medical case study attempted to present and classify phenomena that its author considered to be pathological. Although it was generally aimed at finding meaning in a given case and explaining it, the essence of the genre was constantly being reinterpreted (Ibid.: 2).[1] What made it especially conducive to endless new interpretations was its heterogeneous character (Lejeune 2017; Damousi 2015). The writing strategies employed by physicians and psychiatrists in the late 1800s often consisted in copying lengthy fragments of their patients' autobiographies, creating a biographical narrative, and combining it with scientific discourse. As a result, the genre of the case study emerged at the intersection of medicine, legal sciences, the arts, and literature.

In the second half of the nineteenth century, the medical case study was a platform for the construction and dissemination of a new image of human gender and sexuality.[2] After Michel Foucault, case studies have often been treated as a modern form of disciplinary power. By contrast, I would like to show that psycho-medical literature of the turn of the century gave birth to a poetics of engagement. Therefore, I would like to investigate the writing strategies of three physicians who worked in the German-speaking world: Sándor Ferenczi (Budapest), Richard von Krafft-Ebing (Vienna), and Magnus

DOI: 10.4324/9781003441892-3

Hirschfeld (Berlin). It is worth noting that whereas Krafft-Ebing's *Psychopathia Sexualis* and Hirschfeld's writings have become part of the history of sexology, Ferenczi's early texts have not been received as widely by scholars.[3]

In the decade 1900–1910, Ferenczi became "the Hungarian representative of humanist psychiatry of the age" (Mészáros 2014: 19) in Budapest's artistic and intellectual circles as he called for the liberalization of psycho-medical discourse. As we shall see, his rarely discussed articles – written at a time of rapid socio-cultural changes in Hungary – reveal a gradual exhaustion of the nineteenth-century model of looking at patients, while at the same time pointing to the emergence of a new ideal: the doctor's concern about his patients' fates.

2.1 Modernist cultures: Budapest around the year 1900

John Lukacs wrote that the Budapest of the early 1900s was a city of rapidly flowing ideas, heated scientific debates, and burgeoning art trends (Lukacs 1994; Hanák 1998; Korbel 2020: 220–242). His 1988 book *Budapest 1900: A Historical Portrait of a City* was inspired by a belief that while studies on turn-of-the-century culture in Vienna were growing increasingly popular, the modernization processes of the Kingdom of Hungary (Magyar Királyság) were not sufficiently discussed (Lukacs 1994: 55–56; Csáky 2010).

As Lukacs observed, Budapest in the year 1900 was already a metropolis, and

> foreign visitors arriving in that unknown portion of Europe, east of Vienna, were astounded to find a modern city with first-class hotels, plate-glass windows, electric tramcars, elegant men and women, the largest Parliament building in the world about to be completed.
>
> *(Lukacs 1994: 35)*

In the first two decades of the twentieth century, the swift modernization converged with the golden age of modernist art and literature (Angyalosi et al. 2009; Bálazs 2009; Barki et al. 2012). This is how modernist writers portrayed the former "lost" era:

> time, which flew like a bird of passage, made it so that old people cannot be seen in Pest today – because those who reluctantly and warily watched new inhabitants appear in the capital city have already died out. Gone are the merchants riding through the streets on their way to the countryside, while the lawyers and agents of various sorts have mixed into the crowd of new inhabitants [...] What a humorous phenomenon a Váci street dandy from the eighties would seem today!
>
> *(Krúdy 2019: 300)*

The space of the city became cosmopolitan: English habits, clothing, sports, and literature came into fashion. Soon, the elegant dandy was replaced by "clean-shaven youths with broad shoulders." The portrait of the new man and the new woman – Adam and Eve, whose refinement matched the image of the modernizing city – was painted in 1924 by Sándor Bortnyik.

In the early years of the twentieth century, the revolution of the young and the "worldly" – as Krúdy ironically wrote – was propelled by the slogan "Away with the mustache!" Apart from sports and English small talk in Budapest coffeehouses, the city was – as Lukacs wrote – "a grand place for literature" (Lukacs 1994: 15). It was a bustling cityscape, perfect for writers searching for new ways of literary and artistic expression. Young, debuting creators were now able to publish their works in magazines specially dedicated to that purpose, such as *A Hét* (The Week) or *Jövendo* (Future) – which were modeled on the Austrian *Das Junge Wien* (The Young Vienna) – and later the modernist *Nyugat* (West).

In 1907, the artists of the older and younger generations established the Circle of Hungarian Impressionists and Naturalists (Magyar Impresszionisták és Naturalisták Köre), whose members included Pál Szinyei Merse, József Rippl-Rónai, Károly Ferenczy as well as Károly Kernstok, Béla Czóbel, Ödön Márffy, and Dezső Czigány (Horváth 1993; Markója & Bardoly 2010). Károly Kernstok first presented his manifesto of the new art as a tool for exploring the human psyche at a meeting of the liberal association of young doctors and scientists A Galilei Kör (The Galileo Circle) in his lecture "Explorative Art" ("A kutató művészet"). The young painters surrounding Kernstok were searching for new means of artistic expression and slowly moved further away from the Impressionist aesthetic.

In works by Kernstok, Róbert Berény, Vilmos Perlrott-Csaba, Ödön Márfy, Bertalan Pór, and Béla Czóbel, the human body was typically placed in the idyllic space of nature and freed from the restrictions imposed on it by the process of civilization. For example, Kernstok's 1911 painting *Male Nude Leaning Against a Tree* depicts a young, naked man in a relaxed pose, which highlights his chest and slightly protruding stomach. In his nonchalance, the man resembles both the nineteenth-century dandy, and a child who is unashamed of his or her nudity. The tree is evocative of the paradise lost – a time and space when man was oblivious to any notion of guilt or shame. The modernist Eight's (Nyolcak) penchant for themes of nudity and corporeality did not escape the critics, who reacted with varying degrees of malice. As early as 1911, a caricature of the Eight's first exhibition appeared on the cover of the May edition of the magazine *Fidibusz* (Fidibus). The image showed the exhibition's visitors behaving in a manner relaxed to the point of acrobatics and enjoying portraits of naked bodies twisted in equally unusual, often "indecent" poses. The theme of nudity in Kernstok's, Berény's, and Márfy's paintings could be associated with the queer history of fin-de-siècle Budapest. At that time, gay culture developed primarily in bathhouses:

> During the twentieth century, bathhouses were reserved for men only during certain days of the week and became important social spaces especially for gay men, providing a hassle-free environment in which they could meet and physically interact with one another without raising suspicion.
>
> *(Takács 2014: 192)*

These places facilitated physical proximity between men and supported the culture of the affirmation of the body, which found its way to the visual arts.

In the urban coffeehouse atmosphere of early twentieth-century Budapest, Hungarian literature and art interacted intensely with medicine and psychology. The young generation of creators, intellectuals, and physicians was united in its desire to abandon the patterns established both in scientific literature and *belles-lettres* as well as painting, sculpture, and music. They wanted to create a new language, fit for expressing the ideals of liberalism and cosmopolitanism. The language of turn-of-the-century medicine and literature articulated their search for a new frame of looking at the human being (both as a fictional character and a patient): at the psyche and sexuality. Late-nineteenth-century case studies conveyed a need to create a detailed medical portrait of an individual whose experiences transcended the horizon of established social and moral norms. In novels, novellas, and short stories, there was a growing number of characters who did not follow the norms of the bourgeois society. In post-1900 Hungary, books by bestselling authors such as Arthur Schnitzler, Thomas Mann, Henry James, and Oscar Wilde explored spaces of (sexual) non-normativity (Haralson 2004; Hurley 2008; Glick 2009).

2.2 Miksa Schächter, Sándor Ferenczi, and *Gyógyászat*

John Lukacs asserted that the advent of modernism in Hungary – which could be seen most clearly in the cultural life of early-twentieth-century Budapest – had been brought about by the generation of 1900. In his book, Lukacs specifically named many people of science and medicine (including psychoanalysis), but he did not mention Sándor Ferenczi.[4] In the history of psychoanalysis, Ferenczi is remembered as an eminent theoretician and practitioner as well as a key figure in the development of the international psychoanalytic movement in the first decades of its existence. Sigmund Freud himself viewed Ferenczi this way, writing in 1914: "Hungary, so near geographically to Austria, and *so far from it scientifically* [italics mine], has produced only one collaborator, S. Ferenczi, but one that indeed outweighs a whole society" (Freud [1914] 1957: 1–66). As opposed to Carl Gustav Jung or Otto Rank, Ferenczi became an "internal critic" (Rudnytsky 1996: 13) of Freud and the psychoanalytic movement. In 1933, soon after the Hungarian analyst's death, Freud reminisced on their journey to the United States: "I would ask him to suggest what I should talk about that day and he would sketch out for me what I would then improvise half an hour later." He stressed that in a short time, Ferenczi "made all analysts his pupils" (Freud 1933: 301–304).[5]

As Judit Mészáros said, the Hungarian analyst's early writings "foreshadow not only Ferenczi's character and scholarly and therapeutic orientation as a psychoanalyst, but also the unique perspectives that would emerge in the Budapest School" (Mészáros 2008).[6] In the first two decades of the twentieth century, Ferenczi was Freud's close collaborator and friend as well as the most important advocate of psychoanalysis in Hungary. Earlier, Ferenczi had worked closely with Miksa Schächter (1859–1917), whom he treated as his teacher and mentor. It was thanks to Schächter's influence that Ferenczi became involved in popularizing new trends in the Hungarian medical circles. As Ferenczi's case neatly illustrates, psycho-medical literature in Hungary was evolving as a component of turn-of-the-century culture in general, rather than being an entity separated from literature and art (Buklijaš 2012: 209–244).

In 1897, Ferenczi arrived in Budapest with his diploma from the University of Vienna. He quickly joined the circle of Schächter's collaborators which was centered around the liberal magazine *Gyógyászat* (Therapy).[7] In the final years of the nineteenth century, Ferenczi began his medical practice in St. Rochus Hospital (Szent Rókus Kórház), and then continued in the St. Elizabeth Hospital (Szent Erzsébet Kórház), where he treated patients from the lowest social strata. His early writings demonstrated his interest both in late-nineteenth-century psychiatric trends such as hypnosis, magnetism, and spiritism, and in the budding science of sexology (Mészáros 2014: 15–18).

When the literary magazine *Nyugat* (West) was established in 1908, Ferenczi began publishing his works there alongside leading writers of Hungarian modernism, such as Mihály Babits, Milán Füst, Géza Csáth, Frigyes Karinthy, Dezső Kósztolányi, and Gyula Krúdy, who were interested in contemporary psychology and psychoanalysis. According to Michelle Moreau-Ricaud, Ferenczi was not just a friend to key representatives of the new Hungarian literature: he was a great inspiration (Moreau-Ricaud 2012: 92–94). Ignotus, Kósztolányi, and Karinthy frequently met with Ferenczi in his apartment at the Hotel Royal to discuss Freud's theory, the arts, and literature. After the physician's death, Kósztolányi emphasized in his obituary that as an analyst, Ferenczi was extraordinarily "attracted by the arts and artists" (Ibid.: 88), which translated into his belief in the value of psychoanalysis as an interpretive tool for literature.

Between 1897 and 1908, Ferenczi was seeking a new language for expressing medical knowledge. At that time, apart from reviews and topical essays, he published a case study entitled "Female homosexuality" ("Homosexualitas Feminina") (1902) in *Gyógyászat*, followed by a text on Magnus Hirschfeld's work entitled "On the intermediate sex" ("Sexualis átmeneti fokozatokról") four years later. At the turn of the century, psycho-medical literature developed an interest in the subject of homosexuality. In 1868, the Viennese physician Karl-Maria Kertbeny first wrote the word "homosexual" in a letter to Heinrich

Ulrichs, who was the creator of the term "Uranian" (used in the second half of the nineteenth century to refer to homosexual men) and of the magazine *Uranos*, entirely devoted to the subject of homoeroticism (1870) (Conway 2017: 131–134). In 1897, Magnus Hirschfeld initiated the establishment of the Wissenschaftlich-Humanitäres Komitee in Berlin. In the following years, the *Jahrbuch für sexuelle Zwischenstufen unter besonderer Berücksichtigung der Homosexualität* (Yearbook of the intermediate sex with special reference to homosexuality) was published to present the results of most recent research on that matter.

Ferenczi's "Homosexualitas Feminina" appeared nearly two decades after Richard von Krafft-Ebing's *Psychopathia Sexualis* (in fact, the year 1902 marked its eleventh edition) and Hirschfeld's *Sappho und Sokrates*, which he had published under the pen name "Dr. med. Th. Ramien" at the Max Spohr Verlag in 1896. In the same year, Adolf Brand launched the magazine *Der Eigene* which explored themes of homoeroticism, while a year later Havelock Ellis's *Sexual Inversion* became the first English-language treatise on homosexuality. In 1898, Hirschfeld approached Spohr again with a proposal to publish a pamphlet entitled *Paragraph 175 of The Reich Criminal Code: the question of homosexuality in the judgment of contemporaries* (*§ 175 des Reichsstrafgesetzbuchs: die homosexualle Frage im Urteile der Zeitgenossen*), which included a petition for the abolishment of Paragraph 175 signed by 250 people: physicians, scientists, politicians, artists, and members of the clergy. In 1905, Freud's *Three Essays on the Theory of Sexuality* saw the light of day. Because Ferenczi's "Homosexualitas Feminina" was written at a time of the rapid expansion in sexological discourse, he intended it to be a commentary on the proliferation of psycho-medical literature. However, as we shall see, what the text rather did was to anticipate the exhaustion of the established psycho-medical discursive strategies as tools of portraying patients – a breakthrough which was facilitated by publications like Krafft-Ebing's and Hirschfeld's.

2.3 Ferenczi's art of psycho-medical portraiture

In the 1930s, the German literary critic André Jolles suggested that the case study be treated as a legitimate literary genre and an archetypal example of the narrative form (Lang & Damousi 2017: 2). The case study was usually devoted to one patient's history, and represented an opportunity for authors to present the results of their research.[8] In terms of its form, it was a heterogeneous genre where subjective statements (the physician's personal view of the patient) intertwined with objective ones (the established model of psycho-medical writing).[9] The case study talked about how the doctor saw the patient, but at the same time exposed the emotions that the patient stirred within the doctor.

Ferenczi's "Homosexualitas Feminina" is a medical portrait of Róza K., who was known to Hungarian police officers and doctors as Róbert (Ferenczi 1902: 167–168). Dressed in men's clothes, (Róbert) Róza would be ceaselessly pursued by law enforcement, taken to courts and locked in asylums. Ferenczi began his case study by saying:

> Róza K. also known as Róbert K., a forty-year-old unmarried house maid [...] is one of those unfortunate creatures whose inborn pathological tendencies cause an unbridled desire for people of the same sex, while [...] the heterosexual satisfaction of sexual desire is of no interest to them, while often causing repulsion. Such cases are not at all isolated.
>
> *(Ibid.: 167)*

By describing (Róbert) Róza as an "unfortunate creature" defined solely through their[10] "pathological tendencies," Ferenczi's very first sentences classified his patient as a case of "psychopatia sexualis." However, in the next paragraph, he distanced himself from other medical literature devoted to non-normative forms of sexual expression:

> "Scientific" literature on sexual perversions, which is currently springing up like mushrooms and bringing substantial profit to its authors and publishers, has already ensured that physicians are incomparably more familiar with every detail of this section of psychopathology than other *much more significant* areas of the medical sciences [italics mine].
>
> *(Ibid.: 167)*

Because of his perceived overproduction of texts on sexuality, accompanied by the neglect of "much more significant areas of medical science," Ferenczi felt the need to justify his undertaking by writing: "I am only devoting these few words to the subject because some publications are simply asking for commentary" (Ibid.: 167). Surprisingly, though, Ferenczi did not refer to any other publication further in his case study, concentrating instead on (Róbert) Róza and their experiences. Ferenczi described his patient's life story as a "veritable odyssey" during which they had experienced much undeserved abuse by their family, employers, acquaintances, the police, and the justice system. Fereczi introduced (Róbert) Róza as an extraordinarily intelligent and sensitive person with a great ear for music. They were not to blame for their misfortunes – their surroundings were: their soulless family, the indifferent society, and the stringent law enforcement, which had condemned them to "perpetual vagrancy." Because of police persecution, (Róbert) Róza kept landing in poorhouses, jails, or mental wards. They fell victim to blackmail and the heartlessness of people who did not hesitate to take their last penny.

Their appearance – Ferenczi wrote – caused widespread confusion. Although in Pest and Vienna, they had been thrown in jail for donning men's clothes, in Estergom they were arrested for being "dressed up" as a woman. Because such situations repeated frequently, in Budapest (Róbert) Róza finally received permission to go outside in men's clothing, which – as

Ferenczi stressed – brought them great joy. Despite their lack of contact with their family, (Róbert) Róza returned to their hometown, where they were hired as a server by a tavern. Ferenczi recounted his patient's relationship with the cashier at the tavern. The partners moved in together and led the life of a regular married couple. The relationship ended in a break-up. The patient's further story was one of vagrancy, exclusion, and increasing alienation from society. (Róbert) Róza was banished to Pest, where they were forced to live in a poorhouse. There, they met with the hostility and aggression of its other residents. Ultimately, they were transferred to a mental asylum, where they were kept under permanent psychiatric observation.

From the case study of (Róbert) Róza, the reader does not learn much about the patient's sexuality. Ferenczi did not explain (Róbert) Róza's masculine identity, merely concluding that because of their non-normative desire, they were destined to suffer and experience social exclusion since their childhood. He seemed to be more interested in the coldness of the family and the cruelty of the poorhouse residents than in any potential causes for (Róbert) Róza's "homosexualitas."

Nevertheless, despite his admiration for (Róbert) Róza's talents, Ferenczi depicted them as a degenerate and highlighted the unattractiveness of their face and body. In the conclusion to the first part, he wrote:

> Among the so-called symptoms of corporeal degeneration – or, in other words, innate developmental defects – her high-arched palate comes to the foreground along with her protruding mandible (prognathia), and the disproportionately large size of the teeth in relation to the jaw [...]. The face is rather unsightly, even repulsive. *Such a level of ugliness allows one to talk about degeneration, because the unattractive impression is nothing but the aesthetic impact of the irregularities which consist of numerous details* [italics mine].
>
> *(Ibid.: 168)*

Ferenczi said that the degeneration of (Róbert) Róza's body was also evident in a number of details, but he did not elaborate. The questions about (Róbert) Róza's non-normative sexuality or developmental irregularities remain unanswered by Ferenczi. What he considered more important was the future of people like (Róbert) Róza. Ferenczi gave two arguments for increasing the freedoms of those deemed "degenerate" and "sick" by society. First, he believed that medical institutions should be tasked with caring for and helping those who had been socially excluded for any reason. Second, he thought that (Róbert) Róza was ultimately just a symptomatic example of how existing social policies hurt non-heteronormative people: a talented and intelligent person lost their home, became a vagrant, and lived under constant threat of attack.

Ferenczi wondered about the patient's fate, but he was unable to look at them outside of the sexualized frame of attractiveness/unattractiveness. With their "manly" heavy walk, their "gracelessness," and the "unwomanly" shape of their jaw, (Róbert) Róza appeared both "unfortunate" and unattractive to him. To Ferenczi, their "masculine" interests seemed to elevate the patient's status, while the "unwomanliness" that he observed in their body made them a "degenerate." The normative gaze directed at (Róbert) Róza by the physician starkly contrasted with the new ways of looking at the body that were emerging due to the development of modernist art in Hungary. One of the best examples of an image of gender that transcended the binary oppositions of the feminine/masculine is Bertalan Pór's painting *Yearning for Pure Love* (1911). It shows three characters that bring to mind the three Graces, the ancient Greek patrons of art, which was a recurring motif in the European fine arts (c.f. Sandro Botticelli's *Primavera*, 1477–82; Rafael Santi's *The Three Graces*, 1505; Peter Paul Rubens's *The Three Graces*, 1630–35). Although the people in Pór's painting vary in terms of their sex (one has pronounced breasts, the two others visible male genitalia), they are similarly built and equally muscular. The lack of any difference in the build of their legs, arms, or hips was intended to illustrate the fact that they have been molded from the same clay. Moreover, by showing a strong, well-built woman, not only did Pór reject the bourgeois image of a delicate, fragile lady, but he also renounced the belief in the fundamental difference (or even alienness) of "the woman's nature" from the man's.

While the Hungarian modernists offered a new way of perceiving and representing the human body, the physician's eye remained unmoved. Despite his pursuit of a new psycho-medical language for case studies, it did not occur to Ferenczi to abandon a pathologizing view of the patient and their body. In the second part of "Homosexualitas Feminina," Ferenczi wrote:

> Experience shows that the more serious the degenerate individuals' symptoms of physiological and psychological degeneration are, the less capable of reproduction they become [...]. Sexual perversions similar to those described in the present article *are relatively beneficial to society* (Hungarian: szexuális perverzió előnyös a társadalomra) [italics mine]: the bodily and spiritual signs of degeneration prevent such individuals from having progeny.
>
> *(Ibid.: 168)*

Although this fragment suggests that the author treated homosexuality as a kind of spiritual degeneration (which was also reflected in the imperfections of the body), Ferenczi's further words seem to contradict this. The physician wrote: "Any sexual otherness (Hungarian: szexuális rendellenesség) does not fit the norm *merely because it deviates from those sexual behaviors which contribute to procreation* (Hungarian: mert eltér a nemi szexuális érintkezés azon rendjéről, amely a faj fenntartására alkalmas) [italics mine]" (Ibid.: 168). Here, the word "abnormal" referring to sexual behaviors meant no more and no less than "one that does not lead to reproduction."

Ferenczi stressed that the reason for (Róbert) Róza's misfortunes was neither their homosexual desire nor their masculine identity, but rather their emotional instability resulting from difficult experiences. In the conclusion to "Homosexualitas Feminina," Ferenczi argued after social Darwinism that nature itself – without humans' help – ensured the preservation of the species. By highlighting the authoritarian power of nature, the author could then contend that rather than oppressing "the ill," it should be the duty of medicine and law enforcement to return them to social life. Ultimately, although the text was supposed to comment on the development of sexological literature, it did not discuss research on the "etiology" or "nosology" of homosexuality. Instead, its overarching goal was to appeal to physicians for a more conscious and socially engaged approach to patients.

The story of (Róbert) Róza described by Ferenczi confusingly resembles another case of cross-dressing that was widely publicized by the Hungarian press of the late nineteenth century (Mak 2004: 54–77; Borgos 2011: 220–231). In 1889, the press reported the arrest of Count Sándor (Sarolta) Vay (1859–1918), who was accused of fraud by their father-in-law. Born Sarolta Vay, Sándor had married a woman several years before, and led a "normal" married life without arousing suspicion among their loved ones. Vay's case, first analyzed by C. Birnbacher in 1891, attracted the attention of Richard von Krafft-Ebing and Havelock Ellis (Krafft-Ebing 2011: 539–552; Ellis 1900: 94). Although in Austria – unlike Germany – women were punished for "acts against nature" (from 1852 to 1971), the Hungarian law only covered sexual relations between men. Vay was pardoned, and they returned to their old life.

Unlike (Robert) Róza, Vay was high-born and well-educated. They published their first literary attempts as Sarolta Vay. Later, they used a number of pen names (Vayk, D'Artagnan, Floridor, Celesztin), writing for newspapers such as *Magyar Szalon* (Hungarian Salon), *Pesti Hírlap* (Pest Newspaper), and *Budapest*. By 1918, Vay had also published several literary works (Vay 1909; 1986; 2006). The Hungarian actor Izsó Gyöngyi remembered Sándor as follows:

> It is not this guest performance I want to evoke, but the chevalier servant of the guest artist. Last year I saw her in women's clothes in Miskolcz. She was called Sarolta Vay, and in Fehérvár she appeared at the theater as a pretty suitor, by the name of Sándor Vay! [...] He smoked like a chimney, and chatted and behaved like an enfant terrible. Well, as a boy from Miskolcz I heard that the old count Vay was eccentric, dressing his daughter in boy's clothes and the boy in girl's. But that this countess is now inviting me to carouse in Fehérvár, I didn't dare to dream about – and he didn't back down. To carouse. And where? In a night club! Where one finds women! My eyes goggled; this young lad seated the girls in his lap. After many years, Krafft-Ebing's *Psychopathia Sexualis* has explained what I could not conceive at that time.
>
> *(Gyöngyi 1922: 72–73)*

In *Psychopathia Sexualis,* Krafft-Ebing presented Sándor Vay as a case of hermaphroditism, while providing many interesting details of the writer's emotional life. A comparison of Vay's story with Ferenczi's "Homosexualitas Feminina" shows the extent to which social class influenced the lives of non-normative men and women at the turn of the century. While Róbert (Róza) was forced to spend their life between prisons, poorhouses, and psychiatric institutions, Vay remained free and independent; while the former's voice disappeared in Ferenczi's narrative, the latter was able to speak for themself and have their works published.

2.4 Polyphonic writing strategies in *Psychopathia Sexualis*

Freud began his *Three Essays on the Theory of Sexuality* (1905) with a meticulous review of the latest literature on "sexual aberrations" (*die sexuellen Abirrungen*). He named Richard von Krafft-Ebing, Albert Moll, Paul Julius Moebius, Havelock Ellis, Albert von Schrenck-Notzing, and Magnus Hirschfeld as key representatives of modern sexology (Freud [1905] 1953: 123). In the second half of the nineteenth century, doctors who sought to discover their patients' erotic desires explored a variety of literary genres. They combined psycho-medical discourse with biographical writings (when the physician reconstructed the history of the case) as well as analyzed autobiographical writings by patients who were encouraged to record their life stories and send their answers to the doctors' surveys. Based on the acquired material, the psychiatrists then wrote case studies that were polyphonous texts created at the intersection of scientific discourse and the individuals' subjective experiences (Lejeune 1987: 79–94; Oosterhuis 2012: 152–155).

A prime example is Richard Krafft-Ebing's *Psychopathia Sexualis,* where he included large fragments of his patients' autobiographical accounts. His work opens with a quotation by Ambroise Tardieu:

> No physical or moral misery, no wound, no matter how infected, should frighten someone who had dedicated himself to science of man; and sacred ministry of physician, while obliging him to see everything, also *permits him to say everything* [italics mine].
>
> *(Krafft-Ebing 2011: 36–37)*

The pursuit of the scientific truth was not only supposed to allow the doctor to "say everything" but also to excuse anything that might be said.

In the part devoted to his homosexual patients, Richard von Krafft-Ebing was not only interested in their sexual behaviors, but also their social situations. The biographies he discussed were stories of people who – unlike (Róbert) Róza – originated from the privileged classes. Most cases described by Krafft-Ebing were men, but he also reconstructed the stories of several female patients. They included a young person who had been born into a family of a high-ranking state official. Like (Róbert) Róza, they were only interested in "masculine" sports and games in their childhood. As Krafft-Ebing recounted one of the patient's memories:

> Up to her marriage (at the age of twenty-one) she could not recall to mind a single instance in which she felt herself drawn to persons of her own sex. Men were equally indifferent to her. When matured she had many admirers. This flattered her greatly. However, she claimed that *the difference of the sexes never entered her mind*; she was only influenced by the difference in the dress.
>
> *(Ibid.: 415)*

To the patient, sexual difference only seemed like a social construct. At the age of thirty-six, they fell seriously physically ill. They claimed that the illness resulted in their transformation into a man. Krafft-Ebing painted a portrait of the patient's gender transition, naming the changes they observed in their body: their breasts had atrophied, their voice lowered, their skin roughened, and there had been "a different odor coming from her person" (Ibid.: 417).

Krafft-Ebing also mentions Sándor Vay, reconstructs the story of their emotional life, and comments: "Her movements were powerful, not unpleasing, though they were somewhat masculine and lacking in grace. She greeted one with a firm pressure of the hand. Her whole carriage was decided, firm and somewhat self-conscious" (Ibid.: 549–550). As Anna Borgos points out, "Krafft-Ebing's controversial characterization of Vay as a perverse and at the same time respectable person is remarkable" (Borgos 2011: 227). At the end of the case report, Krafft-Ebing adds:

> S.'s characteristic expressions – "God put love in my heart. If He created me so, and not otherwise, am I, then, guilty; or is it the eternal, incomprehensible way of fate?" – are really justified. The court granted pardon. The "countess in male attire," as she was called in the newspapers, returned to her home, and again gave herself out as Count Sandor. Her only distress was her lost happiness with her beloved Marie.
>
> *(Krafft-Ebing 2011: 551–552)*

In the end, in Krafft-Ebing's eyes, Vay's self-identification was more than justifiable. On the one hand, he indicated that Vay's non-normativity was hereditary, but on the other hand, he acknowledged Vay's right to self-identify.

The author continues with another case (no. 129). This time, he does not paraphrase the patient's story, but he quotes fragments of their autobiography *in extenso*. The author of the essay spoke about their childhood and youth, introducing themselves in detail to the doctor and their numerous readers. "With a very active imagination – my enemy through life – my talents developed rapidly. I could read and write at the age of four [...] I was always simply but very elegantly dressed, and thus developed a taste for beautiful clothing" (Ibid.: 392). The author was bullied at school due to their "girly" movements and delicate facial features. After a difficult period of adolescence, they were able to receive a degree in medicine. They spent their days working and leading a social life. At the same time – they wrote – "I went through life, such as it was, never satisfied with myself, full of dissatisfaction with the world" (Ibid.: 398).

In time, their dissatisfaction had transformed into depression that killed any of their happiness. They recalled: "even on my marriage night, I felt that I was only a woman in man's form, it seemed to me that my place was under the woman" (Ibid.: 398–399). The marriage brought them relative peace and stability. After several years, however, they fell physically ill for a few days, and they recovered in a new body:

> I awoke and found myself feeling as completely changed into a woman; and when, on standing and walking, I felt female genitals and breasts. [...] I feel like a woman in a man's form. [...] I always feel the vulva. [...] The skin all over my body feels feminine.
>
> *(Ibid.: 400–403)*

Krafft-Ebing did not interfere with the text, merely quoting a large fragment of the patient's self-analytical description of their experience of gender transition. The life after their transformation became a constant battle with repressed desires, including the need to start an intimate relationship with a man. At that time, their marriage also underwent a transformation: "Marriage then, except during coitus, where the man feels himself a woman, is like two women living together, one of whom regards herself as in the mask of a man" (Ibid.: 406–407). The patient's life became a sort of actor's performance on which their freedom and the maintenance of social respect depended. Following "the rules of the game" required much effort and numerous acts of self-denial:

> Since the anus feels feminine, it would not be hard to become a passive pederast; only positive religious command prevents it. [...] I have a desire to be sexless, or to make myself sexless [...] Contact with a woman seems homogenous to me; coitus with my wife seems possible to me because she is somewhat masculine, and has a firm skin; and yet it is more an *amor lesbicus.*
>
> *(Ibid.: 407–410)*

Krafft-Ebing selected the most striking self-analytical fragments, leaving space for the patient to tell their autobiographical story. Here, the doctor's commentary was limited to one sentence: "The forgoing autobiography, scientifically so important, was accompanied by the following no less interesting letter" (Ibid.: 412). He quoted the letter *in extenso*:

> Sir [...] your work gave me courage again; and I am determined to go to the bottom of the matter, and examine my past life, let the result be what it might. It seemed a duty of gratitude to you to tell you the result of my recollection and observation, since I had not seen any description by you of an analogous case; and, finally, I also thought it might perhaps interest you to learn, from the pen of physician, how such a worthless human, or masculine, being thinks and feels under the weight of the imperative idea of being a woman. [...] After reading your work, I hope that, if I fulfill my duties as physician, citizen, father and husband, *I may still count myself among human beings who do not deserve merely to be despised* [italics mine].
>
> *(Ibid.: 413)*

For the author of *Psychopathia Sexualis*, the letter constituted an affirmation of the value of his research, which he considered to be of service not only to the development of knowledge, but also to the moral cause – as it encouraged people to self-analyze and learn about their own emotional life.

The Viennese doctor made his patients' voices an integral part of his argument. As a text, *Psychopathia Sexualis* was then equally heterogenous (by mixing diverse genres such as the case study, the autobiography, the letter) and polyphonous (by intertwining the psychiatrist's narrative with his patients' writings) as it was dialogical (in the communication between the psychiatrist and the patient). The fragment of the anonymous non-heteronormative patient's autobiography was the longest personal statement quoted there. In that case, Krafft-Ebing's role was limited to the task of an editor who selected passages from the text and annotated it. Therefore, the author of *Psychopathia Sexualis* remained more of an observer and commentator than an analyst-interpreter.

2.5 Psycho-medical writing and emancipation: a manifesto

In 1901, Magnus Hirschfeld published the pamphlet *Was muss das Volk vom dritten Geschlecht wissen!* (What People Should Know about the Third Sex). It concluded with an appeal to abolish Paragraph 175 in Germany, which – alongside Albert Moll and Paul Adolf Näcke – was also signed by Richard von Krafft-Ebing. In his justification for such a petition, Hirschfeld wrote:

> In view of the fact that the scientific research that has engaged intensively with the question of homosexuality (sensual love for persons of the same sex) in the German-, English- and French-speaking territories within the last twenty years has without exception confirmed what the first scholars who turned their attention to the issue expressed, that this phenomenon which is widely distributed in time and location must, by its very nature, be the product of a deep internal constitutional disposition.
>
> *(Hirschfeld [1901] 2017: 114)*

Although Hirschfeld was referring to medical knowledge and the rapid development of sexological literature, the scientific discourse in his text was limited to a minimum. Adhering to the poetics of a manifesto, the author appealed to emotions more than to the reader's knowledge. In order to encourage their openness, he wrote:

> Every parent should reflect that one or other of their children may be a uranian […] and that the aforementioned paragraph (175) could threaten their dearest one. Among those who have spoken out for the abolition of this law, there is a priest whom we are certain he is himself unaware that one of his sons is uranian.
>
> *(Ibid.: 106)*

The reference to the reader's feelings was aimed at evoking empathy. The author intended to persuade his readers that the subject of homosexuality could affect any citizen in diverse ways, and therefore should not be marginalized.

The new mode of writing – engaged rather than descriptive – resulted from the turn-of-the-century boom of diverse literature on "the third sex." In 1898, Elsa Asenijeff's *The Revolt of Women and the Third Sex* was published, followed by Ernst von Wolzogen's 1899 *The Third Sex*, Aimée Duc's 1901 *Are They Women? Novel of the Third Sex*, Rudolf Quanter's 1902 *Against the Third Sex* as well as Senna Hoy's *The Third Sex* and Johann's Elberskirchen *The Love of the Third Sex* in 1904. The terms used to denote non-normative behavior or desire were as diverse as they were polysemantic. In Hirschfeld's work, "the third sex" referred to at least three groups: (1) homosexual people, (2) transgender people, and (3) intersex people.

What Hirschfeld's pamphlet had in common with literature on "the third sex" was that he did not just discuss non-normative desire: he talked about love. He argued: "The love for one's own sex can be just as pure, tender and noble as that for the other sex, differentiated only in its object, not its nature" (Ibid.: 109). Hirschfeld took the notions of "nature," and "the natural," and redefined them. He began his pamphlet with this statement:

> Everyone should be taught that every physical and mental quality generally regarded as manly is occasionally seen in women, and everything in the structure and functions of the body that one ordinarily considers peculiar to women can […] manifest in men.
>
> *(Ibid.: 104)*

By highlighting the fluidity of boundaries between the masculine and the feminine, Hirschfeld naturalized various forms of gender transgression. Moreover, his reflections echoed the theory of innate bisexuality, which had appeared in German-language psycho-medical literature in the late nineteenth century.

In the early years of the twentieth century, Otto Weininger's (1880–1903) *Sex and Character* (*Geschlecht und Charakter*) gained great popularity in the German-speaking world (Weininger 2005). In it, the young philosopher presented his concept of bisexuality as the human being's natural disposition. In the first part of *Sex and Character*, he wrote:

> Among plants and animals, the occurrence of genuine hermaphroditism is a fact established beyond any doubt. [...] Of human beings however, it may be said with the greatest certainty that psychologically a person must necessarily be either male or female, at least initially and at one and the same time.
>
> *(Weininger [1903] 2005: 69)*

Clearly, Weininger thought that bisexuality (or rather: being of both genders) was natural and innate at the biological level, but at the psychological level the human being had to necessarily be either a man or a woman. At the same time, he wrote:

> I am not talking merely about a bisexual predisposition but about permanent bisexuality, nor merely about those stages midway between the sides, the (physical or psychical) hermaphrodites, to whom all studies of this kind have been restricted until now for obvious reasons.
>
> *(Ibid.: 14)*

For Weininger, the masculine and the feminine constituted not so much empirical reality as two ideal types, which appeared in nature in more complicated forms. His proposal had as many passionate advocates as fierce critics. For example, in response to *Sex and Character*, Paul Julius Moebius published a lampoon entitled "Sex and Immodesty" ("Geschlecht und Unbescheidenheit"), aimed at ridiculing Weininger's hypotheses.

The motif of the androgyne was especially prevalent in German-language literature of that time. After Weininger's premature death by suicide, the magazine *Die Fackel* (The Torch) edited by Karl Kraus defended the criticized philosopher. In 1907, it published a text entitled "The Sex" ("Das Geschlecht"), written by the Polish-German modernist writer Stanisław Przybyszewski (1868–1927) (Przybyszewski 1907: 1–11). As Daniel Steuer rightly noted, Przybyszewski saw gender "as the universal moving principle, in the Nietzschean style and Schopenhauerian vein, ending with a utopian vision of mankind considering sexuality as something beautiful" (Steuer 2005: xxv). In those years, Przybyszewski's works were focused on desire, eroticism, sexuality, and the question of the masculine/feminine. By the 1880s, Przybyszewski had moved to Berlin, where he studied medicine and practiced literature. In 1893, he published his long poem *The Mass of the Dead* (*Totenmesse*), which begins with the famous sentence "Am Anfang war das Geschlecht. Nichts außer ihm – alles in ihm" (At the beginning, there was sex. Nothing but it – everything in it) (Przybyszewski 1893: 7). Seven years later and three years before Weininger's *Sex and Character*, Przybyszewski's piece *Androgyne* was published in Lviv. There, in the form of a prayer, he told a story of a mystical connection of man and woman in one body:

> it will be one and indivisible, God omni-singular, or God who, here, on earth, broke into pieces and particles – inconceivable mysteries will be revealed, all reasons and purposes of being will be undone – and it will reign over all of the earth and all creation. He – She. Amen.
>
> *(Przybyszewski 1900: 80)*

Here, Przybyszewski equated deification with transcending the sexual difference. He invoked the Babylonian myth of the matriarchal, lustful goddess Ishtar (to whom his character constantly prayed), the Platonian myth of hermaphroditism presented in Aristophanes's speech in Plato's *Symposium*, as well as the biblical story of the creation of Adam. In *Androgyne*, sex (Geschlecht) was merely a disposition to be overcome in order to obtain the fullness of humanity. The feminine and the masculine – when experienced separately – limited the human being both in the senso-corporeal and the psychological domain. It was only the androgyne – as a deified human – that could reign over "all of the earth and all creation."

It was no coincidence that in the conclusion of his pamphlet, Hirschfeld pointed to the long history of homoeroticism in Western culture. An argument that was based both on nature and on culture ("God, or nature, made these men-women and uranians alongside men and women") allowed the author to shift emphasis away from questions about the moral law to the real social situation of homosexual men ("Almost all uranians are unhappy, not because of their passion, which they find difficult to imagine themselves without, but because of the persecution, the social devastation, the loss of honor that they potentially face for that which the normal may allow themselves every day with impunity") (Hirschfeld 2017: 110).[11] Towards the end, Hirschfeld made his final appeal to empathy by saying: "Every normally inclined person should try, once, to cast himself in the place of the uranian" (Ibid.: 110).

The paradigm shift that Hirschfeld postulated was not limited to educating the public, but it was also a call to empathy for the socially excluded. In the author's eyes, knowledge about sexuality was meant to be used for real social change. His aim was to create a "safe" space for homosexual people. Therefore, in his conclusion, Hirschfeld added: "The uranian should – and not just when he finds himself in the hands of blackmailers or involved in other such troubles – turn to the Scientific-Humanitarian Committee" (Ibid.: 112).

Hirschfeld's engaged perspective did not go unnoticed in Budapest's medical circles. In 1906, Ferenczi published another article on homosexuality in *Gyógyászat*, this time entitled "Sexualis átmeneti fokozatokról" (On the intermediate sex) (Ferenczi 1906: 310–314). The text was a printed version of a lecture he had given in April of that year in the medical society (Orvosikör). In its entirety, it was devoted to Magnus Hirschfeld's research and the activities of the Scientific-Humanitarian Committee. Ferenczi concluded his article by saying:

> In my brief description today, I have been able to outline sexual transitional states only very incompletely [...] I wanted to draw my colleagues' attention to these biologically so interesting and socially important phenomena. In his letter to the Duke of Weimar, Goethe even wrote that it was hardly possible to write about this subject. We are over this today. *In our contemporary view, all existing social and natural science objects are worth addressing. You can write and talk about everything* [italics mine].
>
> *(Ibid.: 314)*

Like Krafft-Ebing, Ferenczi believed that modern science – including medicine and psychology – opened up a space for an unrestricted development of knowledge, where every socially significant subject should be discussed. In the final sentences of his text, Ferenczi returned to the question of the role of physicians in their homosexual patients' lives. He insisted that if scientists did not disseminate knowledge concerning the diversity of sexual expression, they would become "not just judges but cruel executioners" (Ibid.: 314). He concluded his argument with a quotation from Hirschfeld: "Es gibt kein höheres Recht, als die der Wahrheit" (There is no higher law than that of the truth).

In the following years, Ferenczi did not abandon his attempts to research homosexuality. In the summer of 1910, he was preparing for the annual congress of Hungarian physicians, this time hosted by his former teacher Miksa Schächter. In a letter to Freud, Ferenczi wrote:

> I couldn't absent myself, and I also agreed to give a lecture, with the title *Psychoanalysis and Homosexuality.* But the audience at this congress is not the right forum for this lecture. I will therefore probably cancel or *talk about a less difficult topic* [italics mine].
>
> *(Freud & Ferenczi 1993: 190–191)*

Clearly, in the Hungary of 1910, the subject that interested Ferenczi still remained too "difficult" and controversial for the medical environment. At the same time, the theme of repudiated homosexuality and paranoia will dominate in Ferenczi's early discussions with Freud and their psychoanalytic writings (Ferenczi 1911: 101–119; 1914: 131–142).

2.6 Conclusion

The successive editions of Richard von Krafft-Ebing's *Psychopathia Sexualis* introduced the poetics of polyphony to psycho-medical literature. By interlacing his own narrative with his patients' voices, he was able to connect diverse worlds in one work and join together his patients' horizons of experience. At the same time, the inclusion of large autobiographical fragments created a new space for reading strategies which transcended the author's expected interpretive frame. On the other hand, Ferenczi did not employ the polyphonous narrative in his "Homosexualitas Feminina." Instead, he used the genre of the case study as commentary on the fast-growing medical and sexological literature of his time, while simultaneously distancing himself from it. The text appealed to the doctors' imagination, reminding them about the social dimension of their work. In 1902, Ferenczi underscored his patient's experience rather than their sexuality as a medical case, and thus performed the role of their biographer. While Krafft-Ebing's and Ferenczi's writing strategies introduced an interest in the patients' fates into psycho-medical literature, Hirschfeld explored the poetics of a manifesto and fashioned scientific discourse into a tool of emancipatory struggle. No wonder that Budapest's progressive medical circles took such an interest in his writings as doctors searched for a new frame of looking at and writing about non-normative sexuality in the early twentieth century.

In one of Ferenczi's earliest texts, one can discern both the engaged language of physicians struggling against various forms of social exclusion and the emotional engagement typical of his late reflection. The question of non-normative sexuality and new images of the psyche soon found their place in Hungarian modernism. As we will see in the next chapter, it was no coincidence that the creative practices of Hungarian modernists from Ferenczi's circle oriented around the problems of social exclusion, rapid modernization, and the affirmation of corporeality and bodily pleasures.

Notes

1 On the case study genre see, for example: Anne Sealey, "The Strange Case of the Freudian Case History: The Role of Long Case Histories in the Development of Psychoanalysis," *History of the Human Sciences* 24 (2011): 36–50; Lauren Berlant, "On the Case," *Critical Inquiry* vol. 33, no. 4 (2007): 663–672; Elizabeth Lunbeck and Bennett Simon, "On Reading Psychoanalytic Case Notes," in *Family Romance, Family Secrets: Case Notes from American Psychoanalysis*, E. Lunbeck and B. Simon (New Haven: Yale University Press, 2003). On the analytic process described in Freud's case histories see George Makari, *Revolution in Mind: The Creation of Psychoanalysis* (New York: Harper Perennial, 2008). On Freud's case studies as literary writings see Peter Brooks, *Psychoanalysis and Story Telling* (Hoboken: Wiley-Blackwell, 1992); John Forrester, *Thinking in Cases* (Cambridge: Polity Press, 2017).

2 A significant body of literature on the psycho-sexological discourse in the German-speaking world currently exists in German as well as in English, see: Robert Beachy, "The German Invention of Homosexuality," *The Journal of Modern History* vol. 82, no. 4 (2010): 801–838; Chandak Sengoopta, "Glandular Politics: Experimental Biology, Clinical Medicine, and Homosexual Emancipation in Fin-de-Siècle Central Europe," *Isis* vol. 89, no. 3 (1998): 445–473; Manfred Herzer,

Magnus Hirschfeld. Leben und Werk eines judischen, schwulen und sozialistischen Sexologen (Frankfurt am Main: Bibliothek rosa Winkel, 1992); Elena Mancini, *Magnus Hirschfeld and the Quest for Sexual Freedom: A History of the First International Sexual Freedom Movement* (New York: Palgrave Macmillan, 2010); Ralf Dose, *Magnus Hirschfeld: The Origins of the Gay Liberation Movement*, trans. Edward H. Willis (New York: New York University Press, 2014). For the development of the confessional mode through the Western history, see Michel Foucault, *The History of Sexuality*, 3 vols., vol. 1: *The Will to Knowledge*, trans. Robert Hurley (New York: Penguin Random House, 1978), 61–66; Klaus Müller, *Aber in meinem Herzen sprach eine Stimme so laut: Homosexuelle Autobiographien und medizinische Pathographien im neunzehnten Jahrhundert* (Berlin: Männerschwarm, 1991); Alison M. Moore, *Sexual Myths of Modernity: Sadism, Masochism, and Historical Teleology* (Lanham, Maryland: Lexington Books, 2016); Katie Sutton, *Sex Between Body and Mind: Psychoanalysis and Sexology in the German-speaking World, 1890s-1930s* (Ann Arbor: University of Michigan Press, 2019).

3 On Ferenczi's preanalytic writings, see Claude Lorin, *Le Jeune Ferenczi. Premiers écrits, 1899–1906* (Paris: Aubier Montaigne, 1983); Arnold Wm. Rachman, "Ferenczi and Sexuality," in *The Legacy of Sándor Ferenczi*, ed. Lewis Aron and Adrienne Harris (London: The Analytic Press, 1993), 81–100; Judit Mészáros, *Ferenczi and Beyond: Exile of the Budapest School and Solidarity in the Psychoanalytic Movement during the Nazi Years* (London: Karnac, 2014), 1–22. A selection of Ferenczi's pre-analytic writings (in Hungarian) were recently published as S. Ferenczi, *Ferenczi a pszichoanalízis felé: Preanalitikus írások (1897–1908)*, ed. J. Mészáros (Budapest: Oriold és Társai, 2022).

4 Lukacs only mentions the Hungarian psychoanalyst Franz Alexander (Ferenc Gábor Alexander), see Lukacs, *Budapest 1900*, 298. Born in 1891, Alexander studied in Berlin, where he met Karl Abraham and Helene Deutsch. In the 1930s, he moved to the United States, where he worked in the Chicago Institute for Psychoanalysis. According to Lukacs' terminology, the generation of 1900 includes Hungarians born between 1875 and 1905. Ferenczi was born in 1873, but he undoubtedly was a part of "a cohort whose formative years occurred in or around 1900. It [the generation of 1900] will even include a few people who were born a few years later but who were still formed by the cultural atmosphere of the period, men and women born between 1875 and 1905 – men and women who were very bright, very different, and some of them very successful," Lukacs, *Budapest 1900*, 295.

5 In 1996, Peter L. Rudnytsky argued: "Ferenczi's rehabilitation in recent years has much to do with his position in the early history of the psychoanalytic movement. [...] Apart from Freud, he is the first-generation pioneer who addresses most immediately the concerns of contemporary psychoanalysts; and, in some respects, he has come to represent not only a complement but a powerful alternative to Freud as well," "Introduction," in *Ferenczi's Turn*, 3.

6 For the English translation, see: *Ferenczi and Beyond*, 1. In this context, Mészáros stresses: "It is important to take a closer look at this early pre-psychoanalytic, or pre-analytic, phase because it is in these writings that we uncover traces of the internal process that would eventually give shape to psychoanalytic thinking. The term pre-analytic is, therefore, descriptive, not evaluative; it designates a period which ended on 2 February 1908 with the meeting between Freud and Ferenczi," 1.

7 The magazine was launched in 1861 by Imre Poór and others. Earlier, Poór had been an editor in the more conservative *Orvosi Hetilap* (Hungarian Medical Journal) – the first Hungarian medical periodical established in 1857 by Lajos Markusovszky. Miksa Schächter took *Gyógyászat* over in 1886, making it the second most influential Hungarian magazine on medicine.

8 For example, John Gerring emphasizes the descriptiveness of the case study genre, see: John Gerring, "What is a Case Study and What is it Good for?" *The American*

Political Science Review vol. 2, no. 98 (2004): 347; cf. Izabela Sobczak, "Case Study," *Forum of Poetics* 20 (2020), 86–95.

9 On the paradigmatic shift in medical case study writing see, for example, B. Lang, "Fin-de-siècle investigations of the 'creative genius' in psychiatry and psychoanalysis," in: *A History of the Case Study*, 55–89; Warwick Anderson, "The Case of the Archive," in: *Case Studies and the Dissemination of Knowledge*, 15–30. Although very instructive, these works seem to omit the question of the performative dimension of case writing and the spaces of the authors' involvement in homosexual men's emancipation movement, see also Katie Sutton, "Sexological Cases and the Prehistory of Transgender Identity Politics in Interwar Germany," in *Case Studies and the Dissemination of Knowledge*, 85–103.

10 While writing about (Róbert) Róza and other non-normative cases I will use a gender-neutral pronoun "they," see: https://uwm.edu/lgbtrc/support/gender-pronouns, accessed March 11, 2021. That way I want to stress the yet unnamed forms of gender expression.

11 In this context, it is worth mentioning the English writer, philosopher, and social activist Edward Carpenter (1844–1929). In 1908 he published *The Intermediate Sex: A Study of Some Transitional Types of Men and Women*. His book, both in terms of the subject matter addressed, empathy, and the author's progressive commitment to "Uranians," recalls Hirschfeld's works. In the last chapter of his book ("The Place of the Uranian in Society"), he wrote: "I have said that the Urning [sic] men in their own lives put love before money-making, business success, fame, and other motives which rule the normal man. I am sure that it is also true of them as a whole that they put love before lust. I do not feel *sure* that this can be said of the normal man, at any rate in the present stage of evolution." See: E. Carpenter, *The Intermediate Sex* (New York-London: Mitchell Kennerley 1912, 120). Similarly to Hirschfeld's fin-de-siècle reflections, at the heart of his discussion of non-normative desire, Carpenter placed not the etiology of homosexuality but love between two human beings.

References

Anderson, W. "The Case of the Archive," in *Case Studies and the Dissemination of Knowledge*, New York: Routledge, 15–30.

Angyalosi, G., Csorba, E. *et al.* (Eds.) (2009). *Nyugat népe. Tanulmányok a Nyugatról és koráról*, Budapest: Petőfi Irodalmi Múzeum.

Bálazs, E. (2009). *Az intellektualitás vezérei. Viták az irodalmi autonómiáról a Nyugatban és a Nyugatról: 1908–1914*, Budapest: Napvilág Kiadó.

Barki, G., Benesch, E. & Rockenbauer, Z. (Eds.) (2012). *Die Acht. Ungarns Highway in die Moderne. A Nyolcak*, Wien: Deutscher Kunstverlag.

Beachy, R. (2010). The German Invention of Homosexuality, in *The Journal of Modern History* 82 (4), 801–838.

Berlant, L. (2007). On the Case, in *Critical Inquiry* 33 (4), 663–672.

Borgos, A. (2011). Sándor/Sarolta Vay, a Gender-Bender in Fin-de-Siècle Hungary, in S. Tötösy de Zepetnek & L. O. Vasvári (Eds.), *Comparative Hungarian Cultural Studies*, Indiana: West Lafayette, 220–231.

Brooks, P. (1992). *Reading for the Plot. Design and Intention in Narrative*, Cambridge, Massachusetts/London: Harvard University Press.

Buklijaš, T. (2012). The Politics of Fin-de-Siècle Anatomy, in J. Surman & M. G. Ash (Eds.), *The Nationalization of Scientific Knowledge in the Habsburg Empire, 1848–1918*, London: Palgrave Macmillan, 209–244.

Carpenter, E. (1912). *The Intermediate Sex*, New York/London: Mitchell Kennerley.

Conway, James J. (2017). Afterword, in Magnus Hirschfeld, *Berlin's Third Sex*, Berlin: Rixdorf Editions, 129–150.
Csáky, M. (2010). *Die Gedächtnis der Städte. Kulturelle Verflechtungen – Wien und die urbanen Milieus in Zentraleuropa*, Wien: Böhlau Verlag.
Damousi, J. (Ed.) (2015). *Case Studies and the Dissemination of Knowledge*, New York: Routledge.
Dose, R. (2014). *Magnus Hirschfeld: The Origins of the Gay Liberation Movement*. Translated by E. H. Willis. New York: New York University Press.
Ellis, H. (1900). *Studies in the Psychology of Sex, vol. 1., Sexual Inversion*, London: Cambridge University Press.
Ferenczi, S. (1902). Homosexualitas Feminina, in *Gyógyászat* 11, 167–168.
Ferenczi, S. (1906). Sexualis átmeneti fokozatokról, in *Gyógyászat* 19, 310–314.
Ferenczi, S. (1911). Über die Rolle der Homosexualität in der Pathogenese der Paranoia, in *Jahrbuch für psychoanalytische und psychopathologische Forschung* 3 (1), 101–119.
Ferenczi, S. (1914). Zur Nosologie der männlichen Homosexualität (Homoërotik), in *Internationale Zeitschrift für Psychoanalyse* 2, 131–142.
Ferenczi, S. (2022). *Ferenczi a pszichoanalízis felé: Preanalitikus írások (1897–1908)*, ed. by Judit Mészáros, Budapest: Oriold és Társai.
Forrester, J. (2017). *Thinking in Cases*, Cambridge: Polity Press.
Foucault, M. (1978). *The History of Sexuality, vol. 1: The Will to Knowledge*. Translated by Robert Hurley. New York: Penguin Random House.
Freud, S. (1933). Sándor Ferenczi, in *Internationale Zeitschrift für Psychoanalyse* 19 (3), 301–304.
Freud, S. ([1905] 1953). Three Essays on the Theory of Sexuality, in J. Strachey (Ed.), *The Standard Edition of the Complete Psychological Works of Sigmund Freud*. Vol. 7, London: The Hogarth Press, 125–245.
Freud, S. ([1914] 1957). On the History of Psycho-Analytic Movement, in J. Strachey (Ed.), *The Standard Edition of the Complete Psychological Works of Sigmund Freud*, Vol. 14, London: The Hogarth Press, 1–66.
Freud, S. & Ferenczi, S. (1993). *The Correspondence of Sigmund Freud and Sándor Ferenczi. Vol. 1: 1908–1914*, Cambridge, Massachusetts: Harvard University Press.
Gerring, J. (2004). What is a Case Study and What is it Good For?, in *The American Political Science Review* 2 (98), 341–354.
Glick, E. (2009). *Materializing Queer Desire: Oscar Wilde to Andy Warhol*, Albany: SUNY Press.
Gyöngyi, I. (1922). *Színész egy félszázon át*, Budapest: Hajnal Kiadás.
Hanák, P. (1998). *The Garden and the Workshop: Essays on the Cultural History of Vienna and Budapest*, Princeton: Princeton University Press.
Haralson, E. (2004). *Henry James and The Queer Modernity*, Cambridge: Cambridge University Press.
Hirschfeld, M. (2017). *Berlin's Third Sex*, Berlin: Rixdorf Editions Berlin.
Horváth, B. (1993). *Kernstok Károly*, Tatabánya: Vatera.
Hurley, N. (2008). Henry James and the Sexuality of Literature: Before and Beyond Queer Theory, in G. W. Zacharias (Ed.), *A Companion to Henry James*, Oxford: Oxford University Press, 309–323.
Korbel, S. (2020). Jews, Mobility, and Sex: Popular Entertainment between Budapest, Vienna, and New York around 1900, in *Austrian History Yearbook* 51, 220–242.
Krafft-Ebing, R. von (2011). *Psychopathia Sexualis*, New York: Arcade Publishing.
Krúdy, G. (2019). *Miasto uśpionych kobiet*. Translated by Elżbieta Cygielska. Warszawa: PIW.

Lang, B. (2017). Fin-de-siècle investigations of the "creative genius" in psychiatry and psychoanalysis, in *A History of the Case Study: Sexology, Psychoanalysis, Literature*, Manchester: Manchester University Press, 55–89.
Lang, B. & Damousi, J. (Eds.) (2017). *A History of the Case Study: Sexology, Psychoanalysis, Literature*, Manchester: Manchester University Press.
Lejeune, P. (1987). Autobiographie et homosexualité en France au XIXe siècle, in *Romantisme* 52, 79–94.
Lejeune, P. (2017). *Autobiographie et homosexualité en France au XIXe siècle*, Paris: Éditions de la Sorbonne.
Lorin, C. (1983). *Le Jeune Ferenczi. Premiers écrits, 1899–1906*, Paris: Aubier Montaigne.
Lukacs, L. (1994). *Budapest 1900: A Historical Portrait of a City and Its Culture*, New York: Grove Press.
Lunbeck, E. & Simon, B. (2003). On Reading Psychoanalytic Case Notes, in E. Lunbeck & B. Simon (Eds.), *Family Romance, Family Secrets: Case Notes from American Psychoanalysis*, New Haven: Yale University Press.
Mak, G. (2004). Sándor/Sarolta Vay: From Passing Woman to Sexual Invert, in *Journal of Women's History* 1, 54–77.
Makari, G. (2008). *Revolution in Mind: The Creation of Psychoanalysis*, New York: Harper Perennial.
Mancini, E. (2010). *Magnus Hirschfeld and the Quest for Sexual Freedom: A History of the First International Sexual Freedom Movement*, New York: Palgrave Macmillan.
Markója, C. & Bardoly, I. (2010). *A Nyolcak*, Pécs: Janus Pannonius Múzeum.
Mészáros, J. (2008). *"Az Önök Bizottsága" – Ferenczi Sándor, a budapesti iskola és a pszichoanalitikus emigráció*, Budapest: Akadémiai Kiadó.
Mészáros, J. (2014). *Ferenczi and Beyond: Exile of the Budapest School and Solidarity in the Psychoanalytic Movement during the Nazi Years*, London: Karnac.
Moore, A. M. (2016). *Sexual Myths of Modernity: Sadism, Masochism, and Historical Teleology.* Lanham, Maryland: Lexington Books.
Moreau-Ricaud, M. (2012). Healing boredom, in J. Szekacs-Weisz & T. Keve (Eds.), *Ferenczi and his World: Rekindling the Spirit of the Budapest School*, London: Karnac, 87–96.
Müller, K. (1991). *Aber in meinem Herzen sprach eine Stimme so laut: Homosexuelle Autobiographien und medizinische Pathographien im neunzehnten Jahrhundert*, Berlin: Männerschwarm.
Oosterhuis, H. (2000). *Stepchildren of Nature: Krafft-Ebing, Psychiatry, and the Making of Sexual Identity*, Chicago/London: Chicago University Press.
Oosterhuis, H. (2012). Sexual Modernity in the Works of Richard von Krafft-Ebing and Albert Moll, in *Medical History* 56 (2), 133–155.
Przybyszewski, S. (1893). *Totenmesse*, Berlin: F. Fontane.
Przybyszewski, S. (1900). *Androgyne*, Lwów: Towarzystwo Wydawnicze.
Przybyszewski, S. (1907). Das Geschlecht, in *Die Fackel*, 239–240, 1–11.
Rachman, A. Wm. (1993). Ferenczi and Sexuality, in L. Aron & A. Harris, *The Legacy of Sándor Ferenczi*, London: The Analytic Press, 81–100.
Rudnytsky, P. L. (1996). Introduction: Ferenczi's Turn in Psychoanalysis, in P. L. Rudnytsky, Antal Bókay & Patrizia Giampieri-Deutsch (Eds.), *Ferenczi's Turn in Psychoanalysis*, New York: New York University Press, 1–22.
Sealey, A. (2011). The Strange Case of the Freudian Case History: The Role of Long Case Histories in the Development of Psychoanalysis, in *History of the Human Sciences* 24, 36–50.

Sengoopta, C. (1998). Glandular Politics: Experimental Biology, Clinical Medicine, and Homosexual Emancipation in Fin-de-Siècle Central Europe, in *Isis* 89 (3), 445–473.
Sobczak, I. (2020). Case Study, in *Forum of Poetics* 20, 86–95.
Steuer, D. (2005). A Book That Won't Go Away: Otto Weininger's Sex and *Character*, in D. Steuer & L. Marcus (Eds.), *Otto Weininger, Sex and Character: An Investigation of Fundamental Principles*, Bloomington: Indiana University Press, xi–xlvi.
Sutton, K. (2015). Sexological Cases and the Prehistory of Transgender Identity Politics in Interwar Germany, in *Case Studies and the Dissemination of Knowledge*, New York: Routledge, 85–103.
Sutton, S. *Sex Between Body and Mind: Psychoanalysis and Sexology in the German-speaking World, 1890s-1930s*, Ann Arbor: University of Michigan Press, 2019.
Takács, J. (2014). Queering Budapest, in Jennifer V.Evans & Matt Cook (Eds.), *Queer Cities, Queer Cultures: Europe Since 1945*, London: Bloomsbury, 191–210.
Vay, S. (1909). *Erzsébet királynéról és más krónikás följegyzések*, Budapest: Légrády.
Vay, S. (1986). *Régi magyar társasélet*, Budapest: Magvető.
Vay, S. (2006). *Európa bál*, Budapest: Pont.
Weininger, O. (2005). *Sex and Character: An Investigation of Fundamental Principles.* Translated by Ladislaus Löb. Bloomington: Indiana University Press.
Zepetnek & L. O. Vasvári (Eds.), *Comparative Hungarian Cultural Studies*, Indiana: West Lafayette, 220–231.

3

THE INTERPRETATION OF LITERARY DREAMS

Psychoanalysis, trauma, and painful modernity – the case of Mihály Babits

In previous chapters, I have analyzed selected examples of psycho-medical literature with special attention paid to the dynamics of knowledge transfer between the discourses of psychiatry, sexology, philosophy, life writing, and art. A detailed reading of the correspondence between Sigmund Freud and Wilhelm Fliess (Chapter 1) allowed me to take a closer look at the emergence of Freud's self-analysis in epistolographic practices. Next, an investigation of Sándor Ferenczi's writings in the context of the rapid development of modernism and psycho-medical literature in Hungary (Chapter 2) made it possible to consider the modern *scientia sexualis* as an interdisciplinary discourse suspended between the psycho-medical, literary, and artistic perspectives on the human body and its desires.

In this chapter, I will examine a literary record of a split personality, created in Hungary in 1913 and inspired by psycho-medical discourses.[1] Rather than showing literature's or art's influence on psycho-medical discourses, this case is about the language of literature itself entering in an intimate relationship with psychiatric knowledge and psychoanalysis; about literature which digests and processes psycho-medical discourse in order to produce its own, fiction-based theory of the human (un)conscious and sexuality. A close reading of a novel by Hungary's leading representative of modernism in the light of Sándor Ferenczi's early psychoanalytic writings as well as Otto Gross's reflections on sexuality, aggression, and death will cast new light on how psychoanalytical thought penetrated Hungarian literature in the first two decades of the twentieth century. It will also present literature itself as a key field of influence for psychoanalytic thought as well as a site of its reappropriation and reinterpretation.

Ever since his first encounter with Freud in 1908, Ferenczi made every effort to popularize psychoanalytic thought in Hungarian medical circles. At the same time, as a friend to the most prominent Hungarian writers of

DOI: 10.4324/9781003441892-4

"Generation 1900," he shared his psychoanalytic knowledge with Budapest's foremost literary and intellectual milieus of that time. Shortly after his return from Vienna, Ferenczi began associating with progressive (leftist and anti-nationalist) newspapers and environments: *Gyógyászat* (Therapy), *Huszadik Század* (The Twentieth Century), *Szabad Gondolat* (Liberal Thought), and the Galileo Kör (The Galileo Circle). In the early twentieth century, they became the sites for the transfer of Freudianism into broader Hungarian culture. Importantly, many Hungarian writers were not just learning about psychoanalysis "passively," but also as patients or analysts. The best-known example of a writer-psychiatrist was Géza Csáth/Joseph Brenner (1887–1919) whose own medical practice and inspiration by Freud's discussion of hysteria gave rise to a 1911 work entitled *Diary of a Madwoman* (*Egy elmebeteg nő naplója*). Another example was poet Géza Szilágyi (1875–1958) who also practiced psychoanalysis (until 1941). Attila József (1905–1937) underwent analysis by two students of the Budapest School of Psychoanalysis: Robert C. Bak (1908–1974) and Edith Gyömrői Ludowyk (1896–1987). Frigyes Karinthy (1887–1938) attended therapy with Ferenczi, but quickly abandoned Freudianism especially as a therapeutic technique – nonetheless remaining an inquisitive reader of psycho-medical literature, which is best evidenced by his last novel *A Journey Round My Skull* (*Utazás a koponyám körül*). Although in the 1930s Freud's theories began losing their impact on Hungarian writers, psychoanalysis – particularly the interpretation of dreams – had left a significant mark on the budding Hungarian modernist literature. It remained an important reference point especially for the literary circle around *Nyugat* (West). Through Ferenczi, Freud's newest theories reached writers such as Dezső Kosztolányi, Frigyes Karinthy, Mihály Babits, and Milán Füst. Mihály Babits (1883–1941) penned his first novel influenced precisely by the spread of the psychoanalytic interpretation of dreams.

Ten years Ferenczi's junior, Babits studied philology at the University of Budapest. He specialized in classical languages and later took an interest in English literature. As a writer and literary critic, he quickly became involved with the modernist *Nyugat*.[2] Babits's literary career gained momentum during the Great War (Gál 2003).[3] A short period of liberalization post-1919 was an important time for Hungarian intellectuals of liberal, pacifist, and cosmopolitan orientation. At that time, Babits was appointed a professor at the University of Budapest – a position which (like Ferenczi) he was to lose quickly. He had already begun writing *The Caliph Stork*[4] (*A gólyakalifa*) before the outbreak of the First World War. The novel, completed in 1913, first appeared in *Nyugat* (1913, no. 24, 805–907) as fragments, and in 1916 in its entirety as a book.[5] The title was taken from the German author Wilhelm Hauff (1802–1827) – a writer, theologian, and philosopher whose fairy tale "The Story of the Caliph Stork" was published in 1826 (Hauff 1991). Babits did not only borrow Hauff's title; he also explicitly modeled his protagonist Elmér Tábory's biography on caliph Chasid's. As we will see, *The Caliph*

Stork went beyond Babits's inspiration with psychoanalytic theory as the author offered his own suggestions for understanding dreams, the dynamics of illusion, and the structure of the unconscious. Moreover, dream content and the act of dreaming were localized by Babits in the realm of the kind of phantasmatic production that is typical of paranoid mechanisms, which especially intrigued doctors and analysts at that time.

3.1 Dream theories and multiple personalities: Elemér Tábory as a reader

In *The Caliph Stork*, dream theory occupies a central place in the story of the protagonist and narrator, Elemér Tábory. The moment his nightmares appear, Elemér begins searching for an answer to his burning question about the source of dreams. With the help of a friendly Professor Darvas, he reads extensive literature on dreams, automatisms, and dissociative identity. At the professor's library, he first encounters Morton Prince's (1854–1929) work on Christine "Sally" Beauchamp (Clara Norton Fowler) (Prince 1906).[6] As the narrator relays, she "had four or even six personalities at the same time. [...] One of her selves was good, the other bad" (Babits 1966: 61). The case, which was described by Prince biographically, helps the narrator to self-diagnose while simultaneously revealing Babits's inspiration by the psycho-medical literature of his time. In *The Dissociation of Personality*, Prince presented his patient in the following way:

> Miss Christine L. Beauchamp the subject of this study, is a person in whom several personalities have become developed, that is to say, she may change her personality from time to time, often from hour to hour, and with each change her character becomes transformed and her memories altered.
>
> *(Prince 1906: 1)*

Prince observed that his patient developed multiple personalities. Although they seemed to be independent of one another, they distinctly influenced Miss Beauchamp's "original" self (in the text labeled as "BI"). In one of the key chapters ("Sally as a Subconscious and as an Alternating Personality"), Prince emphasized:

> In the first place, Sally is a distinct personality in the sense of having a character, trains of thought, memories, perceptions, acquisitions, and mental acquirements. [...] Secondly: She is an alternating personality in that during the times when the primary self has vanished Sally is for the time being the whole conscious personality, having taken the place of the other. As an alternating personality so much of the whole field of consciousness as persists belongs to her and there is no other self. At such

> times BI does not become a subconsciousness to Sally but as a personality is wiped out.
>
> *(Ibid.: 144)*

The case study of Miss Beauchamp-Sally closely corresponds with the story of Elemér's split personality. Prince considered the possibility of Miss Beauchamp's dreaming a space for merging her multiple selves. Notably, Sally haunted Miss Beauchamp in her sleep and influenced the content of her dreams (Ibid.: 332).

Prince's work was not the only source of learning about the theory of dissociation. In Professor Darvas's library, Elemér found another work entitled *The Psychological Automatism* (*L'Automatisme Psychologique*) (1889) (Babits 1966: 60).[7] Babits must have known the works of French psychiatrists, whose ideas influenced Hungarian psycho-medical and literary circles at the turn of the twentieth century. French studies of hysteria, hypnosis, and magnetism became popular among Hungarian medical circles. Pierre Janet was one of the first to propose a systematic approach to the dissociation mechanisms he had observed in his hysterical patients. The first theories of the split personality appeared as early as the first half of the nineteenth century in French magnetism. In the 1880s, in works by Janet, Charles Richet, and Frederic Myers in England, dissociation started to be understood as the existence of two selves, two wills, and two streams of thought in one person. It was Janet, though, who, at that time, linked dissociation with the traumatic experience. His case study of Lucy, similarly to Miss Beauchamp's case, could have served Babits as a model for Elemér's biography.

A few important details related to Lucy's analysis are also worth mentioning. In his patient, Janet discovered a second, independent personality, with whom he was able to communicate only in writing. In his article "The personality during induced somnambulism" ("La personnalité pendant le somnambulisme provoqué"), Janet wrote:

> After having had L. write several automatic letters of this kind, I had the idea of questioning her when I made the suggestion to her and of ordering her to answer me in writing. [...] It was enough to suggest to her once during sleep that she answer my questions in writing, so that, once awake, she always did it in the same automatic way. At this moment L., although awake, seemed no longer to see or hear me consciously; she did not answer me and spoke to everyone, but not to me.
>
> *(Janet 1886: 588)*

Janet considered it particularly important that Lucy's second personality (called Adrienne) could reveal itself only through automatic writing. Automatic writing of its own kind also appears in Babits's first novel. Elemér writes his autobiography nearly automatically, in a great hurry, on the verge between reality and sleep.

Another crucial theme in *The Caliph Stork* was the psychoanalytic understanding of dreams. Although Freud's name is not mentioned in the text, Elemér's story shows that the novel's author was no stranger to psychoanalytic dream theory. Babits may have read *The Interpretation of Dreams*, and he certainly must have known about it second-hand as Ferenczi had recently published a text entitled "Psychoanalysis of the dream and its pathological significance" ("Az álom psychoanalysise és annak kórtani jelentősége")[8] in *Orvosi Hetilap* (Medical Weekly) where he outlined the basics of Freudian dream theory. Babits was well-versed in French- and English-language psychological and psychiatric literature. He surely must have known Ferenczi's short essay (nineteen pages) which constituted one of the Hungarian analyst's first popular publications on dreams. With physicians as his target audience, Ferenczi stressed the uses of psychoanalytic dream theory in treating neurotic and psychotic disorders.

His article continued to be the most significant introduction in Hungarian to *The Interpretation of Dreams* until 1915, when a translation of Freud's "Über den Traum" was published as "Az Álomról" ("On the Dream") with Ferenczi's foreword (second edition: 1918).[9] As Ferenczi states in his introduction, Freud's dream theory marked "a new era in psychology" (Ferenczi 2011: 7). The theme of dreams recurred not only in medical journals but also in literary and cultural periodicals, most importantly in *Nyugat*.[10]

In *The Caliph Stork*, the narrator suggests his own definition of a dream: "How closely this dream resembled reality, despite its more adventurous colouring! There was nothing impossible, nothing vague in it, and there were none of the usual abrupt leaps in time" (Babits 1966: 58). A dream converges with reality and is governed by a similar logic. Such a formulation only seemingly contradicts Freudian thought, which understood dreams as phenomena that are meaningless on the level of *explicit* content, but deeply meaningful on the *implicit* level. As a wishful fabrication, a dream has its own logic which does not conform to the order of rationality. The content of dreams is usually heavily distorted in relation to reality and controlled by the dream-censor. In his "A Metapsychological Supplement to the Theory of Dreams" (1915, published in 1917), Freud wrote:

> The dream-wish, as we say, is *hallucinated*, and, as a hallucination, meets with belief in the reality of its fulfillment. It is precisely round this concluding piece in the formation of dreams that the gravest uncertainties center, and it is in order to clear them up that we are proposing to compare dreams with pathological states akin to them. The formation of the wishful phantasy and its regression to hallucination are the most essential parts of the dream-work, but they do not belong exclusively to dreams. They are also found in two morbid states: […] the hallucinatory phase of schizophrenia.
>
> *(Freud [1917] 1957b: 229)*

In the case of hallucinatory confusion, the wishful fabrication itself remains ordered "a perfect day-dream" (Ibid.: 230). Moreover, in a wishful psychotic fantasy, the wish is depicted as fulfilled. Freud adds: "hallucination brings belief in reality with it" (Ibid.: 230). The mechanism of the dream-wish as described by Freud in the light of hallucinatory wish dynamics is reflected in Elemér's story. The author creates an insightful portrait of a psychotic wish-fantasy that follows psychoanalytic reflection on dreams. Elemér's dreams are organized in their own perfect order; they are also accompanied by a "belief in their reality" to the extent that the boundaries between the real and the imagined are blurred. For the narrator, his own life becomes nothing but an objectified self-illusion – a reality where a projected fulfillment of a repressed wish can take place.

Hauff's "The Story of the Caliph Stork" had enjoyed great popularity since its publication. It tells a story of a young ruler of Baghdad named Chasid and his Vizier Mansor. One day, a merchant arrives at Chasid's beautiful palace. Among various tempting wares, a little casket piques the caliph's curiosity. In it, he finds some mysterious powder and a handwritten note in a language he does not understand. As it soon turns out, it is a spell in Latin, allowing a person to transform into an animal of his or her choosing. In order to come back to human form, the animal must never laugh. Chasid and Mansor decide to transform into storks, but – as one can easily guess – they break the rule immediately after their metamorphosis and are doomed to life in a stork's body. Ultimately, the protagonists are able to happily return to human form with the help of an Indian princess enchanted into an owl.

By drawing from a famous fairy tale, Babits added a dimension of a universal narrative on the human condition to Elemér's story, one which touches on the deepest secrets of human life and stems from a search for the sources of the unconscious. A universal message extracted from an individual narrative is a key feature of fairy tales, which, as a genre, are characterized by an unspecified time ("once upon a time…") and location ("beyond seven mountains, beyond seven valleys") of the plot. The story told in a folktale may happen at any time or place. Moreover, oriental themes were thought to enrich the narrative with an element of the uncanny, intensified by depicting what was simultaneously near (e.g. a hierarchical social structure) and far (motifs from Arabic culture). Analysts were attracted by myths and fairy tales from the very inception of psychoanalysis. On the one hand, these genres fascinated them because – in their timelessness – they could be considered as reflections of universal human fears and desires (an emanation of the unconscious). On the other hand, each tale – while seemingly fantastic and detached from the mundane – could say something important about the currently experienced social reality.

Another important context for Babits's psychobiography of Elemér Tábory was English literature, particularly Robert Louis Stevenson's *Strange Case of Dr Jekyll and Mr Hyde* (1886) and the slightly later *Picture of Dorian Gray* by Oscar Wilde (1890). Like many members of the Hungarian intelligentsia, Babits had already become fascinated with English and American culture at university. Before the Great War, due to his "Anglomania," in Hungarian literary circles he was often called "the Hungarian Swinburne" or "the Hungarian Poe." Later, Babits read and translated works by such authors as William Shakespeare (significantly, *The Tempest*, published in Hungarian in 1916), William Blake, John Keats, Edgar Allan Poe, Algernon Charles Swinburne, Oscar Wilde, and William Wordsworth. His (self-)portrait of Elemér Tábory brings to mind both the protagonist of Stevenson's novella and Basil Hallward's painting of Dorian Gray. Both works essentially discussed the duality of human nature (Dr Jekyll and Mr Hyde's was a case of a split personality, like Elemér Tábory's) as well as the tension between beauty and monstrosity. In Wilde's novel, the dirty, evil, and immoral was *externalized* into a painting. Meanwhile, in Stevenson, evil became *internalized* by the protagonist as his second nature.

In psychoanalytic circles, it was Otto Rank who became particularly interested in the literary descriptions of split personality. In his two works *Die Don Juan Gestalt* (1924) and *Der Doppelgänger. Eine psychoanalytische Studie* (1925), Rank analyzed different ways of representing the mechanisms of dissociation. Leporello – as Don Juan's double – played the role of the protagonist's *super-ego*. For Rank, the double (*der Doppelgänger*) as a literary trope reveals the most profound of the inner conflicts existing in the human psyche (Rank 1924: 13–15). In his book, Rank mentions Stevenson and stresses that the theme of double-consciousness allowed the author to shed light on the psychological mechanisms of suppression and disavowal (Rank 2009: 40). Rank goes even further when he argues that the protagonist often plays the role of the author's double. In this light, a literary work can be considered its author's autobiography – a manifestation of their inner life (Ibid.: 80). This tension between autobiography, self-analysis, and psychography finds its expression in Babits's intertextual play with the case study genre.

3.2 Elemér's autobiography as a psycho-medical document

In the first pages of *The Caliph Stork*, the reader learns that the book is an autobiography by Elemér Tábory. Although its author is neither a writer nor a doctor, he resolves to present a detailed, autobiographical study of an illness which he diagnoses as a "multiple personality" (Babits 1966: 60–61). It is the tragic story of a wealthy and ambitious young man who one day decides to record it before he commits suicide – which he justifies in these words:

> I wish to tell the story of my life. Who knows how much time I have left? The step I have decided to take may be fatal. The night is passing slowly but surely. And suddenly, black sleep will come on tiptoe, like a murderer, and will stand silently behind me. Suddenly it will press its palm on my eyes, and then I will no longer belong to myself. Then anything may happen to me. I wish to tell the story of my life before I go to sleep again.
> *(Ibid.: 9)*

Elemér gets his autobiographical notes in order on the last night before his death. Notably, the word "autobiography" cannot be found in the introduction. Instead, the narrator prefers to talk about "the records"[11] of his life and adds: "I have accurate notes on everything. My life was like a dream, and my dream like life…" (Ibid.: 9). In a short self-presentation, Elemér gives a detailed account of his dreams. He describes dreaming itself as a state from which one cannot awaken. Dreaming becomes a figure of death, lurking in the shadows like "a murderer." The idea of associating sleep with death (and the fear of death) did not only appear alongside an interest in the unconscious; rather, it has its sources in antiquity. In the ancient Greek imaginary, Hypnos and Thanatos were twin brothers – sleep was perceived as akin to death, and death was strictly tied to sleep (Pick & Roper 2004). The idea of the special kinship between sleep and death prompts Elemér Tábory to quickly gather "the records of his life" in fear of falling asleep again.

Equating an autobiographical text with a "record" is a sign of inscribing the genre of autobiography into the psycho-medical literature, which, as Philippe Lejeune (2017: 19–49) demonstrated, eagerly relied on personal narratives in the second half of the nineteenth century.[12] In *The Caliph Stork*, the narrator assumes the role of a patient with ease, and treats his personal story as an intimate (autobiographical) case study of a disease. This is confirmed by the addition of a supplement entitled *The author's letter* to the novel's ending:

> Dear friend, it was three years ago that I first spoke to you about Elemér Tábory's writings. That was when the mysterious tragedy took place which made such a sensation in the newspapers: he was found dead in his room, a shot wound in his forehead, but no weapon anywhere. What could have happened? The subsequent investigation was quite futile. I kept these writings concealed for a long time. […] I have changed all the names. You, however, will know who it is. I beg you to accept these tragic pages. I am sending them to you first, I am sure you will read them with interest and sympathy.
>
> *(Babits 1966: 136)*

The reader learns from the note that Elemér (whose name was changed by the writer-editor) died in mysterious circumstances. The protagonist's real identity remains unknown, as does the writer's and the addressee's. The author of the note does not explain why Elemér chose him as his confidant. Nevertheless, he stresses the uniqueness of this self-analytic document which his friend – who is likely very familiar with recent psychological theories – "will read with interest and sympathy (Hungarian: részvét)" towards the afflicted. Keeping in mind Ferenczi's close relationship to Babits's literary circle, one can imagine that the novelist himself may have been the author of *The author's letter*, and Ferenczi – as the famous physician-Humanist – its addressee. The acquired record of a disease – which, as one can infer from the notes, somewhat edited by the writer – was intended to become a source of knowledge about dissociative identity disorder and the dynamics of the dream-wish.

It was no coincidence that Babits decided to tell Elemér's story as an autobiography rather than a biography or a case study. As I have tried to demonstrate in the previous chapter, the quickly developing psycho-medical literature of the late 1800s treated the autobiography as a fundamental source of information about the genesis and course of a given ailment. Patients were encouraged to write memoirs and autobiographies which were then supposed to facilitate the understanding of a given pathological case by doctors. Based on autobiographical accounts, case studies were then formulated where the patients' reflections intertwined with medical narratives. As I have shown with Richard von Krafft-Ebing's *Psychopathia Sexualis*, quotations from the sufferers' autobiographical records could function as the basic material of psycho-medical discourse. In such cases, the doctor's commentary merely accompanied fragments written by the patients themselves. The modernist *Caliph Stork* did not only allude to psycho-medical literature, but it also perfectly followed the convention at the intersection of medical, life writing, and literary discourses. Elemér's autobiography can therefore be viewed as one of many examples of a patient's intimate records meant for the eyes of a doctor-psychoanalyst.

Elemér seems aware of the use that psycho-medical literature may make of his account. In order to facilitate any future diagnosis, he adds:

> I was almost certain that I too had developed a case of split personality, and I could have wept at the thought of the happy, healthy boy whom I had thought myself to be the day before yesterday. *Would I too then become one of those unfortunate cases about whom doctors write books and whom people find objects of pity, a sadly attractive curiosity* [italics mine]?
>
> *(Babits 1966: 62)*

It would seem that Elemér Tábory was born with a silver spoon in his mouth – but he has a secret. His personality is split into two opposite parts: the "good" one, and one that is profoundly depraved. At the beginning of his life story, the narrator is still attempting to maintain an idealized self-image:

> In every way I was much better off than my class-mates. They liked and admired me because I was a handsome, skillful boy, cleverer and stronger than they; [...] but the main reason for their admiration was that I paid absolutely no attention to them and did not give a damn about their friendship.
>
> *(Ibid.: 10)*

A perfect childhood spent in a loving family and the joy of growing up in adoration are suddenly disturbed when the protagonist starts suffering from nightmares. Elemér dreams about himself as someone radically different: a bastard, orphan, and pauper who elicits animosity and derision rather than universal respect. The recurring dreams lead him to reflect on his own psyche and conclude that: "These feelings seemed to be omen of some hidden horror in the depths of my memory – something that would change the whole aspect of the world for me – but I did not know what it was" (Ibid.: 11).

When the narrator wakes up to his "other life," it starkly contrasts with his idyllic childhood. In his dreams, he does not even have a name. What he knows about himself is that he has been an apprentice at a workshop for some time. He recalls:

> All this was like a nightmare. I felt that now I should think of something, remember something, something fine and clean that would comfort me directly. But I was so stupid! So ignorant! My head… and my spirit… so oppressed. […] Could I have been dreaming ever since my early childhood? Was I myself only a dream I was dreaming?
>
> *(Ibid.: 29)*

Although Elemér's "dream" life is happy and glowing, his other self is condemned to suffering. A linear narrative offered by the protagonist gives way to a "repetitive and monotonous" litany of complaints by a man imprisoned in a life that is (not) his own – which could be easily characterized as depressive speech (Kristeva 1992: 33). When Elemér sleeps, his nocturnal self goes through a nightmare. In his self-analytic notes, the following words return like a mantra:

> I felt sudden alarm at my thought, my whole being shuddered as if it had been defiled by some disgusting filth, spilled from who knows where in the world. I felt that my whole life was irrevocably and indelibly soiled by this thought. I, the clean and noble-minded child, who, though everything was clean and honourable about me, had suddenly discovered that all this bright cleanliness, even the alloyed, with hidden disgusting filth in the unknown recesses of my soul. This was so horrible that all at once I could not concentrate and think of anything else.
>
> *(Babits 1966: 46)*

Living through the dream as if it was reality, the narrator writes about an experience of utmost humiliation and befoulment. Like the caliph confined to an animal's body in the fairy tale, Elemér perceives his dream state as de-subjectified, inhuman.

3.3 Painful modernity: the metropolis, the machine, the ability to write

At the turn of the century, Hungary was undergoing a revolution of modernity: cities grew, new roads were built, railways expanded. Budapest became a symbol of urban culture which was forged in the commotion of restaurants and cafés and dictated by the ubiquitous fashion for Englishness and Americanness. The modernizing acceleration in Hungary introduced cultural changes and significantly impacted local inhabitants' daily life. After the unification of Austria-Hungary in 1867, apart from legislative adjustments (for uniformity in the newly created *Gesammtmonarchie*), a number of significant changes in social policy were made, including the acknowledgment of religious liberty and respect for the rights of national and religious minorities (called the Ferenc Deák and József Eötvös laws) as well as a regulation on mandatory elementary education (instituted in 1868 by Eötvös) (Molnár 2014: 201–249).

At the turn of the nineteenth and twentieth century, the Hungarian society was diverse both in terms of nationalities and religions. The country was dominated by ethnic Hungarians (who constituted a little over half of all inhabitants of the Hungarian part of the Empire), followed by Germans, Slovaks, Romanians, Serbs, and Jews (Ibid.: 214–216). Despite the government's open policy towards minorities (especially under the liberal prime minister Kálmán Tisza), the first years of the twentieth century saw an intensification of calls for forcible Magyarization, which resulted in a gradual uniformization of language and the leveling of Hungary's earlier cultural diversity (Ibid.: 222–223).

In 1907, in accordance with the so-called "lex Apponyi," free and open obligatory education was introduced and a network of schools for children from working-class families and those in economic need was established. Meanwhile, Hungarian became the language of instruction in classrooms. The second half of the nineteenth century also brought mass literacy and school enrollment, accompanied by the emergence of new educational centers and universities in smaller towns. In 1872, there were already two universities in Kolozsvár, and a further two began operating in Debrecen and Pozsony. In 1895 in Budapest, Eötvös József College opened, modeled on the Parisian École Normale Supérieure (Ibid.: 221, 223). Alongside these changes, a new kind of "metropolitan" bourgeoisie (the so-called *polgárosodás*) emerged with their own culture and practices. Notably, the lightning-speed industrial development and urbanization did not eliminate social stratification. Astronomically rich landowners and factory capitalists were still separated from destitute workers and peasants by a wide chasm (Ibid.: 226–227).

Babits's novel includes the very modernist trope of social exclusion, linked to urbanization and the bureaucratic machine working at full speed. Babits made the split self-image that his character describes an illustration of the modern subject's condition: the struggle to keep up with the processes of modernization that determine their existence. The narrator summarizes: "my entire life was as if two orchestras played various pieces of music in a dreadful discord" (Babits 1966: 96). From the moment it first appears (soon after the apprentice's escape from the workshop), the city – dirty, rushing, crowded – occupies a central place in *The Caliph Stork*. The protagonist wanders through bustling urban streets possibly for the first time in his life. In his account, excitement mixes with fear and frustration. He recalls:

> It was appallingly noisy. The trams jangled out their crazy melodies. Some long iron bars which were being hauled along with wheels bent, shuddered and screeched horribly. Unwieldy removal vans jolted along in a dignified way, covered with huge letters. Colorful, ragged posters on the hoardings demanded attention. *A chaos of screaming letters filled my head. I deciphered strange, senseless words from the walls, alien, unheard-of, unpronounceable words* [italics mine].
>
> *(Ibid.: 49–50)*

This is a description of a rapidly developing city which has gained access to "the whole world" through mass media and communication (evoked by the advertising posters full of foreign words that the narrator cannot understand). The city assaults the protagonist's senses: it screams, screeches piercingly, burns bright with colors and shapes, smells like coal and oil (Ibid.: 49). The narrator cannot grasp most words; he calls it "dirty Babel," and adds: "Like magic letters in a town of wizards. [...] I shall never understand anything. [...] What is all this for?" (Ibid.: 50). Roaming around the city's streets aggravates his despair, especially when he idles in front of the bright, thick-paned shop-windows as the "fly buzzes constantly at the window-pane, beating itself a hundred times against the glass" (Ibid.: 56). He has no money or food. Nevertheless, he considers his difficulty in reading to be his greatest problem:

> The story of my second self is the story of forgotten words. In this life something always seemed to be at the tip of my tongue – something that I could never quite utter. It was at the tip of the tongue of my soul, and it tormented my soul. [...] I wanted to be a gentleman, a gentleman who could read and write. *The gentleman writes* – this sentence which I recalled from my first-grade primer, rang like a tune through my head. During my long, hungry wanderings as a vagabond I had kept repeating the phrase to myself in different keys and rhythms. [...] *Papers, school certificate* – how much I had pondered over these words, too!
>
> *(Ibid.: 80)*

The seemingly innocent sentence "The gentleman writes" (Hungarian: Úr ír) taken from a children's primer constitutes an allusion to the spread of literacy and school enrollment (Brabant-Gerö 1993; Molnár 2014: 201–249; Rakoczy

2022: 119–196, 261–322). At that time, the ability to read and write as well as further education were signs of social class and they became the way to narrate to oneself the increasingly less understandable world.

The protagonist is also aware that this skill affords the special power of subjectification: an opportunity for social advancement and self-expression. Elemér's other self is met with rejection and malice; he does not even have any identity documents. One day, he manages to steal a school diploma and finds employment in a public office under someone else's name. Since then, he becomes haunted by a vision of building a professional career based on fraud. The idealized image of a respected youth appears to hide a lurking common crook. The narrator concludes gloomily:

> This thought led me to new and still more fantastic thoughts. I formed mysterious theories for myself. [...] Wasn't it possible that all of us, every human being, had in his dreams subconsciously such a copy, a dark shadowy image somewhere in the distance even physically, yes, physically, in a distant world or another planet? Wasn't it possible that there was such another world somewhere in space, a dark pendant, a sad caricature of our own ancient Earth?
>
> *(Babits 1966: 95)*

In his nocturnal life, the narrator is an impostor; he is also frightened by the pressures of the bureaucratic machine that he fails to understand. It is worth noting that the inability to follow social expectations is something that the narrator has in common with Franz Kafka's protagonists.

In *The Caliph Stork*, many of Kafka's characteristic themes can be detected, especially ones that appear in his pre-1916 works. He and Babits were born in the same year (1883). Both matured in the climate of urban changes, which impacted turn-of-the-century literary milieus in Budapest and Prague. At that time, the latter city was home to several literary groups, such as Concordia, Jung Prag, or Prager Kreis; in the former, the enterprising circle of *Nyugat* was just taking shape. Kafka's seminal works such as *The Trial, In the Penal Colony*, and *The Metamorphosis* were created soon after Babits's *Caliph Stork*. The Hungarian writer's novel contains tropes also employed by Kafka, such as the destructive workings of the social, administrative, and family machines. Moreover, both writers drew from the classics, shaping their imagination with works by such artists as Heinrich von Kleist, Friedrich Hebbel, Byron, and Stendhal, members of the younger generation like Arthur Schnitzler, Henrik Ibsen, August Strindberg, and rising stars, including Thomas and Heinrich Mann, Hugo von Hofmannsthal, and Gustav Meyrink.

Babits's and Kafka's work developed at a time when psychoanalysis and anthroposophy were becoming increasingly fashionable in artistic and literary circles. Kafka likely had his first encounter with psychoanalysis in 1912, not much later than Babits. However, while Kafka was only superficially familiar with Freud's theory, Babits was introduced to Freudianism by one of Freud's main collaborators: Ferenczi. In addition, while no formal psychoanalytic societies, associations or circles operated in Prague until the 1930s, Babits had witnessed the birth of a powerful psychoanalytic movement in Budapest, which survived both the First and the Second World Wars. The completion of *The Caliph Stork* coincided with the formal establishment of The Hungarian Psychoanalytic Society.

In the ending of *The Caliph Stork*, Etelka utters the words:

> Look Elemér, that other, the clerk, who spoils your life, who has sinned against you and against me, is only an evil image in a dream, a shadow, which does not deserve pity. Kill him! Kill him, tell him, persuade him to kill himself. Why did you not let him perish long ago?
>
> *(Ibid.: 135)*

After a moment's hesitation, the protagonist is persuaded to follow her idea and adds: "Today it will all be decided. Today the clerk will kill himself" (Ibid.: 136). In Kafka's 1913 short story *The Judgement* – as in *The Caliph Stork* – a caricature of the father figure is accompanied by the theme of a repressed death wish. Nevertheless, the father figure (at times powerful, at other times childish) does not play as significant a role in Babits's novel as in Kafka's short story. From the beginning of his narrative, Elemér rather concentrates on the relationship with his mother and other women – ultimately, they become the object of his love, hatred, cruelty, and submission. The experience of social exclusion was a key theme for both authors. Although Babits was not Jewish, his first novel reveals his sensitivity towards the problem of marginalization and social inequality. While Elemér belongs to the Hungarian society's wealthiest stratum of that time (landowning families) and follows an urban bourgeois lifestyle model, his other self is a representative of the underclass – the hungry and exhausted "worm-breed people" excluded from society both economically and symbolically.[13]

3.4 Elemér Tábory's polyphonic (self-)narratives

In Babits's novel, the narrator identifies with the caliph turned into a stork. He is convinced that he is living in a foreign body, having forever forgotten the spell that would allow him to recover his real identity. At a certain point of self-analysis, as he recalls wandering aimlessly around the city, he explains:

> *It was as if I had known it all once and I could not now recall it;* and this was infinitely, nightmarishly agonizing! Like the caliph of the fairy-tale who had change into a stork and forgot the magic word, that would change him back into man.
>
> *(Babits 1966: 50–51)*

When night falls in Elemér's world, the painful experience of losing humanity is reawakened within him. He explains: "But the most oppressive part of it was that I could not remember my own thoughts … And these were the most agonizing moments of my life. *The moments of the caliph stork*" (Ibid.: 80). The protagonist longs for *another* life – the one that is real, though lost forever. His "exile" strongly resembles that of the caliph and his vizier. After numerous unsuccessful attempts to break the spell:

> The two enchanted birds wandered sadly on through the meadows. In their misery they could not think what to do next. They could not rid themselves of their new forms; there was no use in returning to the town and saying who they were; for who would believe a stork who announced that he was a Caliph; and even if they did believe him, would the people of Bagdad consent to let a stork rule over them?
>
> *(Hauff 1991: 25)*

Chasid and Mansor's curse not only imprisons them in an animal's body, it also deprives them of their high social standing. The same idea is highlighted by Babits in *The Caliph Stork*. The protagonist's curse effaces the memories of his splendid life which contrasted so starkly with his current experiences. The narrator comments: "In reality all that is good and beautiful is in fact enveloped in an aura of wickedness and ugliness" (Babits 1966: 71).

When Elemér "falls" into his nocturnal life, he has no beautiful home, or even his own bedroom; he awakens among other destitute people: "I woke up to the bite of a bed-bug in a revolting wooden bed" (Ibid.: 78). In these moments, the protagonist is haunted by the frightening thought that either he is not Elemér Tábory (whose life is actually the dream), or he is suffering from a split personality: "while in the symptoms of a split personality two souls inhabited the same body, in my case, my soul lived alternately in two different bodies" (Ibid.: 92). As years pass, the narrator begins to engage in self-observation, which leads him to the following conclusions:

> Because in truth these two had the same soul, and although they may have separated from each other for a time, now they mingled, their memories were identical and – this was the horror of it – their character, their inward being was the same, appearing different only on the surface. […] Does everyone have a dark ego, perhaps hidden, perhaps subconscious, the guilty unfortunate dregs of his soul? Perhaps… But my evil ego possessed a body as well. […] For what was the body if not the accumulation of a multitude of remembered sensations, of a great many physical perceptions?
>
> *(Ibid.: 92)*

In his adolescence, while Elemér leads a sophisticated life, spending most of his time in Budapest or abroad, his other self is confined to his violent landlord's workshop. When he is asked to go out and buy cigarettes, he enviously admires shop and restaurant windows. The sight of other people's happiness sparks anger in him. He confesses: "If I met an old school-mate walking happily along the street I felt like pulling out a knife and stabbing him" (Ibid.: 30). The aggression rises gradually, but deepens with each day, and ultimately leads to real acts of violence. The narrator's first victim is a toddler who woke him up from a blissful dream about beautiful Elemér Tábory. He reports:

> Suddenly, I saw red. My mind went blank, I cared for nothing. I had just woken from sweet and warm dreams [...]: a disgusting hateful little dwarf stood in front of me [...]. I felt the blood rushing to my face, my cheeks burnt with a pitiless desire for revenge and the cowardly thought flashed into my mind that with a single jerk of my hand I could break the neck of this ugly little frog. [...] With desperate, cowardly courage, like the soldier who knows death is near and kills mothers and infants in his rage, so I began to strike and beat the little brat whatever I could.
>
> *(Ibid.: 34–35)*

The narrator discloses that he feels a swelling desire to kill the child. The little boy embodies all the "bad people" that the dreamer has encountered. However, the violence inflicted on the toddler does not stem only from despair. Elemér adds: "I am experiencing the most beautiful hour of my life" (Ibid.: 35).

This scene's ambivalence – the euphoria of violence clashing with shame – resurfaces later in the novel. On the following pages, the protagonist recalls:

> For a long time I had found female beauty exciting and I greedily enjoyed all that I was allowed to see of it at home, in the theatre and in the street. My keen sensitivity, nurtured among beautiful gentle ladies, taught me to find delight even in the smaller and more subtle beauties of a woman's dress, and those few charming childhood loves I had known made every part and every gesture of the female body sacrosanct. [...] During one of our longer visits to Budapest I decided that I would overcome my natural modesty and shyness and would visit one of the street-girls. [...] The entire scene was completely devoid of all impression of erotic beauty as I had until then imagined it. It was rather comical and very repulsive.
>
> *(Ibid.: 68–69)*

The subtlety of feminine beauty conflicts with the repulsion at the sight of a "street-girl" as she is only considered through her belonging to a low social class. The spasms of her body are devoid of any "sacrosanctity," whereas the physical encounter makes the protagonist feel defiled rather than allowing him to enjoy the "subtle beauties" of her countenance and dress. However, Elemér recalls that when he was finally able to control his reluctance:

> I smelt the cheap scent in her hair, it seemed a very familiar odour, and at this moment all of a sudden I unexpectedly saw everything in a different light. Suddenly I felt overwhelmed by a mad, savage desire, I forgot the surroundings, and thought no longer of beauty or ugliness, in fact *I saw and felt nothing but naked flesh, female flesh, beside me, under me. All at once I seemed to turn into someone else, and I was nothing but a copulating beast interested only in his lust* [italics mine].
>
> *(Ibid.: 69)*

Sexual desire combined with repulsion and contempt towards the woman (who is reduced to a "female flesh") becomes appealing to Elemér when the smelling of a "cheap scent" reminds him about his nocturnal life. Only then does wild lust rise within him (Ibid.: 69). The omnipresent pressure of repulsion has become the essence of his other, secret existence. The narrator repeatedly stresses his own purity and perfection, thus renouncing what is unclean and yet desired. Anything unpleasant or unseemly incites the narrator to produce an idealized self-image. Subsequently, his self-portrait reflects nothing but a desperate attempt to reverse what he sees as repulsive.

At the same time, abjection is at the very center of the narrator's interest. In one of the novel's final scenes, repulsion and violence merge with sexual desire. One night, Elemér's "other self" goes to a bar, where he meets a young woman. When he finally finds himself alone with her, the scene culminates in murder. This is how he describes the experience:

> I slid my hand along her back, slowly up, up to her neck. Then suddenly I pressed with the palm of my other hand too and then I clutched and squeezed her neck as hard as I could. […] Her eyes bulged toward as if they wanted to leave their sockets […]. Gradually a faint redness flushed her face. Her lips opened. I stood up and standing still I squeezed, I squeezed, I choked, I strangled silently. I felt a vast, slow, dull ecstasy as my five happy fingers lay on the girl's smooth neck, tightly, tightly as if wanting to penetrate her as a lover his mate. I felt that there was no limit to my power […]. I could squeeze the neck of a beautiful girl as I pleased, for ever, to the end, eternally. […] *Oh, what ecstasy it was: an eternity was tightly, tightly packed into those moments* [italics mine].
>
> *(Ibid.: 129–130)*

Only during the murderous act can the narrator achieve fulfillment, which constitutes both sexual and existential satisfaction.

The narrator perceives sexuality as destructive – a phenomenon which must ultimately lead to the obliteration of someone's life. A strikingly similar concept was laid out by the psychoanalyst and anarchist Otto Gross (1877–1920) in his text "On the Symbolism of Destruction" ("Über Destruktionssymbolik") published in *Zentralblatt für Psychoanalyse* in 1914 (525–534). This short article by one of Freud's most controversial collaborators was largely inspired by Sabina Spielrein's (1885–1942) extensive 1911 essay entitled "Destruction as Cause of Coming-into-being" ("Die Destruktion als Ursache des Werdens") (1912: 465–503). Gross set out to answer the question whether sexual relations must always be rooted in the symbolism of rape and follow the dynamics of destruction. Referring to Freud's theory of sexuality, he noted:

> Freud's teaching on "infantile sexual theories" states that sexual intercourse is habitually reflected in children's imagination as some form of rape on the woman by the man; as the image of a sadistic act of any kind [...]. The determinist approach does not allow us to believe in psychological actions that would be causeless, meaningless, or even really insufficiently justified [...] The problem remains why the infantile misjudgment of the nature of the sexual and reproductive event occurs, why it regularly assumes the symbolism of rape and disease, and why the symbolisms of "destruction," in Sabina Spielrein's sense, must regularly develop here.
>
> *(Gross 1914: 525–526)*

The problem discussed by Gross directly relates to the question of the permanent placement of the aggressive drive in the sphere of human sexuality (Heuer 2017). Although children do not understand what a sexual act is, fear appears in their conscious, and with it – as a premonition – an image of rape. In this case, the body becomes the main space subjected to affectation. Depending on the gender, Gross writes, the body recognizes itself as raping or being raped. Apart from the symbolism of rape, a fear of disease also appears: the body is threatened by violence on the one hand and disease on the other. At the psychological level of imagination, illness can connote both a weakness of the body and its defilement. Then, the diseased becomes what is dirtiest and most repulsive.

When Elemér falls asleep and awakens in his other life, everything around him seems loathsome. The constant presence of insects (flies, bedbugs) is a clear sign of the protagonist's repugnance not only at the external world (the workshop, the landlord, the master, and his wife), but also his grubby body and soul. While Elemér's hidden world is depicted as unequivocally bad, his apparent real life is the essence of purity and nobility. The tension between them constitutes an irreconcilable conflict between desire (which is by definition *amoral*) and shame, which inhibits the realization of the wish (which is by definition *immoral*). In this context, Gross adds:

> Psychoanalytic literature has familiarized us with the importance of the moral motive as a component of inner conflicts. But the basic ethical tendency we are talking about here has nothing to do with moral judgments [...] Rather, it is a congenital, primal instinct, specific to humans, which is aimed at preserving one's own individuality and the loving-ethical relationship to the individuality of others, and which can be expressed in concrete terms as the striving not to let oneself be raped and not to rape others.
>
> *(Gross 1914: 528–529)*

In his argument, Gross set the "primal instinct" (der Urinstinkt) against a "loving-ethical" (liebend-ethische) instinct – which could also be described as a conflict between the self and the unconscious. The psychoanalyst continues, writing that the "basic ethical tendency" (die ethische Grundtendenz) radically contradicts "the destruction symbolism of sexuality" (die Destruktionssymbolik der Sexualität) (Ibid.: 529). In this light, Elemér's diurnal world could be considered as a reality of "basic ethical tendency," while the nocturnal world is a space of the unbridled operation of destructive forces. In his dreams, the narrator faces "an irresistible urge (German: Trieb) to rape" (in Gross's words: "Vergewaltigen und Vergewaltigtwerden") (Ibid.: 529); outwardly, he is content with the quasi-platonic contemplation of feminine beauty. He reacts with shame to any erotic wishes – as illustrated by his behavior towards his mother:

> The door opened and my mother looked in, and I, sitting on my bed putting on my clean shirt, suddenly realized that I had started like a frightened deer. My mother was such a young, beautiful and elegant women that I was ashamed to dress in front of her. And yet I was not ashamed in front of the maid-servant. But when I saw that fine, noble face, which mine is supposed to resemble so closely, that impressive figure in the expensive gown, I slipped back under the quilt like a snail into its shell.
>
> *(Babits 1966: 12)*

The narrator looks at his mother as an especially graceful woman whose beauty makes him feel self-conscious to the point that he hides under the covers. Later in Elemér's life, another ideal (a mother-imago) appears: a girl named Etelka. The narrator recalls: "I was overcome by a kind of happy embarrassment" (Ibid.: 72–73). Like many years earlier in his mother's presence, in front of Etelka Elemér remains "clumsy and taciturn" (Ibid.: 73). Meanwhile, his behavior in dreams is completely different. As he writes, "the pure and noble Elemér Tábory had dreams pregnant with the coarsest, most disgusting desires and the most perverse thoughts" (Ibid.: 90). When these obsessions take control, all women appear vulgar, obtrusive, stupid, and naïve. Despite his repulsion, he sporadically reflects on the advantages of marriage which he thinks may allow him to free himself from his "animalistic" passions.

The narrator's despair results from his suspension between sexuality (as a destructive desire) and the ethical instinct (a formative desire). In this context, it is worth rethinking Gross's remarks. In his 1914 article, he adds that the ethical instinct – as a sort of forcible socialization to the life in a given society – requires one to relinquish limitless freedom and accept socio-ethical norms. Gross writes: "The fear of loneliness, and an urge to attach [to others] forces the child to adapt: the suggestion of alien will, which is called education, is absorbed into one's own desire" (Gross 1914: 530–531). Following Gross's suggestions, Elemér could be classified among the type of people who are unable to renounce their "peculiarity." The more perfect he seems to himself in the one life, the more corrupt he is in the other. Despite a growing fear of rejection, he cannot contain his desire to break away from the social order. At a moment of his greatest weakness, he submits to his destruction drive and calls out:

> I was an anarchist, and considered myself a sort of profligate and misunderstood genius, I would have liked to be a murderer, an incendiary, and it was not any innate goodness or will-power that kept me from it – only cowardice, infinite cowardice. […] My desires, my insatiable and cowardly desires, governed me, hatred, pride and coarse sensuality, children of boredom and stupid day-dreaming nurtured by the basest penny thrillers, sensational films and pornographic magazines.
>
> *(Babits 1966: 89)*

Elemér immerses himself in lowbrow literature, spins his fantasies, and at the same time avoids closer encounters with people. One obstacle in his relationships with women is his own body, which he perceives as odious ("indeed in *this* life I was ugly") (Ibid.: 89). When waking up to his other, night life, the narrator blames himself for "disgusting and the most perverse" desires. With time, they intensify to the extent that he cannot liberate himself from them at all.

3.5 Elemér's loss of reality: a psychoanalytic reading

At one point in his account, Elemér realizes that a strange similarity can be observed between his two incarnations: "All this, all this tallied horribly. The shortest moments of my two lives overlapped with ghastly accuracy. Like two sheets of paper, whose figures exactly correspond, there wasn't an hour, there wasn't a minute which did not fit" (Ibid.: 90). In his nocturnal life, both his mother and Etelka appear, having undergone a reversal and become their own opposites. Although the narrator cannot remember his mother's face, he recalls having seen her: "in underpants, in a shift, and even completely naked, and as if it had been cruel torture to think of this" (Ibid.: 40). Digging through his childhood memories, he concludes that his mother never loved him, just abused him and repeated: "Why didn't I get rid of you?" (Ibid.: 40).

In Elemér's diurnal life, his father is an elegant and respected citizen; at night, he is absent ("I… in my dream… did not have a father") (Ibid.: 41). The protagonist considers abandonment by his father as a reason for the greatest shame (Ibid.: 39). Meanwhile, the girl from the bar whom the narrator brutally murders resembles the innocent and delicate Etelka (Ibid.: 135). The narrator's account illustrates Gross's statement that "In all men, whether consciously or unconsciously […], an inner feeling persists that their sexual relations with the woman are rape" (Gross 1914: 534). Elemér's narrative can be read as a record of the painful process of realizing the feeling ("Gefühl") referred to by Gross.

At the beginning of his autobiography, Elemér devotes much space to a mysterious man called Kincses. He begins with a detailed description of his clothing, and eventually moves on to Kincses's "animalistic" gaze which clearly captivates him:

> His shirt was negligently open so that his chest showed when he moved. I sensed something savage in his face, the crudeness of a tradesman. There was something in his eyes that roused you. As I watched him, all the rest of the picnic seemed like something seen in a daze, in a pleasant dream, and I could not concentrate on anything else.
>
> *(Babits 1966: 16–17)*

Kincses's image haunts Elemér. When he encounters Kincses by chance, he gets a thrill of fear. Finally, the narrator recognizes the "wild" man's face in the violent master at the workshop. When Elemér falls asleep thinking of Kincses, he is awakened by "a huge left hand" (Ibid.: 25). The proximity of men in the narrator's nocturnal life is tied to violence, but also some "marvelously scary" intimacy (Ibid.: 36–37). The apprentices' nighttime conversations always turn to sexual matters. The narrator hates the other men's smell while simultaneously fantasizing about being tormented by the violent master-Kincses.

Notably, similar paranoid and homoerotic ideation was described around the same time by Sándor Ferenczi who linked it to repressed homosexual desire. In an article entitled "On the Part Played by Homosexuality in the Pathogenesis of Paranoia" ("Über die Rolle der Homosexualität in der Pathogenese der Paranoia"), which preceded *The Caliph Stork* by two years and was published in *Jahrbuch für psychoanalytische und psychopathologische Forschung*, Ferenczi followed Freud's intuitions on the close connection between homosexual desire and paranoid fantasies (Ferenczi 1911: 101–119). Writing about Daniel Paul Schreber, Freud stressed that delusions of grandeur and persecutory beliefs can be observed in psychotic patients. Ferenczi captured the problem of "losing touch with reality" by psychosis-sufferers similarly. Having distinguished between neurotic and paranoid mechanisms, Ferenczi wrote:

> The neurotic gets rid of the affects that have become disagreeable to him by means of the different forms of displacement (conversion, transference, substitution) […]. The paranoiac also would make an attempt to withdraw his participation (in external interests), but it meets with only a limited success. Some of the desires get happily retracted into the ego – grandiose delusions occur in every case of paranoia – but a greater part of the interest, varying in amount, cannot disengage itself from its original object, or else returns to it. This interest, however, has become so incompatible with the ego that it gets objectified (with a reversal of affect, i. e. with a "negative sign in front") and thus cast out from the ego. The tendency that has become intolerable, and has been withdrawn from its object, in this way returns from its love-object in the form of a perception of its own negative. The feeling of love is turned into the sensation of its opposite.
>
> *(Ferenczi [1911] 1952: 154–155)*

The repressed wish, which Ferenczi describes as "the tendency that has become intolerable," is *projected* outwards by the paranoiac – ejected outside of the self – and starts appearing as an objectively existing part of reality. This way, the psychotic patient creates their own world where the desired (an object of love) materializes as its own opposite (an object of hatred). Similar conclusions can be found in Freud's writings. In his 1924 text titled "The Loss of Reality in Neurosis and Psychosis," the author posited that both psychosis and neurosis are ways of expressing the revolt of the unconscious against the external world (Freud [1924] 1961a: 183–184). Both mechanisms identified by psychoanalysts were believed to result from an affective retreat from reality in which the subject's *impossible* wish is inhibited by the "ethical instinct." However, as Freud underscores, in psychosis reality is "remodeled" and substituted (Ibid.: 185). He adds: "the psychosis is also faced with the task of procuring for itself perceptions of a kind which shall correspond to the new reality; and this is most radically effected by means of hallucination" (Ibid.: 186). Because the imposing reality (including in the form of restrictive moral laws) is still unbearable, it appears as its own opposite at the affective level. Therefore, as Ferenczi wrote, the *feeling* of love may transform into the *experience* of its opposite.

This mechanism – extensively described by Ferenczi – can be discerned in *The Caliph Stork*. It follows from the protagonist's narrative that the hidden content of his life is a sort of a dream-fantasy which reflects a repressed wish. The narrator himself leads his readers to this conclusion when he writes about awakening to his other life and about dreams which seem more real than life. Nevertheless, he sometimes becomes lost in his own story, unable to determine whether he is experiencing a nightmare or a psychotic fantasy. He explains:

> The whole world was a picture for me, a beautiful picture, and I often thought that perhaps it was only a dream; and, indeed, my childhood

> with its easy, even flow and unclouded happiness was like a dream. Whether I wanted to or not, I was always a little afraid of awakening.
>
> *(Babits 1966: 20)*

Reality appears to him as its own representation which has lost its materiality. Elemér is afraid to sleep; with time, he can no longer tell which of his two lives is the real one. Not only does he experience his life as split, but he also feels a constant fear of persecution. In his 1911 article, Ferenczi recounted a similar case of a man tormented by his immediate environment:

> Previous experiences with paranoiacs made it easy for me to infer from these facts alone the extraordinarily important part played by homosexuality in this case. The appearance of the delusion of persecution, perhaps long hidden, was evoked by the sight of a half-naked officer, whose shirt, drawers, and gloves also seem to have made a great impression on the patient. (Let me recall the part played by the bed-clothes in the two cases mentioned above.) No female person was ever accused or complained of, he constantly fought and wrangled only with men, for the most part officers or high dignitaries, superiors. I interpret this as projection of his own homosexual delight in those persons, the affect being preceded by a negative sign. *His desires, which have been cast out from the ego, return to his consciousness as the perception of the persecutory tendency* […] [italics mine].
>
> *(Ferenczi [1911] 1952: 175)*

The patient creates an alternative word in which persecution conceals his homosexual desire. Here, the wish to be intimate with men is replaced with the feeling of hatred. Elemér undergoes a similar process. Kincses-master and other apprentices both fascinate and frighten him ("Softly I stretched my body, rubbing it against the sweat-moistened bedding […]. There was a pleasant mist in my head […] it was good to lie here in the dark in the quiet warmth") (Ibid.: 47). With each passing day, the narrator feels increasingly overwhelmed: by the violent master, apprentices, and the caretaker in his nocturnal life, and by his "other self" in his diurnal life. According to this argument, his fantasies (of a homoerotic and depraved nature) allow him to partially fulfill his repressed desires which are recognized in a distorted form. In fact, the narrator's hidden life – as a wish transformed into "objectified" reality – is not far from the paranoid mechanism described by Freud and Ferenczi.

Elemér experiences encounters with his other self in dreams as a collision with something that is the most foreign yet familiar. The simultaneous experience of strangeness and identity was described by Freud in his seminal 1919 essay "The 'Uncanny.'" With the German term *das Unheimliche* and its etymology as his point of departure, Freud contemplated its perplexing meaning with connotations of both "the foreign" and "the familiar." He wrote: "the uncanny is that class of the frightening which leads back to what is known of old and long familiar" (Freud [1919] 1955c: 220), and continued: "everything is *unheimlich* that ought to have remained secret and hidden but has come to light" (Ibid.: 225). Moreover, the uncanny is something that, though seemingly "foreign," "eerie," "daemonic," "bloodcurdling," is always present, waiting in hiding to rise to the surface, to become conscious. In Babits's *The Caliph Stork*, this is the dynamic that governs the experience of encountering oneself as the *other* which is concurrently strikingly similar to oneself. The uncanny converges with the unconscious.

Whereas the narrator's explicit story involves a split personality and may be treated as a literary depiction of dissociative personality disorder, the implicit layer is an insightful depiction into the workings of the unconscious. In the experience of hair-raising familiarity and intimacy with a caricature of oneself (the "other embodiment"), with which Elemér increasingly identifies, Babits demonstrated the paradoxes of the very structure of human psyche, where what has been once and for all pushed away into the void returns anyway, albeit in a distorted form. Inhibited sexuality and its close link to the symbolism of destruction mark the main axis of the repressed content in *The Caliph Stork*.

3.6 "Nightmares are real"

In the 1930s, psychoanalysts were reflecting on dreams and their relationship to trauma. With the publication of *The Discovery of the Self* by Elizabeth Severn, Ferenczi's patient and an analyst herself, the problem of nightmares became linked to split personality and traumatic experiences. Severn's reflection sheds new light on Babits's novel and may facilitate a better understanding of the protagonist's dreaming as a way of processing the trauma of modernity. In the opening paragraph of the fifth chapter of her book, titled "Nightmares Are Real," Severn wrote:

> I sought for many years for the meaning of dreams, gaining much, though not enough, *from certain Oriental sources*, and even more, though still not enough, from psychoanalysis. [...] I wrote in 1913 [...] that the dream-life was *continuous* and as essential a part of our existence as anything in the waking time; that it was, in fact, but a reverse side of the shield and not different, except in form and configuration, from our known conscious life [italics mine].
>
> *(Severn [1933] 2017: 86)*

Reflection on dreams had led Severn to further considerations of the boundaries between daydreaming and hallucination; psychosis and neurosis. As she emphasized with regard to psychotics: "The dream-life in these people tends to come to the surface and spreads itself over the larger part of the consciousness, so that they see not actual things but mostly their dream-pictures" (Ibid.: 87). Treating the concepts of dreams and hallucinations interchangeably, Severn asserted that dreams were the source of knowledge about the mechanism of psychoses and neuroses. Severn defined the dream as: "the theater wherein [...] facts are dramatically re-enacted" (Ibid.: 88). On the nightmare, she wrote:

> the whole dream-life can be said to be a collection of disturbing or disastrous incidents that one is trying, by fantastic means, to ameliorate and render harmless. [...] But there are dreams entirely lacking even in the "thin veneer" or any form of compensation. The imagination fails utterly to act as a "shock absorber" and what remains is *pure shock*, unadulterated by any fantasies of relief, escape, or amelioration. These dreams are always of painful content and intensity, and constitute what is called *nightmare*.
>
> *(Ibid.: 89)*

In this perspective, the dream symptomatized difficult past experiences that the dreamer was trying to process. As Severn added, nightmares: "are the records of personal catastrophes, the consequence of which was disruption of the whole mental machinery" (Ibid.: 90). The nightmare turned out to be a real trace of the imaginative production of the psyche, "haunted by its tragedy and forever seeking to repair and restore its damaged unity and soundness" (Ibid.: 90). Crucially, the nightmare is a testimony of a person's life. In this light, Elemér's dreams can be viewed not as fantasmatic productions, but as dramatizations of actual traumatic experiences from his past. In other words, Elemér processes past traumatic events in his dreams.

If we look at Elemér's "other" life in the light of Severn's reflections, the protagonist's nightmare proves to be the result of the trauma he experienced. For him, the dream of the poor, socially excluded boy becomes a theater in which past experiences are now replayed. The story of the protagonist's nocturnal life is a product of the unconscious – but, unlike in Freud's understanding, it constitutes a "dramatized tragedy" produced by the unconscious in response to disastrous past experience(s) (Ibid.: 90). Severn stressed the importance of trauma as the source of the nightmare:

> The importance of *trauma* as a specific and almost universal cause of neurosis was first impressed upon me by Ferenczi, who, probing deeply, had found it present in nearly all his cases. He thus resurrected and gave new value to an idea that had once, much earlier, been entertained by Freud, but that was discarded by him in favor of "fantasy" as the explanation of the strange tales or manifestations given by his patients. [...] Experience has convinced me, however, that the patient does not "invent" but *always tells the truth*, even though in a distorted form; and, further, that what he tells is mostly of a severe and specific injury, inflicted on him when he was young and helpless.
>
> *(Ibid.: 91)*

Based on her own research and experience, and Ferenczi's late text "Confusion of Tongues" (1933), Severn argued that psychotic fantasies and neurotic hallucinations must be regarded as the result of previously experienced cruel abuse (Ibid.: 91–92).

As we saw earlier, cruelty was central to Elemér's story. It was represented by the key themes of Babits's novel: the violence and the destructive dimension of human sexuality on the one hand, and the rapid modernization processes in Hungary on the other hand. The rapidly changing city was not perceived positively, but as a major source of shock and trauma. What the protagonist was actually working through – and what appeared in his nightmares – can be described as the trauma of modernity: the effect of an uncontrollable and incoherent technological progress and bureaucratic acceleration. The split personality described by Babits symbolizes the shattering of the coherence and integrity of the psyche as a result of the clash with the modernist machine, which causes an unbearable cacophony of the old and the new within the emotional life of the individual.

3.7 Conclusion

For its author, *The Caliph Stork* was an opportunity to enter into a dialogue with contemporary knowledge on the psychology of dreams, the unconscious, psychosis, and dissociative personality disorder. His selection of the autobiography as the right genre to tell Elemér Tábory's story of disease locates Babits's novel in the realms of both modernist literature and turn-of-the-century psycho-medical discourses. On the one hand, the author refers to psychoanalytic theory. On the other hand, he draws from other contemporary traditions of psychological and psychiatric thought (especially Morton Prince's and Pierre Janet's, as mentioned above) which focused on split personalities more than on the mechanism of repression. This way, Elemér's case becomes a literary variation on themes that were widely discussed in medical and psychoanalytic circles, such as: the wish function of dreams, the seeming realness of hallucinatory formations, the sex drive's close links to the death drive and the symbolism of destruction as well as the (un)conscious as a sphere strictly tied to the dynamics of culturally conditioned morality.

At the same time, in his *The Caliph Stork*, Babits partially applies the model of the *Bildungsroman* only to completely reverse its order. Rather than recounting the protagonist's coming of age, Elemér's (auto)biography tells the story of his regression. By placing the subject's repeated encounters with himself as the *other* at the center of his narrative, Babits created an intimate study of experiencing the uncanny that comes with a conviction about the existence of one's own double. In Elemér's case, his other self is a product and an extension of his unconscious: the poor, uneducated clerk using a stolen identity embodies all of the protagonist's repressed desires. Aggressive impulses, a desire for destruction, and the death drive boil to the surface. In *The*

Caliph Stork, the unconscious becomes the site where a destructive and perverse desire develops, and the wish for sexual ecstasy gains a sadistic and masochistic dimension.

Elemér's socially privileged position (which simultaneously connotes moral innocence) strongly contrasts with the experience of the other self (a crook and impostor from the underclass). By highlighting the violent nature of a society based on hierarchy, exploitation, and repression, Babits showed some kinship not only to Freud but also to Otto Gross, whose work sparked an interest both among psychoanalysts and authors in Central Europe (including Franz Kafka). Babits's emphasis on the relationship between sexuality and destruction also brings to mind Sabina Spielrein's ideas whose seminal text "Destruction as Cause of Coming-into-being" appeared shortly before *The Caliph Stork*. In his *self-psychography*, as I suggest calling it, Babits also brought to light themes related to the processes of modernization (including mass literacy and school enrollment), combining them with a reflection on the human psyche. If Elemér Tábory were to be treated as a model case of the modern subject, his distinguishing feature would be the fact that he lives in an incessant cacophony of a split self which – in its psychotic production – remains jarringly non-hermetic, allowing what is familiar-foreign, clean-dirty, sacred-perverse to enter the conscious. *The Caliph Stork* can be read both as an autobiography of a psychotic patient with diseased dreams and a novel on the psychological condition of the modern subject as reflected in the protagonist's cacophonous plight.

The problem of the double personality (the self as the other) returned in Surrealist art. The fascination with the unconscious, the symbolism of dreams, and the psychoanalytic theory of sexuality proved crucial to the image of the modern man created by the Surrealists in Czechoslovakia. As we will see, the painful experience of modernization gave way to a Surrealist rebellion against oppressive social norms. In the next chapter, I will show that the primary objective of the Czech Surrealists was to invent a new language of thinking about the human body and psyche, about the relationship between the individual and the collective. Using the Czech Surrealist milieu as an example, I would like to address the issue of Surrealist experiments with self-narration and self-analysis, which were closely related to early psychoanalytic writing practices that constituted a crucial component of the modernist turn in Central Europe.

Notes

1 This chapter is a revised and expanded version of an article previously published in Polish in *Wielogłos*, see A. Sobolewska, "Autopsychografia Eleméra Táboryego. Od literackiej interpretacji snów po psychomedyczną diagnoz nowoczesnośći," *in Wielogłos* 2022, no. 4 (54), 17–35.

2 It should be noted though that *Nyugat* was preceded by other important literary and cultural periodicals such as *Jövendő* (Future) 1903, *Magyar Géniusz* (Hungarian Genius) 1902–1903, *Figyelő* (Observer) 1905, *Szerda* (Wednesday) 1906. See: Eszter

Balázs, *Az intellektualitás vezérei. Viták az irodalmi autonómiáról a Nyugatban és a Nyugatról*, 1908–1914 (Budapest: Napvilág Kiadó, 2009); see Mateusz Chmurski, *Figury modernosti. Kategorie modernity v bádání o středoevropské literatuře po roce 1989*, in *Moderna/Moderny*, ed. Tomáš Kubíčrk, Jan Wiendl (Olomouc: Univerzita Palackého, 2013), 314–329.

3 Gál describes Babits's connections with the Galileo Circle, with which Ferenczi also closely collaborated. In 1913 – when he was working on *The Caliph Stork* – according to the daily *Pesti Napló*, Babits gave a lecture for the Galileo Circle entitled *The Metaphysics of Matter*. In it, he mostly referred to Henri Bergson's philosophy. As the example of *The Caliph Stork* shows, he was not only interested in psychoanalytic works of that time but also newly emerged theories of the consciousness, 327–328.

4 The title of the English translation is *The Nightmare*. While it differs significantly from the original (*A gólyakalifa*), in this chapter, I have decided to propose a more literal transcription (*The Caliph Stork*).

5 Babits's first novel enjoyed quick success. Just a year after its publication, a film by the same title premiered, directed by Alexander Korda with the screenplay by Frigyes Karinthy.

6 Prince conducted his examinations of the patient in the period 1898–1904. Cf. Saul Rosenzweig, "Sally Beauchamp's Career: A Psycharcheological Key to Morton Prince's Classic Case of Multiple Personality," *Genetic, Social, and General Psychology Monographs* vol. 113, no. 1 (1969): 15–60.

7 *L'Automatisme Psychologique. Essai de psychologie expérimentale sur les formes inférieures de l'activité humaine* was first published by Pierre Janet in 1889. In 1913, during the XVII International Congress of Medicine in London, Janet presented a paper in which he had criticized Freud and psychoanalysis. See P. Janet, *La psychanalyse de Freud. Suivi d'extraits de L'automatisme psychologique* (Paris: Rivages Poche, 2021); cf. Gabriele Cassullo, "Janet and Freud: Long-time rivals," in *Rediscovering Pierre Janet: Trauma, Dissociation, and a New Context for Psychoanalysis*, ed. Giuseppe Craparo, Francesca Ortu, and Onno van der Hart (New York, London: Routledge 2019).

8 Ferenczi's full article is available online: http://real-j.mtak.hu/11169/12/650.1909.11.07.pdf, accessed May 20, 2021.

9 The first full edition of *The Interpretation of Dreams* (1899/1900) in Hungarian translation was published in 1934.

10 Until 1913, see Milán Füst, "A *Szentivánéji álom* a Nemzetiben" (a review of *A Midsummer Night's Dream*), *Nyugat* 21 (1909); Frigyes Karinthy, "A rossz álom" (The Nightmare) 4 (1913), available online: https://epa.oszk.hu/00000/00022/nyugat.htm, accessed May 21, 2021.

11 The English translation is inaccurate. In the original Hungarian version, the narrator repeatedly says: "Össze akarom állitani életem aktáit." Therefore, a more accurate translation would be "I want to collect the records of my life," see Babits, *A gólyakalifa* (Budapest: Helikon Kiádo, 2018), 5.

12 The cited work is the reedition of Lejeune's article published in the literary review *Romantisme*, 52, 1987, 79–94. This particular text can be read as a polemic with Michel Foucault's understanding of hegemonic role of the modern psychiatric discourse in the emergence of homosexual identity.

13 Another important context for both authors' works was obviously the rise of anti-Semitism in the late 1800s, both in the Czech and Hungarian society. In 1899, the Hilsner Affair erupted when Leopold Hilsner was accused of the ritual murder of a teenage Christian girl. Despite legal support from the later president of Czechoslovakia Tomáš Masaryk, Hilsner was sentenced to life in prison in 1900 and only pardoned after eighteen years. As Sander L. Gilman noted in his book on Kafka, the case was strictly tied to the proliferation of anti-Semitic sentiment in Europe, with the Dreyfus Affair as its symbolic beginning, see S. L. Gilman, *Franz Kafka*

(London: Reaktion Books, 2005), 32. Still, it is worth remembering that incidents of blood libel against the Jewish minority took place all across Central and Eastern Europe in the late 1800s. Before the Hilsner Affair, there was the Tiszaeszlár Affair in Hungary (named after the city) in 1883, when a group of Jewish residents were blamed for ritual murder. Unlike Hilsner, these citizens were acquitted during their trail, see M. Molnár, *A Concise History of Hungary*, 225.

References

Babits, M. (1966). *The Nightmare*. Translated by Eva Rácz. Budapest: Athenaeum Printing House.

Babits, M. (2018). *A gólyakalifa*, Budapest: Helikon Kiádo.

Bálazs, E. (2009). *Az intellektualitás vezérei. Viták az irodalmi autonómiáról a Nyugatban és a Nyugatról: 1908–1914*, Budapest: Napvilág Kiadó.

Brabant-Gerö, E. (1993). *Ferenczi et L'École Hongroise de Psychanalyse*, Paris: L'Harmattan.

Cassullo, G. (2019). Janet and Freud: Long-time rivals, in G. Craparo, F. Ortu, & O. van der Hart (Eds.), *Rediscovering Pierre Janet: Trauma, Dissociation, and a New Context for Psychoanalysis*, New York/London: Routledge.

Chmurski, M. (2013). Figury modernosti. Kategorie modernity v bádání o středoevropské literatuře po roce 1989, in T. Kubíček & J. Wiendl (Eds.), *Moderna/Moderny*, Olomouc: Univerzita Palackého, 314–329.

Ferenczi, S. (1961). *Further contributions to the theory and technique of psycho-analysis*. Translated by Jane Isabel Suttie *et al.* New York: Boni and Liveright Publishers.

Ferenczi, S. (1991). *Lélekgógyászat. Válogatott írások*, Budapest: Kossuth, 1991.

Ferenczi, S. (2011). A forditó elószava, in S. Freud, *Az álomról*, Budapest: Hermin Könyvkiadó, 5–7.

Ferenczi, S. ([1911] 1952). On the Part Played by Homosexuality in the Pathogenesis of Paranoia, in *The International Psycho-Analytical Library* 45, 154–184.

Freud, S. ([1919] 1955c). The Uncanny, in J. Strachey (Ed.), *The Standard Edition of the Complete Psychological Works of Sigmund Freud*. Vol. 17, London: The Hogarth Press, 217–256.

Freud, S. ([1917] 1957b). A Metapsychological Supplement to the Theory of Dreams, in J. Strachey (Ed.), *The Standard Edition of the Complete Psychological Works of Sigmund Freud*. Vol. 14, London: The Hogarth Press, 217–235.

Freud, S. ([1924] 1961a). The Loss of Reality in Neurosis and Psychosis, in J. Strachey (Ed.), *The Standard Edition of the Complete Psychological Works of Sigmund Freud*. Vol. 19, London: The Hogarth Press, 181–188.

Füst, M. (1909). A Szentivánéji álom a Nemzetiben, in *Nyugat* 21.

Gál, I. (2003). *Mihály Babits. Tanulmányok, szövegközlések, széljegyzetek*, Budapest: Argumentum.

Gilman, S. L. (2005). *Franz Kafka*, London: Reaktion Books.

Gross, O. (1914). Über Destruktionssymbolik, in *Zentralblatt für Psychoanalyse* 4, 525–534.

Hauff, W. (1991). *Märchen-Almanach auf das Jahr 1826*, Stuttgart: J. B. Metzlerche Verlagsbuchhandlung.

Heuer, G. M. (2017). *Freud's 'Outstanding' Colleague/Jung's "Twin Brother." The Suppressed Psychoanalytic and Political Significance of Otto Gross*, London/New York: Routledge.

Janet, P. (1886). La personnalité pendant le somnambulisme provoqué, in *Revue Philosophique de la France et de l'Étranger* 22, 577–592.

Janet, P. (2021). *La psychanalyse de Freud. Suivi d'extraits de L'automatisme psychologique*, Paris: Rivages Poche.

Karinthy, F. (1913). A rossz álom, in *Nyugat* 4.

Kristeva, J. (1992). *Black Sun. Depression and Melancholia.* Translated by Leon S. Roudiez. New York: Columbia University Press.

Lejeune, P. (2017). *Autobiographie et homosexualité en France au XIXe siècle*, Paris: Éditions de la Sorbonne.

Molnár, M. (2014). *A Concise History of Hungary*, Cambridge: Cambridge University Press.

Pick, D. & L. Roper (Eds.) (2004). *Dreams and History. The Interpretation of Dreams from Ancient Greece to Modern Psychoanalysis*, London/New York: Routledge.

Prince, M. (1906). *The Dissociation of a Personality: A Biographical Study In Abnormal Psychology*, New York/London: Longmans, Green, and Co.

Rakoczy, M. (2022). *Władza liter. Polskie procesy modernizacyjne a awangarda*, Kraków: Wydawnictwo Uniwersytetu Jagiellońskiego.

Rank, O. (1924). *Die Don Juan Gestalt*, Vienna: Internazionaler Psychoanalytischer Verlag.

Rank, O. (2009). *The Double: A Psychoanalytic Study.* Translated by Harry Tucker Jr. Chapel Hill: The University of North Carolina Press.

Rosenzweig, S. (1969). Sally Beauchamp's Career: A Psycharcheological Key to Morton Prince's Classic Case of Multiple Personality, in *Genetic, Social, and General Psychology Monographs* 113 (1), 15–60.

Spielrein, S. (1912). Die Destruktion als Ursache des Werdens, in *Jahrbuch für psychoanalytische und psychopathologische Forschung* 4 (1), 465–503.

Severn, E. (2017). *The Discovery of the Self*, New York/London: Routledge.

Spielrein, S. (1994). Destruction as the Cause of Coming into Being, in *Journal of Analytical Psychology* 39, 155–186.

4

THE SPECTERS OF PSYCHOANALYSIS IN INTERWAR PRAGUE

Bohuslav Brouk and Jindřich Štyrský

In this chapter, I will concentrate on selected tropes in Czech Surrealist art that have not been sufficiently explored in discussions on the transmission of psychoanalysis to Czechoslovak culture and academia before 1939 (Bžoch 2013; Šebek 1993: 433–439; 1999: 983–988). The psychoanalytic approach to human sexuality and Freud's dream theory made their particular mark on Jindřich Štyrský's (1899–1942) erotic works and on theories by the "wild psychoanalyst" and Surrealist Bohuslav Brouk (1912–1978). This chapter will demonstrate that the language of psychoanalysis allowed Czech Surrealists to rethink their self-narrative strategies and to experiment with self-analysis in their theoretical and artistic practices. As art historian Marie Langerová aptly observed:

> Bringing dreams, oneiric images and events to light became part of a new way of looking at language […]. The goal of accessing the sense of the unconscious was pursued wholeheartedly by surrealism, which also used to this end some of the methods of psychoanalysis. Thus in parallel with developments in the philosophy of language, linguistics and semiology the human imagination was explored from the standpoint of psychiatry. Artists drew on these new medical discoveries, on the opening up of pathways to the unconscious…
>
> *(Bílek, Vojvodík, & Wiendl 2011: 163)*[1]

To "unlock" the unconscious, Surrealists used various techniques such as automatic drawing and automatic writing based on free associations. Unlike the Prague group of psychoanalysts who directly collaborated with Freud, Brouk and Štyrský treated psychoanalysis as a polyphonic tool for creating (self-)analytical images of the human being, immersed in a constantly

DOI: 10.4324/9781003441892-5

changing reality – the internal (psychological, emotional, affective) and the external (cultural, social, and political).

Here, I will concentrate on the role of Freudian thought in the development of a new type of self-analytic writing, emerging in the 1930s, in which the story of the self is constructed out of the imagined rather than the "real." I will also emphasize the importance of other traditions among Czech intellectuals that had developed in the psychoanalytic movement in the 1920s. This chapter will shed new light on Brouk's unorthodox theories and Štyrský's erotic works which involved psychoanalytic thinking. In their Surrealist writings from the 1930s, both Štyrský and Brouk developed utopian readings of Freudianism understood as a theory of social revolution based on the refusal of (re)production, violence, and war. As I will show, Brouk's comments on Surrealist art should be seen as precursory to Herbert Marcuse's and later José Esteban Muñoz's reflections.

4.1 The heyday of Freudianism in Czechoslovakia

The transmission of psychoanalysis to Czech and Slovak culture dates back to the immediate aftermath of the First World War. The translation of Freud's works had begun by 1926, when Ladislav Kratochvíl and Ota Friedmann prepared the first-ever Czech edition of *The Interpretation of Dreams* with the help of psychoanalyst Emanuel Windholz. At that time, Freudian thought was developing and spreading in medical, academic, and artistic circles (Nikolai Ossipow, Jan Šimsa, Rudolf Souček, Vilém Forster, Alfred Bem) (Davydov 1998: 35–38; Conci 2013: 221–227; Hristeva 2013: 511–525). Representatives of the psycho-medical sciences in Czechoslovakia were also interested in other newly emerging theories in psychology, neurology, and psychiatry (including those by Carl Gustav Jung[2] and Pierre Janet, whose works were being translated by Rudolf Souček at the time). However, with the growing interest in psychoanalysis, virulent criticism of Freudianism was also put forward and advocated by important Czech intellectuals and politicians of the time, including Tomáš Masaryk (1850–1937) (Šebek 1993: 433–434; Bžoch 2013: 35–62).

The formation of the Surrealist Group in Prague (Vojvodík 2011: 27–29)[3] coincided with the establishment of the first Czech psychoanalytic study group under the auspices of the Vienna Psychoanalytic Society.[4] Pre-World War II, psychoanalysis in Czechoslovakia was developed primarily by Freud's close collaborators, who had settled in Prague shortly before the outbreak of the war. Many of them, such as Otto Fenichel, Frances Deri, Annie Reich, and Heinrich Löwenfeld shared openly leftist views and linked psychoanalysis with Marxism.[5] Otto Fenichel, who was to become the central figure of the Czech psychoanalytic group in the 1930s, closely associated with Wilhelm Reich in the 1920s. This way, the so-called "Freudian Left" that had developed earlier in Vienna and Berlin reached Prague.

In 1935, in a lecture given in Prague entitled "On the Psychoanalytic Method," Fenichel stressed: "Anyone who has not himself looked through the microscope may, for instance, criticize logical contradictions in the utterances of a user of the instrument, but not the facts which the latter asserts he has seen" (Fenichel 1953: 567–568). In Fenichel's view, psychoanalysis was a ground-breaking method of understanding oneself and the other. For him, it was at once a theory of self-revelation and self-liberation. In Prague, Fenichel also wrote about society's destructive influence on the individual psyche. He argued:

> The strong suicidal tendency of depressions on the one hand reflects the powerfulness of the destructive impulses directed against the (introjected) object, and, on the other, is an attempt by the ego to attain a discharge which is unattainable and to placate a superego which is implacable. "Moral masochism" and similar phenomena also only show us once again alterations of instinct through experiential vicissitudes and regressions.
>
> *(Ibid.: 683)*

For Fenichel, the suppression of sexuality was synonymous with the "moral masochism" that he believed characterized the privileged social strata. He stressed that masochism had become a tool for the bourgeoisie to suppress sexual potency – which, as a result of repulsion, was transformed into resentment against excluded social groups (such as the proletariat). This problem was also recognized by Bohuslav Brouk.

It is worth noting that Brouk had no formal psychoanalytic training; he was – in Freud's words – a "wild psychoanalyst." Because Brouk belonged to a wealthy family, he was able to finance the publication of his own texts and those by other Surrealists, including the Surrealist manifesto sent in 1934 to the Czechoslovak Communist Party (Kommunistická Strana Československa, 1921–1992).[6] In the 1930s, Brouk worked closely with Jindřich Štyrský, whose photomontages were later used in some of Brouk's psychoanalytic books.[7] In his writings, Brouk was particularly interested in employing psychoanalysis for social critique and the utopian projects of a new world, liberated from oppressive norms that suppress varied expressions of human sexuality. In his intuitions, Brouk was close to both Wilhelm Reich and Otto Gross.[8]

In the early 1930s, Brouk began publishing numerous studies in which he introduced readers to psychoanalytic theory. Among his most important publications were: *Psychoanalysis* (*Psychoanalysa*) (1932), *Psychoanalytical sexology* (*Psychoanalytická sexuologie*) (1933), *Autoeroticism and Psychoeroticism* (*Autosexualismus a psychoerotismus*) (1935), and *Balance of Psychoanalysis* (*Bilance psychoanalysy*) (1936).[9] Written on the occasion of Freud's eightieth birthday, *Bilance psychoanalysy* illustrated how the process of psychoanalysis's transmission in Czechoslovakia was perceived by Czech Surrealists (Klingenberg 2021: 120–140). In his essay, Brouk argued: "The fate of psychoanalysis in our country is sealed, it is becoming a Moravian specialty" (Brouk 1936: 9). Only as the work of "a great Moravian" could psychoanalysis be accepted and seen as "the fruit of the Moravian spirit" (Ibid.: 6). To Freud's critics, Brouk responded ironically:

> Finally, the discovery of the Moravian spirit in psychoanalysis will not be such a difficult task as it might seem because psychoanalysis [...] does not in any way sin against the Aryan, unspoiled spirit of the Moravian people. In no case is it necessary to see these teachings as a Jewish force, destructive and demoralizing, as we have been told so far.
>
> *(Ibid.: 7)*

Brouk was referring directly to the criticism of psychoanalysis as a Jewish science (Dobroczyński 2021: 27–32). As a "dangerous" method, psychoanalysis could also shatter the oppressive social structures. That is why Brouk so strongly emphasized the revolutionary character of Freudianism. In *Bilance psychoanalysy*, he also pointed to some weaknesses of the psychoanalytic movement that he was seeing:

> The improper popularization and promotion of psychoanalysis resulted in a situation where Freud, instead of having several original collaborators, found a group of dull but dependable [...] people who left the development of psychoanalysis [...] on the shoulders of their teacher.
>
> *(Brouk 1936: 10–11)*

The fact that Brouk accused Freud's closest collaborators of mediocrity is significant in the context of Brouk's own professional biography. His criticisms of the psychoanalytic movement show that he deliberately stayed out of the official (formalized) psychoanalytic circles. Rather than following in Freud's footsteps, Brouk was interested in the theoretical juxtaposition of psychoanalysis with the unrestrained plasticity of the Surrealist imagination.

4.2 Psychoanalysis between revolution and utopia

In the early 1930s, in his commentary to Štyrský's erotic literature published in the Surrealist Edition 69 (Edici 69) series, Brouk stated:

> Our humanity, culture, and civilization are nothing more than an effective way to utilize neurotic conflicts. [...] The sublimation of the neurotic libido is creative, while the normal libido leads only to playfulness. Both libidos, therefore, participate in the creative process motivated by obscenity. The neurotic libido determines the work's content, while the form of its method is conditioned by the normal libido.
>
> *(Brouk 2020: 123)*

Brouk linked the creative process to two kinds of libido: the neurotic, which influences the content of the artwork, and the normal, which determines its form. Sexuality – which manifests itself in the uncontrollable genital desire – is considered the source of any artistic production. In this context, Brouk added: "If the normal libido looks to instant gratification for a surrogate, it will use obscenity to create kitsch, but if its needs are sublimated, then the result is a work of art" (Ibid.: 123). Therefore, while pornography can be reduced to an obscene representation of sexuality, it can also be creatively transformed. Brouk used precisely this argument to defend his Surrealist friends (Jindřich Štyrský, Toyen, Vítězslav Nezval, and František Halas), who were facing charges of obscenity due to pornographic photographs used in their works.[10]

In his commentary on Štyrský's *Emilie Comes to Me in a Dream* (*Emilie přichází ke mně ve snu*), Brouk referred to his friends as "pornophiles" and argued: "In pornophilic works of art the sex is liberated from its actual biological function and envisaged purely in terms of pleasure devoid of its reproductive consequences" (Ibid.: 120). By exposing "animalism" and focusing on the biological dimension of the sexual act, pornographers did not deprive sexuality of its psychological and affective dimension. On the contrary, they sought to liberate it. In their hands, sexuality was "devoid of its reproductive consequences" and only served pleasure. In his analysis, Brouk treated the visual representation of sexuality as a kind of sublimation that replaced sexual gratification with the scopic pleasure, derived from viewing pornographic materials:

> By divorcing sex from its biological aspects and excreta from its content, pornophilic art does not conceal the sadistic nature of its stark obscenity, it merely curtails how its bellicosity is projected. Pornophilically motivated art, therefore, battles the haughty through sex's pleasure principle instead through its biological purpose...
>
> *(Ibid.: 121)*

According to Brouk, pornophilic art liberated (pure) sexual pleasure from reproduction, and, as a consequence, could be used as a tool of collective revolt against false morality. The idea of reclaiming Eros and returning it to the economically and symbolically underprivileged strata constituted the main axis of Brouk's essay. Subsequently, he juxtaposed the impotence of the bourgeoisie and the insincere "guardians of morality" with the joyful, free carnality of the excluded. For Brouk, sexuality was a fundamental category that revealed how the social reality relied on exclusion and structural inequalities.

4.3 Reclaiming Eros

The desire to break the link between productivity-destruction and freedom-repression later returned in Herbert Marcuse's *Eros and Civilization* (1955).

Like Freud in *The Future of an Illusion* (1927) and *Civilization and Its Discontents* (1929), in his seminal book Marcuse discussed the ambivalence of technological and scientific progress. As he noted:

> The continual increase of productivity makes constantly more realistic the promise of an even better life for all. However, intensified progress seems to be bound up with intensified unfreedom. Throughout the world of industrial civilization, the domination of man by man is growing in scope and efficiency. […] And the most effective subjugation and destruction of man by man takes place at the height of civilization, when the material and intellectual attainments of mankind seem to allow the creation of a truly free world.
>
> *(Marcuse 1966: 5)*

Instead of leading to greater freedom, violent technological progress had brought about "the most effective subjugation and destruction of man by man" (Ibid.: 5). This destructive process, typical of Western societies, was described by Marcuse in the following way: "Neither the mechanization and standardization of life, nor the mental impoverishment, nor the growing destructiveness of present-day progress provides sufficient ground for questioning the 'principle' which has governed the progress of Western civilization" (Ibid.: 4). Marcuse understood the rise of authoritarian policies and nationalism as strategies for governing the human libido: the ways of channeling sexual urges so that they would reinforce the politics of exploitation. In *Eros and Civilization* and *One-Dimensional Man: Studies in the Ideology of Advanced Industrial Society* (1964), he attempted to conceptualize a new, liberated society (Ibid.: 8). For him, a "non-repressive civilization" meant the rejection of productivity and the collective rebellion against capitalism. As Marcuse argued, such a revolution could likely erupt among the underprivileged strata or in societies less developed than those of the West:

> The historical chance of the backward countries is in the absence of conditions which make for repressive exploitative technology and industrialization for aggressive productivity. The very fact that the affluent warfare state unleashes its annihilating power on the backward countries illuminates the magnitude of the threat. In the revolt of the backward peoples, the rich societies meet, in an elemental and brutal form, not only a social revolt in the traditional sense, but also an instinctual revolt – biological hatred.
>
> *(Marcuse 2002: 101–102)*

According to Marcuse, a greater degree of freedom could be found in less modernized societies where desire could still escape the mechanisms of production-exploitation. Therefore, the revolutionary reorganization of society would consist in the reclamation of Eros (understood as life itself) by all of the underprivileged. Clearly, Marcuse was thinking along the same lines as Brouk.

The main idea of the Czechoslovak Edition 69 series was to consider art and literature as instruments of social revolution. Similarly, it was the reclamation of Eros from under the yoke of production (capitalism) and destruction (war) that would later become a key point of José Esteban Muñoz's reflection centered around the question of homoerotic desire and queer utopia. Writing about the "grand refusal" and queer aesthetics, Muñoz explicitly drew on Marcuse's and Ernst Bloch's thought. As he explained:

> Both these writers were invested in the power of the aesthetic dimension and, specifically, the utopian force of aesthetics. Utopia, in the way in which Bloch and Marcuse employ the term, is decidedly different from the dismissive invocation of naive utopianism that we encounter nowadays. Utopia in the German idealist usage is a critique of a present order, and of the overarching dictate of how things are and will always be in an unyielding status quo.
>
> *(Muñoz 2019: 132–133)*

Muñoz saw queer aesthetics as a path to the "great refusal" – the refusal of destruction, exploitation, and reproduction understood both literally (as biological reproduction) and symbolically (as the reproduction of the social system and structure). From Brouk and Štyrský to Marcuse and Muñoz, art has been conceived of as a tool for reclaiming Eros and liberating it from the destructive power of civilization. As Brouk wrote: "The body is the last argument of those who have been unjustly marginalized and ignored" (Brouk 2020: 117). The universal dimension of sexual desire makes the body a space of free expression and the eradication of any artificial social divisions. In this vein, Brouk added:

> Pornophilia thus collapses the illusions the high and mighty harbor of their divine nature while exposing their physical decrepitude, the inferiority that they have brought upon themselves through their contempt for the body. [...] With the body, pornophiles not only abolish social barriers between people, through the vigor the non-incapacitated body they also elevate themselves above those who in return scorn them from other angles. *From this perspective, pornophilia could, above all, serve as a potent weapon for the socially powerless, the materially and culturally oppressed, who might, in this context at least, assert their strength and significance through the potency of their non-degenerate body* [italics mine].
>
> *(Ibid.: 117–118)*

On the one hand, pornographic art forces those who repress sexuality to confront the potency of their bodies. The visual representation of the sexual act is a mirror in which its viewer is reflected. On the other hand, it becomes a space for the recovery of the body-as-the-center-of-pleasure by the excluded, who is perceived as rotten and "degenerate."

An important role in enlarging the perception of the body-as-the-center-of-pleasure was played by the changing image of human sexuality in the interwar period. Beginning in the 1930s, Brouk would regularly introduce his readers to the most important theories of proto-sexology, including psychoanalysis. His publications from that period allow us to not only trace psychoanalytic knowledge transmission to the Czech Surrealist milieu, but also see how sexological knowledge was used to liberate Eros by talking about various forms of human desire and sexual expression in a free manner. According to Brouk, psychoanalysts and Surrealists brought to the surface what had previously been repressed and forbidden. By placing the body-expecting-pleasure and the body-experiencing-pleasure at the center of their theories and art, these creators ripped the labels of pathology and reproduction off sexuality. For Surrealists, bodily pleasure became the most important symbol of human liberation from the power of capitalism, which was based on the reproductive dynamics of enslavement and exploitation. Brouk wrote explicitly about this:

> the artist whose work is not bound to reality sees no need to have naked girls urinate into a chamber pot when he could place them in an alpine valley instead. An ejaculation need not became a yellow stain on the bedding – it can be transformed into a bolt of lightning to cleave a Gothic cathedral. The bed of lovers can be replaced by the cosmos and the globe inserted under a woman's buttocks. And from her pudenda a sun then emerges, the most marvelous of miscarriages.
>
> *(Ibid.: 124)*

The artist's imagination, when liberated from the principle of rationality, turned sexual organs into signs of transgression and rose above oppressive social norms. The affirmation of the carnality made it possible to see in sexuality a universal source of rebellion against the brutal exploitation of the body (of the worker or the soldier). As Brouk proclaimed: "The artist, on the other hand, spans the entire world. They piss a sea, shit a Himalayas, give birth to cities, masturbate factory chimneys [...]. Nothing is sacred, everything linked via sexual association" (Ibid.: 125). Pornophilia was meant to allow its viewers to see their own bodies in the light of pleasure. This way, it became a unique art of understanding the world through the bodily experience and the body's capacity for experiencing pleasure. Aestheticizing the genitals – elevating them to the rank of work of art – was a gesture of soiling the sacred, an act of the shameless reversal of the normative order in which the body was perceived pejoratively. The first step towards the social revolution, according to Brouk, was to create a visual catalog of human sexuality.

4.4 The monstrous poetics of dreaming

The central idea behind interwar Czech avant-garde art was summarized by Josef Vojvodík as follows: "To immerse oneself in the current of the world, which now has no unifying sense, order or aim, which is sphere of endless possibilities and whose principle is constant self-destruction and self-creation" (Vojvodík 2011: 26). The first and most important sphere in which the mechanism of "self-destruction and self-creation" could be revealed was the space of the dream. For Surrealists, dreams testified to the unlimited power of imagination and symptomatized the plasticity of mind shaped by the unconscious. Jindřich Štyrský presented his dreams in the graphic-visual form: in texts, collages, and photomontages. Dream dynamics also preoccupied Vítězslav Nezval, who published his oneiric sketch *Sexual Nocturne* (*Sexuální nocturno*) in 1931 and in 1935 completed the novel *Valerie and Her Week of Wonders* (*Valerie a týden divů*) (published 1945), which was entirely maintained in the poetics of a dream and ironically alluded to *The 120 Days of Sodom or the School of Libertinage* (1785, published 1904).[11]

Štyrský's *Emilie Comes to Me in a Dream* (1933) can be read as an extended recording of one dream. The structure of the work is built on a series of freely flowing dream images. As a result, their sequence is not logical.[12] The figure of Emilie occupies a central position. The narrator sees female bodies multiplied, including particularly their eyes "contorted in convulsions of orgasm" (Štyrský 2020: 82). Multiplication is the central motif in *Emilie...* The short text, only a few pages long, is accompanied by twelve photomontages that loosely allude to the presented content of the dream. The narrator tells the story of his former lover, Emilie, who appears to him not so much as a flesh-and-blood person, but as a hazy and indistinct memory. Not only is Emilie gone, but the feelings that once bound them lose their previous intensity. The narrator's imagination transforms his beloved into a sculpture. At the same time, he exaggerates some of her features: the upper lip evokes royalty (superiority), while the lower lip is compared by the narrator to "the foliage of a brothel" (inferiority) (Ibid.: 82). In his imagination, Emilie's body no longer appears in its entirety, but only in fragments.

In Štyrský's twelve photomontages, several key themes suggest interpretative tropes connected with the psychoanalytic understanding of sexuality. Štyrský points to man's inherently sexual and animalistic nature (I, III, V, VII, XI); he elevates the genitals, making them objects of special interest in art (II, XI); he reveals the ambivalent dynamics of desire suspended between Eros and Thanatos (IV, IX, XII); exposes the sexual difference (V), only to abolish it later (VII), and emphasize the multidirectionality of human desire and the variety of sexual expression (IV, VI, VII, VIII, XII); affirms autoeroticism (VI, VIII); finally, he ascribes universal value to bodily pleasures – abolishing the boundaries between man and nature, man and the universe (VIII, X) as well as liberating man from space-time limitations. These photomontages can be connected with elements of the psychoanalytic theory: the genital orientation of sexual desire (I, II), castration anxiety (II), the primal scene, and sexual difference; the conjunction of sexual pleasure with destruction and death.[13]

The body-expecting-pleasure and the body-experiencing-pleasure remain the main actors in Štyrský's photomontages. The artist multiplies bodies and subjects them to fragmentation. He plays with the tension between exposing and covering the genitals (with a nightgown or a fan), at times prudishly veiled, at other times shamelessly exposed (IX). Advocating for pornophiles, Bohuslav Brouk stressed:

> Pornophiles use sadistic methods to attack the supercilious psyches of the ruling peacocks. Finding their dreams frustrated, those who are attacked counter in like manner with a sadistically motivated prudishness, a puritanical persecution of the "depraved." You can verify for yourself the reason for pornophilia's emergence: When in the company of these pompous snobs you will have the overwhelming urge to disrupt their prevailing idiotic idyll [...]. Inasmuch as the biological consequences of one's sex ultimately has an adverse effect on pornophiles as well – since they, too, prefer to deny their mortality – the predilection for pornophilia assumes a particular trait that camouflages the general unpleasantness of being reminded of our animality.
>
> *(Brouk 2020: 118–119)*

Czech Surrealists blamed the imposition of a taboo on sexuality on the socially privileged: the elites ("pompous snobs") and the rich ("nabobs"). Like Wilhelm Reich, Brouk argued that class struggle and the sexual revolution were inextricably linked. Pornophilia was to serve as a reminder of the constantly repressed possibility of enjoying the unlimited potency (both sexual and creative) that bodily pleasure can lead to.

Brouk argued that the creative act was a form of drive sublimation (Ibid.: 123). While the "normal" libido is associated with play and the enjoyment derived from it, the "neurotic" libido is at the root of all artistic activity. Among the various forms and types of art, pornophilia occupies a special place. It draws strength from the affirmation of obscenity, which is placed at its center. As Brouk added: "a work of obscenity may serve as a surrogate to sexual gratification, as a direct sexual charge" (Ibid.: 119). Without leading to actual sexual gratification (unlike pornography), pornophilia at once provokes and fulfills scopic pleasure. Its paradox, however, is that it leads to the partial discharge of sexual desire (through obscenity), while simultaneously redirecting and sublimating it (into aesthetic contemplation). Writing about obscenity as "a surrogate to sexual gratification," Brouk pointed to the fetishistic aspect of pornographic representation. Štyrský's photomontages are dominated by genitalia detached from the body and orbiting in space, juxtaposed with something resembling them (e.g. a flower) or complemented by objects associated with the intimate sphere (underwear, a blindfold) or directly with fetishes (a foot, a stocking, a slipper, a shoe).

In 1927, Freud published a short article entitled "Fetishism" ("Fetischismus"), in which he treated fetishism as a psychic mechanism based on substitution: as a replacement for genitals, the fetish would make sexual intercourse possible. As Freud explained:

> It seems rather that when the fetish is instituted some process occurs which reminds one of the stopping of memory in traumatic amnesia. As in this latter case, the subject's interest comes to a halt half-way, as it were; it is as though the last impression before the uncanny and traumatic one is retained as a fetish.
>
> *(Freud [1927] 1961b: 155)*

The fetish emerges on the way to the discovery of the genitalia. Significantly, the fetish establishes itself as a veil for female sex organs, which are unconsciously seen as undesirable. The paradox between the fetishist's desire and the genital-oriented desire can be observed in one of Štyrský's photomontages, in which the artist juxtaposes a skeleton (a decomposed body) with a young female body dressed in lingerie (IX). The artist directs the viewer's attention to the inevitability of aging and death. The woman's healthy body – still capable of experiencing pleasure – is contrasted with human remains (death) and war (destruction), evoked by army boots artificially attached to the skeleton. Štyrský adds two other elements to his photomontage: male and female genitalia. The viewer's eye, stimulated by the bare bones on the one hand, and a naked female body on the other, is suddenly assaulted by these two added images of sex organs. The genitalia, lurking behind women's underwear and the human remains, strike the viewer – who could be so horrified by the obscenity of the work that they would stop "halfway" from discovering female/male genitalia.[14]

In his text on fetishism, Freud found a potential explanation for the mechanism of fetish formation:

> We can now see what the fetish achieves and what it is that maintains it. It remains a token of triumph over the threat of castration and a protection against it. It also saves the fetishist from becoming a homosexual, by endowing women with the characteristic which makes them tolerable as sexual objects. In later life, the fetishist feels that he enjoys yet another advantage from his substitute for a genital. The meaning of the fetish is not known to other people, so the fetish is not withheld from him: it is easily accessible and he can readily obtain the sexual satisfaction attached to it. *What other men have to woo and make exertions for can be had by the fetishist with no trouble at all* [italics mine].
>
> *(Ibid.: 154)*

Fetish as a defense against castration anxiety becomes a theme eagerly exploited in Štyrský's pornophilic works. In one of the photomontages, female genitalia appear in a mirror that resembles a framed painting. Next to them, the artist placed a fish with menacingly bared teeth, ready to bite. The scene might be depicting either the moment before (potential) castration, or the situation immediately following it – the disintegration of the child's image of the phallic mother. As Freud wrote: "the fetish is a substitute for the woman's (the mother's) penis that the little boy once believed" (Ibid.: 152–153). Štyrský's photomontage evokes the moment in a child's life when he or she discovers the sexual difference. The clitoris exposed in the image can be seen as indicating both castration anxiety and the omnipotence of female genitalia – a sign of symbolic domination over the boy-man.

In the 1920s, Karl Abraham wrote about the phallic mother. In his article "The Spider as a Dream Symbol" ("Die Spinne als Traumsymbol"), he proposed an interpretation of dreams about spiders as a symptom of the fear of an evil mother who weaves a web to imprison and then devour her children. According to Abraham, dreams about spiders revealed the ambivalence of the dreamer's feelings toward his mother. This part of his analysis was followed by an interesting detail: the spider did not just symbolize the evil mother but also the phallic mother:

> The spider's falling down in the dream represents the fall of the mother's penis, which becomes detached on the patient going to the cupboard (mother symbol). The patient's joy at not having come in contact with the spider, i.e. the maternal genitals, is in accordance with his horror of incest. The sight of the female sex-organs in real life gives rise to feelings of horror in him, which are increased by manual contact with them. The subsequent increase in size of the spider, which quite unnecessarily rises up and flies in a semi-circle through the air, is an obvious symbol of erection; the maternal phallus attacks the dreamer.
>
> *(Abraham 1923: 315)*

The mother's omnipotence is symbolized by the penis-spider, while the web is a clear reference to the female genitalia. These two aspects – the spider and its web – reveal the simultaneous love for and fear of the mother who is "formed in the shape of a man, of whose male organ and masculine pleasure in attack the boy is afraid" (Ibid.: 315). The spider symbolizes power and lack thereof, while the woman personifies what is closest (the mother's body) to the child and, at the same time, most alien (the female genitalia). The theme of the phallic mother and the giant mother was further developed in the 1940s by the Hungarian psychoanalyst Imre Hermann. In his article "The Giant Mother, The Phallic Mother, Obscenity" (1949), he wrote:

> Memories of the *large size of the mother's pelvic region* are not infrequent, especially in men. These recollections may concern either the mother herself or a mother-substitute (mother's sister). It is a short step from here to the assumption of huge genital organ as belonging to the mother. In obscene talk huge genital organs are sometimes attributed to women who are particularly desirable sexually. The image of the mother emerging from behind these memories perfectly corresponds to the first sculptures of the paleolithic age: huge breasts, a huge pelvis and huge external genitals. In one case a rather small woman emerges with huge thighs; he dreams of a woman whose external genitals protrude in the form of a prepuce or piece of bowel.
>
> *(Hermann 1949: 303)*

Hermann tried to describe the formation of the phallic mother's imago, in which – due to a significant shift (illusionary misinterpretation) – female organs were replaced by the image of a penis ("the imagined penis"). In other words, contrary to Freud's approach, the child/fetishist does not expect to see the male genitalia in place of the female genitalia (as proof of castration). Instead, under the influence of the incest taboo at the imaginary level, he transforms the monstrous genital organ into a more familiar formation – the male organ (that is, in this sense, easier to accept). Hermann argued that the unconscious retained the idea of an omnipotent mother (with monstrous genitalia) whom the subject desired, admired, and feared. With the primacy of the child's relationship with its mother in mind, Hermann pointed to the persistence of images associated with the maternal body in adult human life. In one of Štyrský's dreams described in *Emilie Comes to Me in a Dream*, female genitalia are depicted as terrifying and monstrous:

> One night I awoke just before daybreak [...] Marta lay next to me [...] I saw her sex swell and spill out from her womb, increasing in size until it overflowed up my room. I quickly got up and ran from the house like a madman. I stopped in the middle of a deserted town square. When I looked back, Marta's vulva, resembling a giant, monumental tear of unnatural color, was surging out my window.
>
> *(Štyrský 2020: 87)*

The lover's genitals are detached from her body and gain their own subjectivity. Martha's enormous and overflowing vulva also suggests her ability to experience superhuman pleasure. In the scene that follows, the protagonist – like the poet traveling through the circles of hell in *The Divine Comedy* – descends to the catacombs, where he meets an apocalyptic monster. He is horrified by a creature made of women's vaginas, with which, despite their monstrosity, he finally has intercourse:

> I came to the catacombs in complete innocence. [...] I saw a cluster of comely naked girls knotted together into a single teeming mass, like a monster from the Apocalypse. Their vaginas opened mechanically, some vacant, others swallowing their own juices. I noticed one in particular whose labia moved like mute lips trying to speak, like someone's petrified tongue attempting to crow. Another smiled like a flower bud [...] It was the sex of my dead Klára [...] I took out my cock and without a moment's hesitation impassively thrust it into that teeming mass at random, telling myself that vice and misfortune are always united by death.
>
> *(Ibid.: 88)*

The monstrosity of female genitalia is associated with the theme of necrophilia, and at the same time calls attention to the inseparable bond of desire and destruction. As if in response to the fear of Thanatos, the narrator takes on the role of God and creates his own microcosm, woven out of memories and the scraps (waste) of everyday life. As he recalls:

> Later I placed an aquarium in the window. In it I cultivated a golden-haired vulva and a magnificent penis specimen with a blue eye and delicate veins on its temples. Yet in time I threw in everything I had ever loved: shards of broken teacups, hairpins, Barbora's slipper, light bulbs, shadows, cigarette butts, sardine tins, my entire correspondence, and used condoms. Many strange creatures were born in this world.
>
> *(Ibid.: 89)*

Significantly, the world created by the narrator is devoid of women: "still my eyes needed something to feast on" (Ibid.: 89). Driven by desire, the protagonist eventually discovers a childhood memory of finding himself in bed with his sister. In the final paragraphs, the themes of incestuous love with his sister as well as her relationship with her father, which the narrator (as a child) witnessed, come to the fore. The narrator comments: "I finally had a chance to witness how one makes love" (Ibid.: 90). In all the women who appear in his story (Klára, Cecil, Marta), the protagonist sees Emilie, the lover whose face peeks out from under the memory of his sister's image. *Emilie Comes to Me in a Dream* ends with the coupling of sexual potency and pleasure with death and decay. After all, as the narrator points out, Emilie's beauty, of which he has become a slave, "decays" rather than "fades." A young body, which constantly desires and receives pleasure, is underpinned by an image of human remains, pointing to the inevitable transience and decay of what was once beautiful, and to the decay of what was innocent as a result of breaking the taboo of incest. Thus, the narrator's every form of sexual desire is marked by the abject encounter with uncontrollable lust (represented by the father who seduced his own daughter) and by the horror of the decaying body.

In *Emilie Comes to Me in a Dream*, the entire human body is subjected to fetishization, and its representation becomes a particular kind of substitute for the actual sexual act. This happens not only because of libidinous depictions of genitalia and sexual acts, but also because the body-experiencing-pleasure is liberated from the chains of urban everyday life and the social order that suppresses sexual desire (bodies suspended in space, bodies "returned" to nature). In his photomontages, Štyrský attempts to extract "pure" pleasure, which he locates in the body – in the bodily experience (which is free of social inhibitions). Herein lies an important difference between the psychoanalytic and the Surrealist understanding of the fetish. For the Surrealists, what hindered the sexual act and led to its fetishization were not sexual organs (whether male or female), but the bourgeois everyday life that channeled desire and sculpted it to fit social expectations. Brouk wrote about this explicitly:

> The libido needs a space to play in, a space that diverts the senses from the dismal post-coital condition and deters those rational speculations poisoning our pleasure. Our eroticism must be rid of its depressing connection to plump wives and conjugal beds under which a chamber pot lurks.
>
> *(Brouk 2020: 126)*

The libido needs a space for free play in which the promise of continued pleasure would be sustained despite the gratification achieved.

At the same time, pointing to the connection between desire and play, Štyrský places sexuality itself in the field of spectacle. It is not far from giving the sexual act a theatrical dimension; it becomes a kind of game that needs certain rules in order to be effective (to bring pleasure). In the case of pornographic art, it is the libido that assumes the role of the director and main actor of the fantastical performances of the body. Bodies once decontextualized – torn away from their everyday reality and placed in cosmic space – ultimately fall back into a reality filled with violence. In Štyrský's photomontages, the constellation "war-death-destruction" functions as a stage on which the spectacle of the body takes place. The body-experiencing-pleasure is presented by pornographic art as a tool directed against the oppressive capitalist machine of bourgeois domination and bourgeois morality. However, the body fails to escape the violence and destruction that cast a shadow over it. The sphere of the body and sexuality affirmed by the Surrealists is clearly marked by the specter of the recent war. This radical form of destruction is inscribed into the dynamics of the death wish as well as the preservation and the reclaiming of Eros.

By linking destruction with desire, Štyrský came close to Freud's reflections of the early 1920s. In his treatise *Beyond the Pleasure Principle*, Freud argued:

> A condition has long been known and described which occurs after severe mechanical concussions, a railway disasters and other accidents involving a risk to life; it has been given the name of "traumatic neurosis." The terrible war which has just ended gave rise to a great number of illnesses of this kind [...]. "Anxiety" describes a particular state of expecting the danger or preparing for it, even though it may be an unknown one. "Fear" requires a definite object of which to be afraid. "Fright," however, is the name we give to the state a person gets into when he has run into danger without being prepared for it.
>
> *(Freud [1920] 1955c: 12)*

All of the affects mentioned by Freud – anxiety, fear, and fright – emerge in Štyrský's photomontages from the image of the body-experiencing-pleasure. Especially those works in which the body-experiencing-pleasure is contrasted with the body-in-decomposition or linked with the signs of death (such as a coffin or a catafalque) evoke the clash between "ego-instincts" and "sexual instincts" (Ibid.: 44).

Štyrský's emphasis on the tension between Eros and Thanatos as the real source of sexual desire brings him close to Sabina Spielrein's thought. As Spielrein wrote: "Pleasure is merely the affirmative reaction of the ego to these demands flowing from the depths. We could feel real pleasure in displeasure or in pain, which we assume is strongly tinged with displeasure" (Spielrein 1994: 160). These words echo Freud's recognition of the ambivalent dimension of human sexuality and its masochistic-sadistic expression as well as the wishful function of nightmares. Significantly, in Štyrský's pornophilic imagination, the desire for pleasure also merges with the sensation of pain, while the beauty of the sexual act fuses with repulsion (as the effect of breaking the taboo of incest). The simultaneous desires for the pleasurable and the painful converge in the space of the body itself – exactly as it is reconciled by the artist in his photomontages.

4.5 Štyrský's dream diary

At the start of the 1930s, Štyrský was searching for the possibility of a complete synthesis of word and image. He started using paper, lines, and colors as a space of experimentation with possible forms of (self-)expression, intended to accurately portray the hidden world of dreams and fantasies. Štyrský saw the image and the word equally important components of his works. As Josef Vojvodík perfectly summarized this "synthetism" of avant-garde art:

> The correlation between individual media (text and image; theatre, choreography and scenography; photography of art and scenography; music, photography, film, typography, design), the subject's aesthetic experience and how that affects his perception of reality and how it is interpreted

> [...] all these aspects may [...] be considered the main constituent features of the Czech avant-garde.
>
> *(Bílek, Vojvodík, & Wiendl 2011: 24)*

Belief in the omnipotence of art in its totality prompted avant-garde artists to probe the boundaries between painting, sculpture, theater, and music.

The dream as a trace of Štyrský's self-analysis was foregrounded in his works from the early 1930s, such as *The Death of Orpheus* (1931), *Milan Nights* (1931–1932), *From My Diary* (1933), and *Čerchov* (1934). The leading representative of Czech Surrealism, Karel Teige, wrote about these key aspects of Štyrský's late work in 1948:

> The objectifying and concretizing of fantastic visions, the representation of which adopts the authenticity of the tangible so that the painting becomes a realistic representation of an ideal object, a depiction of a fantastic object, further evolved to the point where the painting was no longer merely a realistic depiction of fantasy but a fantastical configuration of real objects, in other words, a fantastical reality subjected to the dictates of desire. This shift from the reified to the real, from the actualization of imagination to an imaginative reality, from the clustering of fantastical objects to the fantastical clustering of everyday objects, selected and juxtaposed by desire as a form of hidden tension, was accelerated by a series of photographs and hyperbolic collages that should be considered more than experimental marginalia as they were critical for Štyrský's development.
>
> *(Teige 2018: 15)*

The stark reality was turned upside down in a series of fantastic photographs, collages, and photomontages that visualized and revealed what had so far remained hidden – the hyperreal world of desires and phantasmagorical imaginings. The hyperreality allowed the artist to turn towards himself, and – consequently – to turn away from the external world. In his analysis, Teige paid particular attention to the transgressive and transformative power of Surrealism:

> The growing intensity of the real and the unalloyed surreality of lyrical fantasy in the final period of Štyrský's work suggests that its interrupted trajectory would lead from [...] the depiction of fantastical objects to the fantastical juxtaposition of real objects [...] to the conversion of utopia into reality, to the transformation of life to align it with the ancient dream of humanity.
>
> *(Ibid.: 18)*

Teige stressed the creative power of imagination, which in the 1930s brought utopia into the reality of human experience. Emphasizing the importance of unexplored paths, disappointed hopes, and finally Štyrský's premature death (at the age of forty-three), Teige described his work as simultaneously escaping the surrounding reality, processing it, and drawing its creative force from the matter of everyday life. In this light, the oneiric nature of Štyrský's poetic images also becomes the clearest sign of their suspension between the subjective (autobiographical) and the universal (archetypal).

Vojvodík suggested that the distinguishing feature of the Czech Surrealists' work in the period shortly before 1939 and in the turbulent years of the war had been their play with the binaries taken for granted or considered as natural in their cultural and social reality. The exposure of contradictions between matter and form, the male and the female, the good and the bad led not only to the denaturalization of these categories, but also to their reconfiguration. What seemed inconceivable suddenly becomes part of the same limitless spectral richness of the human psyche. However, such a constantly expanding world-without-boundaries creates anxiety. Following this pattern, Vojvodík considered Štyrský's works from the 1930s (especially *Emilie*... and *From the Dungeons of Sleep*... from 1941) to be the result of "a self being consumed by fear," one that is trying to rebuild "the uprooted, destabilized, dehumanized, ravaged world, incomprehensible in its irrationality" (Vojvodík 2007: 71–72). A confused and lost man can find hope and a sense of security only by creating his microcosm made of the captured scraps of dreams. As Vojvodík adds in this context: "The enclosed world *en miniature* – the space of dream (daylike) and intimacy, memory, recollection, and creative imagination – is contrasted with the unfriendly surrounding world of unlimited spaces, monstrosity, and incoherence" (Ibid.: 74). Thus, Štyrský's fantastic and phantasmic worlds would be a reaction to the overwhelming sense of the threat of the annihilation and disintegration of the familiar reality. In fear of decomposition and fragmentation, the subject takes refuge in his own miniaturized world, transforming himself into a solitary monad, dreamt into existence.

As the examples of *Emilie* and Štyrský's dream "diary" show, a dream turns out to be a space for absorbing and confronting the monstrous, the unlimited, and the incoherent. The complex and variation-prone dynamics of the dream itself show it to be an imaginative formation that continually expands the boundaries of the known world, opening up infinite associative possibilities before the dreamer by lifting bodily limitations and overcoming the order of rationality.[15]

In the opening passage of *Dreams*, Štyrský evokes a blurry memory of his mother and sister. He writes:

> As a young child I saw in the color supplement of a magazine the image of a woman's head, exquisite with golden hair [...]. The head was perverse, yet full of compassion, damned, yet full of kindness. It was head of Medusa, the whole of it in a pool of blood. Blood streamed from its neck, and its hair was a cluster of vipers, erect, ready to penetrate the

> woman through her mouth, nose, and ears. […] Head of Medusa. It kept recurring in my dreams.
>
> *(Štyrský 2018: 23)*

The image of the Medusa's monstrous head haunts the author and merges with the image of his mother and sister. As Štyrský adds: "The head was a perfect fit on my sister" (Ibid.: 23). The sister with her bloodied face and writhing vipers causes horror in him as an association with death and castration – but also with unsurpassed love. He calls the image of his sister in agony "my chimera" – a "phantom object" on which he fixates. It is no accident that Štyrský dedicated one series of dreams he recorded to his sister (Ibid.: 23). For him, she occupied the position of an object both desired and feared, near and far – a form of an uncanny fetish.

In his analysis, Vojvodík also mentioned the sister's mask of the Medusa. He writes: "At the same time, [the protagonist] also puts this imaginary, virtual mask on himself – both to hide behind it, and to look at it as a different reality he must face" (Vojvodík 2007: 76). It is worth asking whether the artist really hides behind the image of Sister-Medusa, or whether, as he himself declares, it constitutes a fetish – an uncanny imago which he places between himself and another person. The Sister-Medusa – as a fetish and an object of fear – mediates the image of every subsequent object of affection in the narrator's adult life and overlaps with it. It stops the narrator "halfway" to his discovery of the sexual difference and his fear of the sexual act (blood=wound=death). The dreamt head of the jellyfish can be treated as a symbol of the female genitalia. For the dreamer, the imago of the Sister-Medusa or the Mother-Medusa triggers an oneiric journey into the female body – which is simultaneously monstrous, omnipotent, bloodthirsty, and deliriously beautiful.

The protagonist's spiritual and physical proximity with his sister also recurs as an important theme in *Emilie…* In the concluding scene, the narrator, like Freud's "Wolf Man," observes the sexual act – with the difference that this primal scene does not involve the creation of a new image of the mother and father, but of the sister and father. Thus, the primal scene – visualized in the form of the Medusa's head – is associated with both the discovery of the sexual difference and the breaking of the taboo of incest. The following words by Štyrský can be read in this light: "Thus I instinctively created my CHIMERA, my PHANTOM OBJECT, on which I am fixated and to which I dedicate this work" (Štyrský 2018: 23). The image of the kinship between sister and brother is a sign of the unity of their bodies. In the narrator's imagination, they incarnate both the modernist ideal of man as an androgyne and the suprasexual power of Eros. In this context, Otto Rank's words apply:

> The threat of castration hits not only the vaguely remembered primal trauma and the undisposed-of anxiety representing it, but also a second

> trauma, consciously experienced and painful in character, though later obliterated by repression, namely weaning, the intensity and persistence of which falls far short of that of the first trauma, but owes a great part of its "traumatic" effect to it. […] the natal anxiety-affect as guilt feeling, which, as in the meaning of the biblical fall of man, actually proves to be connected with the differentiation of the sexes, the difference in the sexual organs and the sexual functions. The deepest Unconscious which always remains sexually indifferent (bi-sexual) knows nothing of this and knows only the first primal anxiety of the universal human act of birth.
>
> *(Rank 2010: 59–60)*

The discovery of the sexual difference implies the original unity (suprasexuality) of man, irretrievably lost at birth. The union of bodies (and souls) so eagerly emphasized by Štyrský embodies the modernist ideal of the androgyne.[16]

Some of Štyrský's dreams refer to the mother's body shown in the form of the ruptured earth (genitals, womb) or the maternal breast – safe bodily spaces in various temporal and spatial configurations. In others, women's bodies are transformed into animal-human creations: Emilie grows snake-like hands, and the body of Cinderella (another girl appearing in *Dreams*) is covered with snails emerging from between her legs, breasts, and under her arms. In the dream about the ruptured snake, there is a clear reference to bisexuality. The appearance of a snake as a symbol for the phallus marked by an oval rapture (which often stand for female genitalia) produces one male-female organism. This dream, as well as Štyrský's drawings *Infinite Snake and Gutted Snake* (1931), are reminiscent of the artist's later painting *Hermaphrodite* (1934), which features the same image of a ruptured/dissected snake (alongside a "miraculous pear") as in *Dreams*. Whereas the head of the Sister-Medusa or the father's long stilts frighten the protagonist with the threat of castration, the broken, endless snake unites what was (wrongly) separated, thus freeing the dreamer from the dynamics of sexual difference and the trauma associated with its discovery.

4.6 Jokes and pornographic fantasies

As David Bates wrote, the Surrealist imagination of French writers and artists had combined the images of pleasure born of pain, the objectification of the female body (a misogynistic fixation), and the predilection for an idealized image of pure love (Ibid.: 148). The search for true love had become the antithesis to sadistic imagination. Pure love, transcending the taboo of incest, is governed by the logic of kinship – it makes siblings into two halves of a broken unity.

As already mentioned, Štyrský began to record his dreams in the 1920s. At that time, he created oneiric sketches, painted and composed photomontages which directly referred visually to the textual records of his dreams. *Dreams*

(*Sny*), which were only published after the artist's death, contain many clues that were also found in *Emilie Comes to Me in a Dream*.[17] The writer was haunted by dreamlike fantasies of snakes, women's breasts, alabaster hands, a father, a mother, a sister, snails hidden in intimate parts of the human body, overflowing excrement, and butterflies. The dream in Štyrský's Surrealist work had a free visual dynamic; verbal poetics were governed by visual representation, whereas the dream imagery demanded translation into text. Following established psychoanalytic ideas, Surrealists believed that dreams both had a wishful aspect and were products of complicated psychic activity. Freud's belief that a child with its infantile desires still lives in our dreams could serve as a motto for Štyrský's *Dreams*.

In the dreamer's psyche, a repressed wish is fulfilled in a distorted manner (appearing under a false form and name). The images pressing on the dreamer often resist interpretation. In his "dream diary," Štyrský does not analyze his dreams but instead tries to faithfully express and visualize them using lines and colors. The scenes range from the abject, frightening, and grotesque to the joyful and innocent. Some of the paintings and sketches produced at that time, such as *The Omnipresent Eye* (1936), *Liquid Doll*, and *Man Carried by the Wind* (1934), followed a psychoanalytic sensibility and also fit well with Štyrský's typical absurdist-humorous dynamic. A man, made not of clay but excrement, a breast full of milk artificially hanging from the Statue of Liberty, an alabaster hand, decorated with greens and served on a tray – all these images, meaningfully composed of multiplied fragments of human and animal bodies left in the strangest spatial configurations, approximated the structure of the joke as described by Freud. By replicating and arranging ordinary objects in surprising compositions, the joke provides a sensation of pleasure obtained by recognizing the familiar which appears different, transformed.

In 1905, Freud considered the relationship between humor and the unconscious. He pointed to a convergence of the processes that shape them: condensation, the appearance of substitute formations, the use of absurdity and opposites. In the joke and the unconscious, displacement also plays an important role, causing the accumulation and exchange of one image for another. Unlike a daydream, a joke does not replace a repressed wish. Rather, it tries to escape the action of the censor by undertaking a (seemingly) meaningless play on words and absurd visual association. Freud adds in this context:

> Nonsense, absurdity, which appears so often in dreams and has brought them into so much undeserved contempt, never arises by chance through the ideational elements being jumbled together, but can always be shown to have been admitted by the dream-work intentionally and to be designed to represent embittered criticism and contemptuous contradiction in the dream-thoughts. […] But besides this, it must not be

> forgotten that the nonsense in a joke is an end in itself, since the intention of recovering the old pleasure in nonsense is among the joke-work's motives.
>
> *(Freud [1905] 1960: 175–176)*

In both cases, delight flows directly from the affirmation of the irrational and the surreal. Freud returned to the problem of rejecting the principle of reality in 1927 in a text on humor. He argued: "Humour is not resigned; it is rebellious. It signifies not only the triumph of the ego but also of the pleasure principle, which is able here to assert itself against the unkindness of the real circumstances" (Freud [1927] 1961b: 163). A sense of humor, then, is a state that brings man out of his reality, a reversal of the dynamics of his everyday functioning which replaces the principle of productivity with the principle of enjoyment (along the lines proposed by Brouk).

Returning to considerations from *Discomfort in Culture,* Freud asserted:

> Its fending off of the possibility of suffering places it [humour] among the great series of methods which the human mind has constructed in order to evade the compulsion to suffer – a series which begins with neurosis and culminates in madness and which includes intoxication, self-absorption and ecstasy.
>
> *(Ibid.: 163)*

The source for Štyrský's surreal imagination lies precisely in the demolition of the order of rationality and the replacement of seriousness with absurdity: a synthesis of wit, humor, and dream-work. As in anxiety dreams, pleasure is derived in a less obvious way, that is, from the painful (masochistic aspect) and the cruel (sadistic aspect). In this respect, Štyrský's take on humor differs from Freud's. The Czech Surrealist did not use humor to "reject suffering" but to confront suffering in a sado-masochistic way. The instance of the "super-ego" (*das Über-Ich*) also plays a completely different role in this case. While, in Freud's understanding, it serves the purpose of relieving tension (like an affectionate father who remains in his function and upholds the Law he has established), in Štyrský's work one could rather speak of the creative-satisfying role of "it" (das Es) standing in the father's way.

In *Dreams*, the author's sister plays a prominent role. He calls her Emilie: both here and in *Emilie Comes to Me in a Dream* her name is at the center of the incest taboo shaping the artist's imagination. Emilie-Medusa thus acts as a clear sign of the fear of incest. The blood spilling around her head refers to female genitalia (menstrual blood=birth) and castration anxiety (castration as punishment for incest). The writer's daydream fantasies reverberate successively as the imago of mother, sister, and father. The bloodthirsty jellyfish at first gives way to a vision of a warm mother-earth body (a return to the maternal womb), soon to be replaced by a fantasy of the father shooting at his son with a revolver or pursuing him in a mad chase on makeshift stilts made out of chairs. In psychoanalytic terms, castration anxiety can also appear in the form of the totemic animal. As Freud stated:

> If the totem animal is the father, then the two principal ordinances of totemism, the two taboo prohibitions which constitute its core – not to kill the totem and not to have sexual relations with a woman of the same totem – coincide in their content with the two crimes of Oedipus, who killed his father and married his mother, as well as with the two primal wishes of children, the insufficient repression or the re-awakening of which forms the nucleus of perhaps every psychoneurosis.
>
> *(Freud [1913] 1955a: 132)*

In *Totem and Taboo*, describing a type of choice in a man (mother-sister), the author noted that in the neurotic desire is trapped in a "family affair" (Ibid.: 17). For example, Štyrský's dream about the marten can be read in this light. Dreams – on the imaginary level – appear to be the product of neurotic fantasy; the same fantasy that in *Emilie Comes to Me in a Dream* made the artist depict death and destruction as the negative of love and carnal pleasure. In writing about the fear of incest, Freud drew attention to the close connection between the social prohibition of incest and the prohibition against "sodomy." This is particularly relevant in the context of Štyrský's work. In *Dreams*, the incestuous fantasy (about the mother and the sister) is entangled in an anal fixation. Štyrský seems fond of describing scatological fantasies in which the excrement takes the shape of a man, mountains, lakes, and so on. This is also depicted in his paintings from 1934 such as *Liquid Doll* or *Man Carried by the Wind*.

The subsequent fantasies described by the artist are arranged in a catalog of word-pictures depicting the pregenital stages of human sexuality: the oral (butterflies perching on the protagonist's face), the anal (scatological fantasies), and the phallic (snake) phases. This interpretative intuition is confirmed especially by the dream about the tattooed child. Štyrský writes: "Around us in an orgy of dance are ten- to twelve-year-old TATTOOED BOYS. They are armed with sticks and make threatening gestures at us. In their midst we also see an infant TATTOOED WITH PORNOGRAPHIC images" (Štyrský 2018: 60). Erotic content materializes on the surface of the child's body, a blank page on which sexual intercourse is visualized. Štyrský portrays the child as a sexual being, while underscoring the long duration of childhood sexual fantasies, which still live in the adult, just as the child lives in the adult (awakened to life when the adult sleeps).

Another key trope in *Dreams* is autoeroticism. In one dream, an alabaster hand appears in the artist's imagination. Štyrský recalls: "I see a delicate white hand slide out of from the bushes growing right next to the house and hold back the left window and shut it easily" (Ibid.: 54–56). The motif of the alabaster hand is also used in *Emilie Comes to Me in a Dream*. In one scene, the narrator turns to himself and states: "You will feel an intense fear […], a fear similar to the pleasure you felt in childhood at your first convulsive erection and the terror you felt when your sister taught you to masturbate with her tiny alabaster hand" (Štyrský 2020: 86). The alabaster hand used for masturbation acts as a prosthesis of the human hand; it indicates both the prohibition of autoerotic forms of sexual pleasure and is associated with the use of various objects in autoerotic play. Autoeroticism became Bohuslav Brouk's main focus in his 1935 book *Autoeroticism and Psychoeroticism*. He pointed out the inseparable connection between eroticism and masturbation (treated as a permanent element of sexuality as well as its key imaginative dimension, which he referred to as psycho-eroticism). The desired and the loved are linked both to stimuli coming from the outside and from within – what "exists in our imaginations" (Brouk 1935: 16). The phantasm is in no way inferior to reality, just as it is impossible to draw a clear line between the reality of dream and the waking reality. Štyrský counterbalances socially managed eroticism – sexuality subjected into the order of productivity – with autoerotic human-animal body in which the clear boundary between nature and culture is blurred. Dream recording may prompt the writer to self-analyze – to reflect on the deeper meaning of his dream fantasies. Yet, Štyrský does not undertake interpretation, leaving the hermeneutic practice to future viewers/readers. His goal is not to explain the contents of a dream, but to find the right way to express it in the language of art. The aim is not to guess the meaning of a dream, but to bring out the dream content itself in all its non-linearity, fragmentary, heterogeneity, and hybridity. It is in this sense that Štyrský's *Dreams* can be read as the artist's microhistory, woven out of projections rather than reality.

4.7 Conclusion

By infusing their works with psychoanalytic themes, Czech Surrealists as a group played a key role in transmitting psychoanalytic knowledge into Czech culture. They combined the Freudian understanding of dreams and theory of sexuality with their own unorthodox interpretations of psychoanalysis, connecting it with Marxism and treating it as a path toward social revolution. Artworks by Jindřich Štyrský and writings by Bohuslav Brouk discussed in this chapter illustrate that knowledge transmission does not end at the implementation of certain notions and meanings in a new cultural context. Rather, it transforms foreign ideas creatively, giving them new meanings in a new social and political context.

Czech Surrealists saw reclaiming sexuality and the body's right to experience unlimited pleasure as the best tools to combat bourgeois morality, capitalist exploitation, and the chaos and destructiveness of war. Štyrský's works from the 1930s brought the dream dynamic to the surface. The same images, themes, and objects recurred in his collages, photomontages, texts, and notes. In dreams, the artist saw a space for the activation of repressed Eros. The oneiric game played with the taboo of incest as well as the clichés of decay and death superimposed on the bodies-experiencing-pleasure allowed Štyrský to reveal the deepest layers of human desire. Moreover, his works added an emotional and loving dimension to the socially unwanted and condemned phenomenon of incest.

Štyrský's exposure of death, destruction, and devastation visualized the progressive decomposition of culture and society in the years leading up to the outbreak of World War II, while also allowing the viewer to process of the trauma of the Great War.

The repulsive memory of war-as-destruction found an outlet, actualizing itself in the surreal space of the dream. At the same time, the specter of war-as-total-destruction reinforced the desire to reclaim life itself – to liberate Eros through artistic creation. The problem of reclaiming Eros, the right to free expression, is a central theme of the next chapter. In it, I will return to the issue of gender identity and psychosexual orientation in the context of modern *scientia sexualis.* As the example of Piotr Odmieniec Włast will demonstrate, the individual's rebellion against the oppressive social norms produced and reproduced by the patriarchal family required creating self-analytic language. As we shall see, the manifesto of the queer identity was subject to constant negotiations between the individual, their relatives, psycho-medical discourses, and life writing, with freedom and human dignity at stake.

Notes

1 Cf. Lenka Bydžovská and Karel Srp, *Jindřich Štyrský* (Prague: Argo, 2007), 425–450 (especially the chapter: "řeč bez gramatiky").

2 Fragments of Jung's writings were published in the Czech avant-garde magazine *Kvart.* Jindřich Štyrský, Toyen, and František Halas closely collaborated with the journal in its early period, see J. Vojvodík, "The Czech Avant-Garde: Evolution, Groupings, Transformations," in: *A Glossary*, 28–29.

3 On Czech avant-garde groups developed before 1930s, see J. Vojvodík, *The Czech Avant-Garde*, 27–29. It should be noted that psychoanalysis became a very important point of reference for Czech avant-garde artists before the actual establishment of the Surrealist Group in 1930s. For instance, Teige wrote about the importance of the psychoanalytic understanding of the unconscious and creative forces in the second manifesto of Poetism. He also stressed the continuity between Poetism and Surrealism, 45–46. On Czech underground avant-garde groups and the idea of supranational Central-European artistic movements, see: Weronika Parfianowicz, "Czeski underground wobec awangardy," in *Awangarda/Underground. Idee, historie, praktyki w kulturze polskiej i czeskiej*, ed. Agnieszka Karpowicz, Weronika Parfianowicz, and Xawery Stańczyk (Kraków: Wydawnictwo Uniwersytetu Jagiellońskiego, 2018), 53–76.

4 In 1934, the Czech Surrealist Group was founded. The manifesto *Surrealism in Czechoslovakia* was signed by the following members: Konstantin Biebl, Bohuslav Brouk, Imre Forbath, Jindrich Honzl, Jaroslav Ježek, Katy King, Josef Kunstadt, Vincenc Makovsky, Jindrich Štyrský, Toyen. Cf. *A Glossary*, 45.

5 Before he came to Prague, Fenichel had organized open sexological seminars in Vienna and had closely collaborated with Wilhelm and Annie Reich, and others (e. g. Helene and Felix Deutsch). At the time, he was already known for his Leftist beliefs, see Elke Mühlleitner, *Biographisches Lexikon der Psychoanalyse: die Mitglieder der Psychologischen Mittwoch-Gesellschaft und der Wiener Psychoanalytischen Vereinigung, 1902–1938*, 93–95.

6 I am using the Polish translation of this document available in *Głuchy brudnopis. Antologia manifestów awangardy Europy Środkowej*, ed. Jakub Kornhauser and Kinga Siewior (Kraków: Wydawnictwo Uniwersytetu Jagiellońskiego, 2014), 119–129.

7 Štyrský's works decorated some of Brouk's covers, for instance *Psychoanalytická sexuologie* and *Bilance psychoanalysy.*

8 Not only Reich's and Gross's reflections were important for Brouk, but also those by Otto Rank. Rank's work *The Trauma of Birth* (1924), which breaks with Freud's theory, also had a significant influence on him. See Bydžovská and Srp, "Trauma zrození," in *Jindřich Štyrský*, 363–374. It should be noted though that Bydžovská and Srp only mention Rank and his seminal book in the context of Štyrský's sojourn in Paris. They also give the wrong date of its publication, 364. The same mistake can be found in Libuše Heczková's and Alžběta Plívová's chapter titled "The Body, Physicality, Anthropological Constants," in *A Glossary*, 118.

9 More on Brouk and his relationship with the Czech Surrealist Group can be found in Vladimir Borecky, "Bohuslav Brouk a psychoanalyza v českém surrealismu v letech 1930–1947," in *Česky surrealismus 1929–1953. Skupina surrealistů v ČSR. Události, vztahy, inspirace*, ed. L. Bydžovská and K. Srp (Prague: Argo, 1996), 66–75.

10 On the pornographic materials used in Štyrský's and Toyen's works, see *A Glossary*, 122–123; *The Dreaming Rebel*, ed. Anna Pravdová, Annie Le Brun, and Annabelle Görgen-Lammers (Prague: Národní galerie v Praze, 2021), 305–313 (especially the chapter: "Luxury in the Wild. Toyen and Eroticism").

11 Works by the Marquis de Sade gained particular recognition in French and Czech Surrealist circles. In his *Manifesto of Surrealism* (1924), André Breton even wrote of de Sade's "Surrealist sadism" (Bates 2003: 145) *avant la lettre.* The nobleman's turbulent biography condemned his work to decades of oblivion. Finally, Guillaume Apollinaire found de Sade's manuscripts at the Bibliothèque Nationale in Paris and introduced them to his milieu of the French avant-garde. De Sade's texts soon appeared on the pages of *La Révolution surréaliste.* Man Ray paid tribute to the rebellious writer in his work *Monument à D.A.F. de Sade* published in *Le Surréalisme au service de la révolution.* Luis Buñuel's famous films *L'Âge d'or* and *Un chien andalou* contain clear references to and quotations from *120 Days of Sodom.* Štyrský and Toyen happened to visit Paris while the French Surrealists were discovering de Sade. Upon their return to Prague, the Surrealist duo brought this fascinating finding with them.

12 On visual associations in Czech surrealist art, see *A Glossary*, 85–86.

13 My analysis is based on the English edition of Štyrský's *Emilie Comes to Me in a Dream*, trans. Jed Slast (Prague: Twisted Spoon Press, 2020).

14 On the Czech avant-garde art's play with the male-female binary as well as on gender conservatism within avant-garde groups, see *A Glossary*, 48–51. Cf. "Coral Islands 1919–1929," in *The Dreaming Rebel. Toyen*, 32–86.

15 It should be noted, however, that the Czech Surrealists took over and reinterpreted Freud's dream theory, according to which dreaming lifts human beings out of the order of linear temporality rather than detaching them from the surrounding reality.

16 On homosexuality and non-normative sexuality in the context of Czech Surrealist art, see: *A Glossary*, 49, 118–119; More on Toyen, *A Glossary*, 54, 62.

17 The first unfinished collection of dreams was prepared by Štyrský himself in 1941. The first full publication came out in 1970. Cf. *A Glossary*, 170–171.

References

Abraham, K. (1923). The Spider as a Dream Symbol, in *International Journal of Psychoanalysis* 4, 313–317.

Bates, D. (2003). *Photography and Surrealism. Sexuality, Colonialism and Dissent*, London/New York: I. B. Tauris.

Bílek, P. A., Vojvodík, J. & Wiendl, J. (Eds.) (2011). *A Glossary of Catchwords of the Czech Avant-Garde. Conceptions of Aesthetics and the Changing Faces of Art 1908–1958*, Prague: Charles University.

Borecky, V. (1996). Bohuslav Brouk a psychoanalyza v českém surrealismu v letech 1930–1947, in L. Bydžovská & K. Srp (Eds.), *Česky surrealism's 1929–1953. Skupina surrealistu v ČSR. Události, vztahy, inspirace*, Prague: Argo, 66–75.

Brouk, B. (1935). *Autosexualismus a psycherotismus*, Praha: Edice Surrealismu.

Brouk, B. (1936). *Bilance psychoanalysy*, Praha: K 31. Prosinci.

Brouk, B. (2009). *O funkcích práce a osobitosti*, Prague: Volvox Globator.

Brouk, B. (2020). Untitled, in F. Halas, V. Nezval & J. Štyrský, *Edition 69*, Prague: Twisted Spoon Press.

Bydžovská, L. & Srp, K. (Eds.) (2007). *Jindřich Štyrský*, Prague: Argo.

Bžoch, A. (2013). *Psychoanalyse in der Slowakei. Eine Geschichte zwischen Enthusiasmus und Widerstand*, Gießen: Psychosozial Verlag.

Conci, M. (2013). Freud, Ossipow and the Psychoanalysis of Migration, in *Psychoanalysis and History* 15, 221–227.

Davydov, S. (1998). Alfred Liudvigovich Bem (1886–1945?), in *Pushkin Review* 1, 35–38.

Dobroczyński, B. (2021). *Polskie zmory. Psychoanaliza w międzywojniu*, Kraków: Universitas.

Fenichel, O. (1953). *The Collected Papers of Otto Fenichel*, New York: Norton & Company.

Freud, S. ([1913] 1955a). Totem and Taboo, in J. Strachey (Ed.), *The Standard Edition of the Complete Psychological Works of Sigmund Freud*. Vol. 13, London: The Hogarth Press, 1–162.

Freud, S. ([1920] 1955c). Group Psychology and the Analysis of Ego, in J. Strachey (Ed.), *The Standard Edition of the Complete Psychological Works of Sigmund Freud*. Vol. 18, London: The Hogarth Press, 7–64.

Freud, S. ([1905] 1960). Jokes and their Relation to the Unconscious, in J. Strachey (Ed.), *The Standard Edition of the Complete Psychological Works of Sigmund Freud*. Vol. 8, London: The Hogarth Press.

Freud, S. ([1927] 1961b). Fetishism, in J. Strachey (Ed.), *The Standard Edition of the Complete Psychological Works of Sigmund Freud*. Vol. 21, 147–158.

Freud, S. ([1927] 1961b). Humour, in J. Strachey (Ed.), *The Standard Edition of the Complete Psychological Works of Sigmund Freud*. Vol. 21, 159–166.

Heczková, L. & Plívová, A. (2011). The Body, Physicality, Anthropological Constants, in P. A. Bílek, J. Vojvodík & J. Wiendl (Eds.), *A Glossary of Catchwords of the Czech Avant-Garde. Conceptions of Aesthetics and the Changing Faces of Art 1908–1958*, Prague: Charles University, 113–123.

Hermann, I. (1949). The Giant Mother, The Phallic Mother, Obscenity, in *The Psychoanalytic Review* 36, 302–306.

Hristeva, G. (2013). A Dream of Freedom: The Correspondence of Sigmund Freud and Nikolay Y. Ossipov 1921–1929, in *Journal of the American Psychoanalytic Association* 61, 511–525.

Klingenberg, I. (2021). Psychoanalysis in exile: early migration in the shadow of the Holocaust and the psychoanalytic study group in Prague, in K. White & I. Klingenberg, *Migration and Intercultural Psychoanalysis: Unconscious Forces and Clinical Issues*, London: Routledge, 120–140.

Kornhauser, J. & Siewior, K. (Eds.) (2015). *Głuchy brudnopis. Antologia manifestów awangard Europy Środkowej*, Kraków: Wydawnictwo Uniwersytetu Jagiellońskiego.

Marcuse, H. (1966). *Eros and Civilization: A Philosophical Inquiry into Freud*, Boston: Beacon Press.

Marcuse, H. (2002). *Towards a Critical Theory of Society: Collected Papers of Herbert Marcuse*. Vol. 2, London/New York: Routledge.

Mühlleitner, E. (1992). *Biographisches Lexikon der Psychoanalyse*, Tübingen: Edition Diskord.

Muñoz, J. E. (2019). *Cruising Utopia: The Then and There of Queer Futurity*, New York: New York University Press.

Parfianowicz, W. (2018). Czeski underground wobec awangardy, in A. Karpowicz, W. Parfianowicz & X. Stańczyk (Eds.), *Awangarda/Underground. Idee, historie, praktyki w kulturze polskiej i czeskiej*, Kraków: Wydawnictwo Uniwersytetu Jagiellońskiego, 53–76.

Pravdová, A., Le Brun, A. & Görgen-Lammers, A. (Eds.) (2021). *The Dreaming Rebel*, Prague: Národní galerie v Praze.

Rank, O. (2010). *The Trauma of Birth*, Connecticut: Martino Publishing.

Šebek, M. (1993). Psychoanalysis in Czechoslovakia, in *Psychoanalytic Review* 80, 433–439.

Šebek, M. (1999). Psychoanalytic Training in Eastern Europe, in *Journal of the American Psychoanalytic Association* 47, 983–988.

Spielrein, S. (1994). Destruction as the Cause of Coming into Being, in *Journal of Analytical Psychology* 39, 155–186.

Štyrský, J. (2018). *Dreamverse*, Prague: Twisted Spoon Press.

Štyrský, J. (2020). Emilie Comes to Me in a Dream, in *Edition 69*. František Halas, Vítězslav Nezval, Jindřich Štyrský. Translated by Jed Slast. Prague: Twisted Spoon Press.

Teige, K. (2018). Introduction, in J. Štyrský, *Dreamverse*, Prague: Twisted Spoon Press, 11–18.

Vojvodík, J. (2007). Świat strachu i strach przed światem w czeskim surrealizmie lat 30. i 40. Translated by Hanna Marciniak, in *Teksty Drugie* 6, 50–77.

Vojvodík, J. (2011). The Czech Avant-Garde: Evolution, Groupings, Transformations, in P. A. Bílek, J. Vojvodík & J. Wiendl (Eds.), *A Glossary of Catchwords of the Czech Avant-Garde: Conceptions of Aesthetics and the Changing Faces of Art 1908–1958*, Prague: Charles University, 15–64.

5

THE QUEER CASE OF PIOTR ODMIENIEC WŁAST

(Psycho)biography, psychoanalysis, and the origins of anti-psychiatric discourse in Poland

Piotr Odmieniec Włast (Maria Komornicka) (1876–1949) was one of the most promising modernist poets in the history of Polish literature (Dernałowicz 1977: 75–88; Krasuska 2012).[1] He had gained recognition in Polish literary circles at just eighteen years old with his work *Forpoczty* (Vanguards, 1894), a modernist manifesto co-written with Wacław Nałkowski and Cezary Jellenta. In the years that followed, Włast worked on a play called *The Hurt* (*Skrzywdzeni*) (1895), a volume of poetry *Fairytales. Psalmodies* (*Baśnie. Psalmodie*) (1900), an epic poem *The Devils* (*Biesy*) (1902), and a translation of Edward Bulwer-Lytton's *Zanoni* (published in Poland in 1906 as *Zanoni. Powieść z czasów rewolucji francuskiej*). In 1903, when he was in Paris, Włast experienced his first nervous breakdown. In 1907, he began identifying as Piotr Odmieniec Włast. As a result of his decision to assume a male identity, he was committed to mental institutions by his family. It was only in 1918 that Włast returned to his family home, where he survived the Second World War distanced from the literary milieu. He died in 1949 at a sanatorium in Izabelin near Warsaw.

In the history of Polish literary history, the case of the modernist writer Włast has exposed the struggles and aporias which have been present in Polish literary science for the recent three decades. Mateusz Chmurski aptly wrote that "works on Komornicka−Odmieniec Włast [...] give insight into the attitudes of literary and cultural historians and the degree of their engagement not only in the subject matter of their work, but also in the contemporary socio-cultural reality" (Chmurski 2015: 133). Writing about Włast has become an opportunity to maintain or transcend the established norms of academic discourse on gender and non-normative sexuality. Similar conclusions were reached by the editors of the first anthology of Polish queer literature: "Maria Komornicka/Piotr Odmieniec Włast, the paradigmatic

DOI: 10.4324/9781003441892-6

changeling of Polish culture, has become a sort of litmus test for shifting methodological paradigms within engaged literary criticism in Poland" (Amenta, Kaliściak & Warkocki 2021: 29). It is no coincidence that one of the most commonly asked questions in research on Włast's work concerned the issue of the poet's gender transgression. Paradoxically, the search for "the truth" on Maria Komornicka's transition into Piotr Włast eclipsed the problem of the cultural dimension of psycho-medical literature in Włast's times.

In order to continue to expand our understanding of what I call the cultural history of non-normative sexuality and identity, it is necessary to return to the historical moment when psycho-medical literature took shape – a process which was closely tied to Włast's biography. In this chapter, I will treat sexological knowledge at the turn of the twentieth century as a result of dynamic interactions between the language of medical sciences, psychology, philosophy, and literary discourses as well as life writing. With the question on "the changing social and discursive conditions in which the desires of historical subjects are constructed" (Halperin 2002: 2) as my point of departure, my aim is to revisit the very dynamics of psycho-medical writing which made such constructions possible at all.

5.1 Piotr Odmieniec Włast and (the) psychiatric institution(s)

The eighth volume of the Polish literary periodical *Literary Archive* (*Archiwum Literackie*), published in 1964, contained a work entitled "Materials on the Life and Work of Maria Komornicka" ("Materiały dotyczące biografii i twórczości Marii Komornickiej"), edited by Stanisław Pigoń (1885–1968), a renowned Polish literary historian, rector of the University of Vilnius in 1926 −1928 and the Jagiellonian University in 1931−1939 and 1945−1960 (Pigoń 1964: 294–382). For many years since then, the document was treated as a literary, (auto-)biographical, and psychiatric compendium of information on the modernist poet Piotr Odmieniec Włast.

The body of life writing (the biographical essay, letters, and memoirs) collected in "Materials" was an attempt to explain the "illness" that shattered Włast's literary career. A selection of the poet's correspondence with his mother, prepared by Aniela Komornicka, shed light on Włast's life after his first nervous breakdown in 1903 (Ibid.: 329). By 1907, when the artist was living with his family, "the necessity of systematic treatment [had become] clear" (Ibid.: 332) The poet's sister narrated her own version of Włast's transition: "in July 1907 in Poznań, on our way to a seaside resort, my sister categorically demanded masculine garments" (Ibid.: 332). Aniela judged Włast's transformation as a "demented worldview, based on erroneous assumptions and surprising associations," which required a medical intervention. However, she added that "Our faith in the effectiveness of psychological therapy, which was in fact incredibly crude at that time […] against our intentions, did not produce the recovery that we wanted so desperately, *but caused* […] *harrowing experiences* [italics mine]," which the poet related in the letter to his mother (Ibid.: 332).

In "Materials," Włast's transformation was deemed by the poet's sister "an ailment," "a demented worldview," "the wrong concept of internal and external development," "an insane hallucination" (Ibid.: 334). On June 17, 1909, Włast begged his mother to take him back from an institution for the mentally ill in Opawa:

> What do I want? – I want to be able to develop my innate capabilities in all domains of human activity. This is my will and my right. In the name of this right, I demand to leave this wretched place of a madman in this institution. *My sexual underdevelopment is not a reason to torment my soul, which is healthy and needs room for activity* [italics mine].
>
> *(Ibid.: 333)*

At the same time, Włast did not conflate his spirit with his sexuality, which sharply distinguished his idea on the relationship between the self and the sex from the turn-of-the-century norm. The dominant conviction was most fully expressed by Otto Weininger in his work *Sex and Character* (1903), in which the feminine gender was a synonym of an incomplete and unformed soul (Weininger 2005: 215–217). In a letter from June 27, 1909, Włast wrote:

> I have read your letter and noticed that many passages require a comment. The sentence: "There aren't and weren't any mysteries or peculiarities in your life" sounds simply offensive to a man who could not know that he was a man until he was 31 years old […] You are tormenting me, but you have no right to do it. This is the sad truth.
>
> *(Pigoń 1964: 333)*

At that time, Włast believed he was on his way to "masculinity and exaltation" (Ibid.: 337).

Like Judge Schreber, Włast framed his spiritual development in a narrative of a gender transgression, while at the same time inscribing his individual experience into a broader theological and historical project. In this context, Aniela Komornicka mentioned that Włast practiced "steadfast and systematic gymnastics of her limbs," believing that he would improve his "underdeveloped" body (Ibid.: 337).[2] Any attempts at intervention by doctors were perceived by the poet as physical violations and a sort of "murder on his soul" (Freud [1911] 1958: 14). In the same letter, Włast added:

> I do not understand what this is all about, what you are calling "nerves" and "balance." […] Mother, did you mean "nerves" as a synonym of SEX and "balance" as an equivalent of complete formation? – And you

> are promising me torture until I am fully *formé* – which would be very stupid. Allow me to develop myself in peace.
>
> *(Pigoń 1964: 334)*

A "confusion of tongues" arose between Włast, his family, and his doctors. In 1907, his mother and his loved ones' attitude towards Włast was an extension and reinforcement of the medical narrative on "diseased nerves" and the poet's supposed insanity. Włast's words directed at his mother are the best indication that he was aware what his family meant by psychological "balance": his sex ("as a synonym" of nerves) was reason enough to take away his freedom and condemn him to imprisonment in a series of psychiatric institutions.

The late-nineteenth-century history of psychiatry saw key changes in the approach to patients and new techniques of therapy. With a rapid development of psychiatry starting in the 1800s, the earlier asylum model, based on isolating the mentally ill from society, gradually gave way to varied therapeutic methods ("the psychotherapy period") until the second half of the twentieth century (Shorter 2005: 3; 10–11). Post-1870, institutions evolved and expanded swiftly, offering treatments for their patients' bodies and souls. In late 1907, Włast found himself in a small institution for the mentally ill called Dr. Lewaldsche Heil- und Pflegeanstalt für Nerven- und Gesuntskranke in Oborniki Śląskie (Obernigk). The poet's placement in a lock-down facility happened shortly after his announcement to his mother that his "period of femininity [had] ended" (Komornicka 2011: 375). Lewald's infirmary was founded in 1879. It functioned as an institution for the "nervously ill" until 1895, managed by Dr. Josef Löwenstein and his assistant Marian Ehrlich.[3] Włast called the institution, which housed under twenty patients at that time, "a miserable ruin" run by a "donkey" (Ibid.: 372). In 1908, his mother made the decision to transfer Włast to a private clinic in Kraków, owned by Dr. Karol Żuławski, professor of psychiatry at Jagiellonian University and head of the psychiatric ward at St. Lazarus Hospital in Kraków. The small clinic mainly attracted members of the intelligentsia and representatives of creative professions (patients included poet and painter Karol Wyspiański and Teodora Matejko, the painter Jan Matejko's wife).

From there, Włast traveled to a large institution in Opava, Moravia (Schlesische Landes-Irrenanstalt). The hospital, headed by Ernst Boeck (1857 –1924) who was assisted by Stefan Felkl, Rudolph Franz, Karl Fauster, and Alois Neumann, opened in 1889 and was continually expanded since then. In 1906, it housed 712 patients (357 men and 355 women) (Ibid.: 374). In letters to his mother from Opava, Włast wrote about his stay there as "an agonizing farce of misery" and "a lethal nightmare" (Ibid.: 376). He called Anna Komornicka, who committed him to the misery, a "shrew" (Ibid.: 377–379). As a result of his mother's cruelty, he was forced to reside "among Opavian prostitutes and pederasts" and "false women" (Ibid.: 378, 384). From what he wrote to his family, it is evident that the poet was quartered with other non-normative patients – but he did not want anything to do with them (Ibid.: 386). In one of his letters, he wrote

> as long as I was ill, you kept me *at home, but when I recovered my sound senses, you pated* [put] *me in mad houses*, where I am sowing the seeds of my fundamental health like a biblical peasant à *tous les ronts* (to all sides).
>
> *(Ibid.: 381)*

As we can conclude from the formula that appears repeatedly in his letters: "I am packed and ready to leave," the mother ignored Włast's requests. In 1910, the poet was finally discharged from Opava and transferred to a smaller institution (with just twenty-two beds at that time) in a village called Micin near Łódź. Shortly before the outbreak of the First World War, he left the institution along with the other patients. He spent the following years in his hometown of Grabów, where he led a "completely free, but lonely lifestyle" (Ibid.: 337).

The letters from institutions show that epistolographic practice was Włast's way to maintain agency and influence over reality. He wrote to his mother for her approval of his return to the family home. The poet used the form of a letter as the only available tool for defending his cause, and simultaneously an opportunity to cast himself in a significant role ("I will stand in front of you with my new Sermon on righteousness, on manhood, on the faith in Providence") (Ibid.: 378–379). In what Włast's family treated as mental illness and "the wrong concept of internal and external development," the poet saw his way to "Angelization" (Pigoń 1964: 332–337). The religious dimension of Włast's notes shows that his transition was closely linked to a mystical experience and a faith in contact with higher powers. The poet apparently understood gender as fluid and overflowing in a process of constant development. In a letter from July 27, 1909, he persuaded:

> I assure you that no diet, no pulling, no tugging, or no other torment [...] is necessary. My body would only benefit from me being able to stretch out spiritually and work. *After all, sex is a gentle beast* [...], *and it contributes to the wellbeing of the rest of the organism* [italics mine].
>
> *(Komornicka 2011: 397)*

By "tugging" and "pulling," Włast probably meant the treatment methods used in the institutions of that time, such as electrotherapy (as a remedy for neurasthenia), baths, forced bed rest, massages, inventive diets, as well as regular conversations with patients (Braslow 1997; Horwitz 2002: 37–47). The mother failed to understand these references and treated them as another piece of evidence testifying to the poet's illness. The family noticed the first symptoms of "a nervous disorder" and delusions of grandeur in Włast's 1903 letters from Paris:

> My creation reflects the wandering of my thoughts and impressions; – you will find that I am learning and developing from my writings and from when you see me [...] I must pay my respects to the Forefathers with one of whose names, the oldest, the greatest, you, dearest Mother, christened me in a moment of inspiration! – You may not yet understand the significance of that fact, the nobility of that choice [...] through your lips, the will of our entire Dynasty spoke – and I took the name from your hands upon myself and in myself, and will carry it until I die – or perhaps after I die, too – and without fault. I am yours; I am your Włast.
>
> *(Komornicka 2011: 319–320)*

According to Włast, assuming a new name was a sign of "the highest sacrifice" and was related to the establishment of a new order for humanity. For the poet, the spirit of the Dynasty whose presence filled the meaning of history was a figure of perfection understood as constant becoming. In a letter from Opava, he urged:

> I am begging you, dear Mother, please do not hesitate in guiding me out of this trap and explaining the whole secrecy around me ... UNKNOWING is NOT INSANITY and I, even if I never get to the bottom of all of this secrecy, *WILL NEVER BE A MADMAN, – even if you piled an entire heap of the most authentic "evidence" in front of me* [italics mine].
>
> *(Ibid.: 389)*

Through his identification with his greatest forbear Włast, the poet gained knowledge on his ancestry and the history of his family, which he needed for self-articulation as it lay at the foundations of his (self-)narrative strategies. Thus, the history of the individual gained a historical dimension, allowing him to "dissolve" the self in something that seemed greater. The question of the essence of the self remained at the core of Włast's self-reflection. However, from that moment on, it was permanently linked to the history of the family, the nation, and ultimately all of humanity. In the correspondence from the period of his institutionalization, this question was left unanswered. At the same time, rather than understanding self-knowledge as something one possesses, he saw it as a state which one pursues endlessly. The lack of knowledge, Włast emphasized, is not and will not be the same as madness, even with "a heap of the most authentic evidence." The poet confronted the truth of psycho-medical science voiced by his mother with a higher truth which – although unable to provide "the most authentic" evidence – manifested itself in the language of poetry and literature.

5.2 Psycho-medical images of Włast

Pigoń supplemented the family's recollections on Włast with observations by his doctor and cousin, Aleksander Oszacki (1883–1945), entitled "A confession of the misborn. Some notes on Maria Komornicka's psyche by a physician" ("Spowiedź niedorodzonej. Kilka uwag lekarza o psychice Marii Komornickiej"). Oszacki was seven years older than Włast and remembered his cousin from his childhood and early youth. He earned his medical doctorate at Jagiellonian University. In 1910–1914, he had internships in Vienna and Innsbruck, where he specialized in cardiovascular diseases. During the First World War, he worked as a doctor in the Austrian army. He was awarded habilitation at Jagiellonian University in 1920. The essay on Włast, written shortly before Oszacki's death, is the only psychographic text among the doctor's publications as he was not professionally interested in mental health (Oszacki 1925; 1929; 1930). However, writing about Włast from the perspective of a family member and physician proved to be an opportunity to construct an image of non-normative sexuality which was deeply rooted in turn-of-the-century medical case studies. As we will see, Oszacki's argument made Piotr Odmieniec Włast into a case of a masculinized woman, similarly to (Robert) Róza K. and (Sándor) Sarolta Vay – two protagonists of fin-de-siècle psycho-medical literature whom I described in Chapter 2.

Oszacki's essay constitutes an intriguing combination of a biographical narrative with philosophical reflection as well as psychiatric and psychoanalytic discourse. Importantly, Oszacki was not a Freudian and never belonged to the psychoanalytic movement. Nevertheless, in his study on Włast, he saw hope for Western culture to free itself from "excessive individualism" in "an increasing awareness of the significance of 'subconscious life'" (Pigoń 1964: 349).[4] A close reading of Oszacki's psychographic essay will allow me to look at it as a perfect example of how psychoanalytic thought infiltrated Polish medical sciences and literary criticism, even if its paths were obscured and difficult to retrace.

In extensive first part of "Materials," a biographical essay on Włast by his sister Aniela Komornicka, "Maria Komornicka in her letters and my memory" ("Maria Komornicka w swych listach i mojej pamięci"), discussed a selection of intimate correspondence with their mother, Anna Komornicka, which illustrated the poet's gradual decline into mental illness. In the second part, Pigoń presented "Three testimonies on Maria Komornicka" ("Trzy świadectwa o Marii Komornickiej"), which included Oszacki's psychographic essay, Włast's own 1937 letter to Pigoń with information on the poet's recent work, and a short recollection about Włast by Jan Komornicki. The third part contained literary-critical remarks by the poet himself. Oszacki's psychographic text was the center of Pigoń's textual archive of Włast's life and works. As we will see, it is also a representative example of the psycho-medical gaze directed at non-normative people, which was embedded in medical professionals' attitudes to queer subjects at the turn of the century.

Pigoń's strategy of combining aspects of psychographic discourse with passages of life writing (letters, memoirs, biography) situates "Materials" in a tradition of psycho-medical writing characterized by the hybridity of employed literary form and the polyphony of literary and discursive genres, which emerged in the second half of the nineteenth century. The document was met with largely critical comments. The editor was reproached for not recognizing the value in Włast's later works, which Pigoń had considered as "a sad testament to [his] ruin," while the doctor was accused of an attempt to make the poet an example of a woman's madness (Janion 2006: 186, 237, 304–395; Helbig-Mischewski 2010: 39–49).[5] Oszacki's strategy for describing Włast's psyche was nothing out of the ordinary on the map of nineteenth- and twentieth- century psychographic and psycho-medical literature developed by physicians. Psychography as a genre evolved throughout the nineteenth century. Proving medical doctors' particular interest in great artists (such as poets, writers, or painters), it discussed a potential relationship between genius and madness.[6]

Notably, none of the recent publications on Włast include an attempt to read Oszacki's essay in the broader context of psychographic writing at the turn of the nineteenth and twentieth century.[7] This sort of a close reading can help transcend the idea that psycho-medical discourse was built on a supposed opposition between the violent language of the physician and Włast's queer identity. The first stage of such a reading of his text is contextualizing the discourse used by Oszacki which feminist scholars writing on Włast considered as hurtful, pseudo-scientific, and harmful. It should be noted that images of the non-normative sexuality did not emerge out of thin air at that time, but were shaped at the intersection of medical, psychological, and psychoanalytic expertise as well as at the nexus of life writing, literary and artistic creation, and the diverse forms of gender expression visible in the public sphere. Written during World War II, the physician's essay provokes reflection on the complicated and non-linear transmission paths of knowledge on human sexuality into Polish science and – due to Pigoń's editorial work – into Polish literary criticism.

5.3 Aleksander Oszacki's notes on Włast

Stanisław Pigoń met Aleksander Oszacki in the Sachsenhausen concentration camp where both men were incarcerated as a result of the 1939 *Sonderaktion Krakau* – a Nazi action targeting Polish intelligentsia (a so-called *Intelligenzaktion*). Before the war, Oszacki enjoyed the renown of a respected scholar and professor of the Jagiellonian University. Pigoń's notes show that the people of Kraków talked much about the fame that the doctor had gained in Vienna. It was Pigoń who ultimately persuaded Oszacki to write a text about

"Komornicka's incredible personality" (Pigoń 1964: 341). The fact that Oszacki only left behind several pages of the essay, which were found posthumously along with his other notes, attests to the difficulty of the task (Ibid.: 342). Throughout the text, Oszacki referred to Włast's piece entitled *The Devils* (*Biesy*) which had been published in the monthly *Chimera* edited by Zenon Przesmycki.[8]

At that time, *Chimera* was a leading literary magazine for Polish modernists. In 1901–1907, it published works by such authors as Stanisław Wyspiański, Stanisław Przybyszewski, Stefan Żeromski, Jan Kasprowicz, Bolesław Leśmian, and Zofia Nałkowska. Włast's *The Devils* conjured a well-known figure of Romantic literature and art: the alienated individual, a misfit rejected by society, a suffering genius. The long poem also featured a key figure of fin-de-siècle literature: the lonely individualist suffering from maladjustment and rejecting bourgeois values.

In accordance with the psycho-medical literary tradition, Oszacki treated the literary work as appropriate material for examining its creator's psyche. He was especially interested in self-analytical passages which he thought revealed the secrets of Włast's psychological life:

> While looking for an example of the author's introspective self-analysis, I remembered Maria Komornicka's *Biesy*. [...] The pathological sharpness of the shapes in the personality's entire interior facilitates the identification of traits which are *much more difficult to grasp in so-called normal persons* [italics mine].
>
> *(Ibid.: 342)*

Oszacki believed that frayed nerves and a pathological personality were characteristic of creative individuals. Such a conviction guided many nineteenth-century psychiatrists who were glad to write psychological portraits of great artists.[9] Cesare Lombroso, who explored the relationship between genius and madness, was followed by people such as Paul Julius Moebius. The Leipzig-born neurologist published a series of pathographic studies on famous poets, philosophers, and composers: Jean-Jacques Rousseau, Johann Wolfgang Goethe, Arthur Schopenhauer, Friedrich Nietzsche, Robert Schumann, and others. Moebius's texts were read by the first psychoanalysts who were looking for new strategies of writing about the psychological lives of great artists. Freud's closest collaborators, such as Ernest Jones, Otto Rank, Wilhelm Stekel, Fritz Wittels, Theodor Reik, and Isidor Sadger published essays on Romantic poets: Goethe, Heinrich von Kleist, Franz Grillparzer, Friedrich Hebbel, and Conrad Ferdinand Meyer.[10]

In his influential *Psychopathia Sexualis*, Richard von Krafft-Ebing used works by the Austrian writer Leopold von Sacher-Masoch (1836–1895). The Viennese psychiatrist not only eagerly cited the writer's works and biography, but he also coined the term for the phenomenon of masochism he was interested in out of the name printed on the cover of *Venus in Furs* (1870).[11] Following that trend, Oszacki compared Włast to the Romantic poet Juliusz Słowacki and drew the following conclusions:

> For all of his powerful imagery and the unparalleled vividness and grace of Słowacki's imagination, for all of his grand artistic scale, I cannot resist a sense of a lack of something I would call: a living warmth, a pulse and richness of real life. [The same lack] can be felt in the language of *Biesy* to an even greater extent. A subtle barrier existed between the author and the material reality – which may have been made of glass, of a soap-bubble, or perhaps of a fog of stifling vapors.
>
> *(Pigoń 1964: 342)*

Oszacki believed that Włast's writings lacked "warmth" and "the richness of real life" (Ibid.: 324). In the poet's work, he detected "a fog of stifling vapors," which had supposedly prevented Włast from having "an emotional approach to people" and condemned him to "a martyr's path" (Ibid.: 342, 346). Oszacki treated Włast's writing as part of the poet's introspection and added:

> It is the matter of the era in which she lived that she was guided by the light of Nietzscheanism in her self-analytic enterprise, and held the scalpel of the somatism and determinism of natural sciences in her hand.
>
> *(Ibid.: 342)*

Moreover, he compared the poet's reclusive lifestyle to the worldview of such playwrights as August Strindberg and Henrik Ibsen, accusing them of "excessive individualism" (Ibid.: 349). Oszacki's understanding of modernity as an aggregate of subjectivism and individualism stemmed from the beliefs of turn-of-the-century philosophers, sociologists, and writers. Friedrich Nietzsche, Georg Simmel, Sigmund Freud, Thomas Mann, Robert Musil, Stanisław Brzozowski, Stanisław Przybyszewski, and Piotr Odmieniec Włast were hearing a painful dissonance between the individual and society. In this spirit, *The Devils* drew out key tropes of fin-de-siècle literature, such as loneliness, feeling misunderstood, and frayed nerves.

In *The Devils*, Włast wrote from a position of a wretched genius about an existence filled with anxiety and suffering (Pigoń 1964: 344). According to Oszacki, the poet's recurring opposition of the outstanding individual against a nameless crowd was proof of "the pathological premises of the author's being." As Gustave Le Bon argued in *The Crowd: A Study in Popular Mind* (1895), the "unconscious action of crowds" began dominating over "the conscious activity of individuals" (Le Bon 2001: 7–8).[12] In Włast's *The Devils*, the crowd, ever unthinking and unfeeling, destroys the artist's sensitive psyche: "The indifference of the crowd affected my frayed nerves [...] destroying my sense of value and power" (Pigoń 1964: 343). The experience of his own estrangement from the crowd resulted in a hatred against "one's own being" – a state that Oszacki quickly associated with Włast's supposed "infantilism" and a "paranoid attitude" (Ibid.: 343, 344).

The tradition of the psychological analysis of literary works was present in Polish literature as early as in the second half of the nineteenth century. The work of art was perceived as a record of human suffering by the prominent psychologist and inventor Julian Ochorowicz, who – in his *Poetry as Viewed by Psychology* (*Twórczość poetycka ze stanowiska psychologii*) – analyzed "the psychological conditioning" of great artists (Ochorowicz 1877; 1914). Ochorowicz assumed that poetic works are intended first and foremost as "the exploration of the depths of the human soul," and therefore constitute a self-analytic activity from their very inception. At the same time, apart from art or literature, Ochorowicz also read the same introspective dimension into scientific work. He argued: "everything we admire in art and science is a product of that spiritual workshop which can only be entered by the priest, the poet and… the psychologist" (Ochorowicz 1914: 4). Many years later, Oszacki operated on the same assumption as he searched for "the psychological conditioning" of Piotr Odmieniec Włast.

Oszacki inherited the belief on poetry as a "sequence of internal metamorphoses" from nineteenth-century psychologists who contended that a literary work opens up the space of its author's "unending internal struggle" to the reader (Ibid.: 9). Some Polish modernist authors, including Stanisław Przybyszewski, thought along the same lines. In *My Contemporaries* (*Moi współcześni*), the writer asserted that any work can be read as the effect of its author's emotional experiences:

> I could seem too jovial in imagining my spirit's path in its various essences: on the contrary! I live by all of these spirits until this very day – and I live by a thousand of other souls, […] and the capacity to advance one soul against the other, to juggle them like a juggler juggles wood saws, the capacity to live first in this soul, and then another … indeed, this constitutes a creator – this is the secret of his creative power.
>
> *(Przybyszewski 1926: 5–6)*

In Przybyszewski's eyes, literature is a site of the potentiality of experience in its infinite variety. The role of the writer-creator consists in developing a work which will become "a reality more genuine than reality itself" (Ibid.: 6).

These remarks from *My Contemporaries* resemble Freud's earlier assertions in "Creative Writers and Day-Dreaming" (1908) in many ways. Although the reflection on psychology of creative writing itself surprised few at the turn of the century, in 1908 Freud introduced a new perspective on thinking about the psychological mechanisms of the creative process. While Ochorowicz and Przybyszewski were convinced about the innateness of a particular emotionality to poets, Freud suggested that creative sensibilities are universal. The poet has an element of a child in him, while the child manifests traits and behaviors which are typical of a creator. Such an assumption allowed Freud to associate the creative act with child's play:

> The creative writer does the same as the child at play. He creates a world of phantasy which he takes very seriously – that is, which he invests with large amounts of emotion – while separating it sharply from reality. Language has preserved this relationship between children's play and poetic creation. It gives [in German] the name of "*Spiel*" ["play"] to those forms of imaginative writing which require to be linked to tangible objects and which are capable of representation. It speaks of a "*Lustspiel*" or "*Trauerspiel*" ["comedy" or "tragedy": literally, "pleasure play" or "mourning play"] and describes those who carry out the representation as "*Schauspieler*" ["players": literally "show-players"].
>
> *(Freud [1908] 1959a: 144)*

Freud made a clear distinction between reality and the world of fantasy and play. Conversely, for many modernist writers – including Przybyszewski and Włast – the creative process was far from innocent play or pleasure derived from day-dreaming. In *The Psychology of a Creative Individual* (*Z Psychologii jednostki twórczej*), Przybyszewski wrote: "in the painful tension of his defective nerves, the afflicted creative individual rises all the way up to that mysterious frontier where joy and sorrow transcend from one into the other in human life" (Przybyszewski [1892] 1966: 7). Thus, suffering and living in a constant "painful [nervous] tension" is the great artist's baseline experience according to Przybyszewski (Ibid.: 7).

In his essay, Oszacki decidedly followed Przybyszewski's intuitions, shared by nineteenth-century psychographers. Meanwhile, in the second part of "A confession of the misborn," he developed his reflection on Włast's "illness" and "persecutory mania." Although Oszacki did not make direct references to Freud's writings and replaced the term "psychoanalysis" with "the study of the subconscious," his considerations intersect with the early psychoanalytical understanding of androgyny, female masculinity, and non-normative sexuality.

5.4 Aleksander Oszacki's psychographic fever

Oszacki began his analysis with the following diagnosis: he believed that Włast was "of infantile nature" (Pigoń 1964: 348) which manifested itself in the incomplete development of "feminine" traits such as emotionality and intuition (Ibid.: 346). Having attributed egotism to Włast, Oszacki added that the poet's self was "lit […] with the bright shine of a paranoiac attitude to her introspective interior" (Ibid.: 345). In Włast's case, self-analysis supposedly led to a "persecutory mania" rather than to self-discovery. Włast was "a misfit" in whom pathological immaturity coincided with excessive individualism and the "sexlessness" of the soul:

> [There is a] lack of any sexual properties in this strange personality. Had it not been for the feminine grammatical form of verbs and nouns, no one would be able to suspect *Biesy*'s author of the femininity of their soul. So sexless, or rather so "masculine," is she in the dryness and rationality of every concept. The lack of the feminine element compounds her incapability of an emotional approach to people all the more strongly.
>
> *(Ibid.: 346)*

Włast chose *masculine* action over *feminine* feeling. Oszacki's attention was drawn precisely by the passage in *The Devils* where the protagonist described the desire for the constant pursuit of life as her "bounty [...] never won forever," her "idol" (Ibid.: 347). In Włast's 1902 piece, the category of "life" encompassed the entire wealth of human experience and was contrasted with the misfit's estrangement. Oszacki read *The Devils* as nothing but Włast's confession:

> The "life": sex, family, "others," and "things" – everything stood around her, but it was separated with a glass wall which was cast out of her "misbirth": her deficiencies, her atonement for the overgrowth of intellect, for which she paid with the underdevelopment of the other parts of her soul, her infantilism which precluded the harmonious fullness of life, although it has already given the world so many geniuses and one-sided talents... and, so often, at the price of a tragic, premature end.
>
> *(Ibid.: 347)*

Oszacki limited the life that the poet described to his gender and family. Interestingly, earlier in his essay, the doctor interpreted the modernist *Biesy* through Friedrich Nietzsche's philosophy and the vitalist notion of life as an unbridled creative force. Ultimately, he reduced that to Włast's gender, which also became a suspect category for Oszacki. "The Misbirthed" is someone who is not alive, lost in the abyss of her own intellect and distanced from people. While Oszacki did not mention Włast's sexual orientation directly, the idea of "being unable to love" in accordance with "feminine" nature recurs in his essay. As an "infantile" individual with a "sexless" soul, Włast was perceived by Oszacki as a woman who lacked "greenery, the scent of flowers, and most of all, she lacked smile and lyricism" (Ibid.: 346).

The poet's psychological portrait by Oszacki corresponds with Freud's study on an eighteen-year-old homosexual patient (Margarethe Csonka/Sidonie Csillag). In his "The psychogenesis of a case of homosexuality in a woman" (1920), Freud wrote:

> A spirited girl, always ready for romping and fighting [...]; she had developed *a pronounced envy for the penis*, and the thoughts derived from this envy still continued to fill her mind. *She was in fact a feminist*; she felt it to be unjust that girls should not enjoy the same freedom as boys, and rebelled against the lot of woman in general [italics mine].
>
> *(Freud [1920] 1955c: 169)*

Like young Komornicka, Freud's patient longed for the freedom which was then only available to men. However, Freud believed that in order to achieve her goal, she needed to *become* masculine. He argued:

> Some of her intellectual attributes also could be connected with masculinity: for instance, her acuteness of comprehension and her lucid objectivity, in so far as she was not dominated by her passion. But these distinctions are conventional rather than scientific. What is certainly of greater importance is that in her behaviour towards her love-object she had throughout assumed the masculine part.
>
> *(Ibid.: 154)*

In Freud's eyes, the patient was a suffragette and a woman who loved in a "wholly masculine way." Although the analyst noticed to a certain extent that categories such as "masculinity" or "femininity" were constructed, he treated her lesbian love and the desire to free herself from underneath her father's authority as a symptom of "penis envy" and the patient's internal conflict.[13] In turn-of-the-century psycho-medical discourses – which relied on an evolutionary notion of human development – homosexuality was often equated with infantilism and androgyny.

In the second half on the nineteenth century, physicians investigated "cases" of hermaphroditism with increasing interest (Mak 2013: 165–166, 172–176). In 1908, Franz (Franciszek) Ludwig van Neugebauer (1856–1914) published a comprehensive study *Hermaphroditism in Humans* (*Hermaphroditismus beim Menschen*), where he collected 1,257 cases of hermaphroditism (Mak 2013: 3–5).[14] The diversity in case studies made it difficult to write a consistent definition of hermaphroditism. While in the 1800s medical professionals investigated the person's body for signs of the doubting sex, turn-of-the-century psycho-medical literature introduced a new concept: psychologic hermaphroditism ("der psychische Hermaphroditismus") perceived as a form of androgyny. Richard von Krafft-Ebing was also interested in cases of women living as men. He wrote in *Psychopathia Sexualis*:

> individuals of antipathic sexuality in whom not only the character and all the feelings are in accord with the abnormal sexual instinct, but also the frame, the features, voice, etc.; so that the individual approaches the opposite sex anthropologically, and in more than a psychical and psycho-

> sexual way. This anthropological form of the cerebral anomaly apparently represents a very high degree of degeneration; but that this variation is based on an entirely different ground than the terotological manifestation of hermaphroditism, in an anatomical sense, is clearly shown by the fact that thus far, in the domain of inverted sexuality, no transitions to hermaphroditic malformation of the genitals have been observed.
>
> *(Krafft-Ebing 2011: 492)*

Even though, after Valentin Magnan, Krafft-Ebing described hermaphroditism as an anomaly, he also devoted much space to cases of psychological hermaphroditism that he illustrated using the example of the Hungarian aristocrat and poet Sarolta/Sándor Vay's life story, which was well-known at the time (case 166) (Ibid.: 539).[15] As proof of Vay's masculinity, Krafft-Ebing cited his penchant for "masculine sports," independent travel, frequent café visits, as well as "a wholly masculine" love for women (Ibid.: 540–542).

In 1920, Freud could not help but comment on the conflation of hermaphroditism with homosexuality which he observed in psycho-medical writing. In a polemic with earlier claims, he stressed:

> The literature of homosexuality usually *fails to distinguish clearly enough between the questions of the choice of object on the one hand, and of the sexual characteristics and sexual attitude of the subject on the other, as though the answer to the former necessarily involved the answer to the latter.* […] The mystery of homosexuality is therefore by no means so simple as it is commonly depicted in popular expositions – "a feminine mind bound therefore to love a man, but unhappily attached to a masculine body; a masculine mind, irresistibly attracted by women, but alas! imprisoned in a feminine […] body" [italics mine].
>
> *(Freud [1920] 1955e: 170)*

The emphasis on the close ties between the dynamics of desire and a person's individual history (their childhood and relationships with their loved ones) allowed Freud to present a critical view of the dynamics between the subject and object of desire.

As early as 1905, Freud associated hermaphroditism and androgyny. At the time when Oszacki wrote his essay, selected works by Freud had already been available in Polish translation for years. In 1911, Freud's *Five Lectures on Psycho-Analysis* given in the United States were published in Polish translation; two years later, it was *The Psychopathology of Everyday Life* (Psychopatologia życia codziennego) (1913), then *On Dreams* (O marzeniu sennem) (1923) and *Three Essays on the Theory of Sexuality* (Trzy rozprawy z teorii seksualnej) in 1924, *Introduction to Psychoanalysis* (Wstęp do psychoanalizy) in 1935, and *An Autobiographical Study* (Wizerunek własny) in 1936. Just a year later, the medical printing house "Eskulap" published a multi-volume

Encyclopedia of Sexual Knowledge edited by Stanisław Higier (1894–1942) and Max Marcuse (1877–1963). In addition, Oszacki spoke German fluently, so he could have familiarized himself with Freud's and other German authors' publications as they came out.

In *Three Essays on the Theory of Sexuality*, Freud argued that "inversion and somatic hermaphroditism are on the whole independent of each other" (Freud [1905] 1953: 142). In the same book, he added:

> It is popularly believed that a human being is either a man or a woman. Science, however, knows of cases in which the sexual characters are obscured, and in which it is consequently difficult to determine the sex. [...] The importance of these abnormalities lies in the unexpected fact that they facilitate our understanding of normal development.
>
> *(Ibid.: 141–142)*

For Freud, reflections on the doubting sex also proved to be an opportunity to point to the universal character of human ambisexuality ("For it appears that a certain degree of anatomical hermaphroditism occurs normally") (Ibid.: 141). Referring to the concept of natural bisexuality as simultaneously developed by Wilhelm Fliess, Herman Swoboda, and Otto Weininger, Freud saw the human being as a hybrid composed of the masculine and the feminine element. Just three years later, the psychoanalyst repeated his assumptions on the bisexual disposition, this time in juxtaposition with day-dreaming and the structure of human thinking. In "Hysterical Fancies and Their Relations to Bisexuality," he wrote "To resolve it one has to have *two* sexual phantasies, of which one has a masculine and the other a feminine character" (Freud [1908] 1959a: 164). Stressing the significance of the bisexual meaning of symptoms, Freud inscribed bisexuality into the very structure of human thinking. The evolutionary model of human psycho-sexual development returned in "Female Sexuality." After Helene Deutsch, Freud argued: "Their sexual life is regularly divided into two phases, of which the first has a masculine character, while only the second is specifically feminine" (Freud [1931] 1961a: 228; Deutsch 1932: 219–241). As early as in "The psychogenesis of a case of homosexuality in a woman," the psychoanalyst associated infantilism – understood as psycho-sexual underdevelopment – with *masculine* rationality which was superior to *feminine* emotionality as well as with his patient's emancipatory struggle. In the conclusion, he stated: "the girl had brought along with her from her childhood a strongly marked 'masculinity complex'" (Freud [1920] 1955e: 169).

The tension between images of female masculinity and notions of effeminacy at the turn of the twentieth century occupied a key space in the psychoanalytic discourse (Boyarin 1995: 117–147). In the case of his homosexual patient, Freud wrote about her assuming an active (male) position which was inconsistent with her physical sex. The reversal of his patient's psychological shift from the feminine to the masculine was described by Freud in "Psycho-Analytic Notes on an Autobiographical Account of a Case of Paranoia." Freud interpreted Schreber's fantasies as follows:

> The most essential part of his mission of redemption is that it must be preceded by his *transformation into a woman.* [...] The psycho-analyst, in the light of his knowledge of the psychoneuroses, approaches the subject with a suspicion that even thought-structures so extraordinary as these and so remote from our common modes of thinking are nevertheless derived from the most general and comprehensible impulses of the human mind; [...]. For we learn that the idea of being transformed into a woman (that is, of being emasculated) was the primary delusion, that he began by regarding that act as constituting a serious injury and persecution, and that it only became related to his playing the part of Redeemer in a secondary way. *There can be no doubt, moreover, that originally he believed that the transformation was to be effected for the purpose of sexual abuse and not so as to serve higher designs* [italics mine].
>
> *(Freud [1911] 1958: 16–18)*

Freud understood the desire to become a woman as the patient's assuming a passive position towards another man. In the second part of the study, he contended:

> We shall therefore, I think, raise no further objections to the hypothesis that the exciting cause of the illness was the appearance in him of a feminine (that is, a passive homosexual) wishful phantasy, which took as its object the figure of his doctor. An intense resistance to this phantasy arose on the part of Schreber's personality, and the ensuing defensive struggle, which might perhaps just as well have assumed some other shape, took on, for reasons unknown to us, that of a delusion of persecution.
>
> *(Ibid.: 47)*

Freud explained the desire for sexual intercourse with God through Judge Schreber's repressed homosexual desire ("Thus in the case of Schreber we find ourselves once again on the familiar ground of the father-complex. The patient's struggle with Flechsig became revealed to him as a conflict with God, and we must therefore construe it as an infantile conflict with the father whom he loved") (Ibid.: 55). Interestingly, the analyst repeated that argument in 1920, writing about his female patient:

> This libidinal position of the girl's, thus arrived at, was greatly reinforced as soon as she perceived how much it displeased her father. After she had been punished for her over-affectionate attitude to a woman she realized

> how she could wound her father and take revenge on him. *Henceforth she remained homosexual out of defiance against her father* [italics mine].
> *(Freud [1920] 1955e: 159)*

Whereas Freud symbolically associated Schreber's case with loss (castration), his patient became a figure of the phallic woman (masculinity=penis envy) and at the same time a synonym of aspirations and ambitions which women were prevented from having. An analogous interpretative dynamic can be found in Oszacki's psychography. Writing about Włast, Oszacki read infantilism into both in the poet's appearance and his "spiritual constitution" (Pigoń 1964: 346). "Short, slim, petite," Włast tried to liberate himself from the limits that his environment imposed on him: "The struggle for herself, for her 'self' as early as this, must have also been conducted firmly on her part" (Ibid.: 346).[16] However, as a result of her innate (over)sensitivity and reading "inappropriate" books ("Nietzsche's era was able to express [...] egocentrism"), Włast fell victim to "a persecutory mania." It is no coincidence that Oszacki's psychographic essay links the poet's personality traits to paranoia. "The Misborn" becomes a case of female masculinity, which at the turn of the century found its negative in the effeminate, passive man.[17]

5.5 Conclusion

The 1964 publication of Oszacki's essay and the fragments of Włast's correspondence introduced the letters to his mother into the field of Polish literary criticism as well as Polish psycho-medical literature.[18] The poet's voice, which was initially addressed privately to Anna Komornicka, gained a public dimension in "Materials" as it became a platform for expressing dissent against oppressive psycho-medical practices. Starting in the mid-nineteenth century, the field of anti-psychiatric literature encompassed works published by the authors under their own name (such as Schreber's *Memoirs of My Nervous Illness*); biographical fragments presented anonymously or under a pseudonym, first given to psychiatrists by their patients, and then printed as part of their treatises (such as Krafft-Ebing's *Psychopathia Sexualis*); and quasi-literary texts directed against psycho-medical discourses (e.g. André Gide's *Corydon*).

One distinguishing feature of such works – which were most often fragmentary and reached the wider public only after interference by the psychiatrist-editor – was a polemic against the psycho-medical theories and discourses of that time which were aimed at demonstrating, describing, and interpreting non-normative gender and sexual expression. Pigoń's "Materials," which are situated at the intersection of psycho-medical literature and literary criticism, allow us to take a close look at a clash of conflicting discourses in life writing, psychoanalysis, and psychiatry as well as literary criticism. After many years of silence, the publication created a space for the emergence of a hybrid (self-)portrait of a modernist poet, with one indispensable component being the anti-psychiatric voice of Włast himself. As I will show in the next chapter, autobiographical strategies suspended between impersonal and personal discourses were at the center of psychoanalytic literature after the Great War. At the same time, writing about one's queer sexuality in the field of psychoanalysis involved new self-writing strategies, which developed at the intersection of lifewriting genres, psychoanalytic theory, and literary modernism.

Notes

1 Because Polish nouns and verbs have gendered endings, an important linguistic layer of the decades-long scientific and personal discussion on Włast's gender is lost in translation. It is worth noting that as a rule, Włast's contemporaries, his family, and early scholars used feminine endings when referring to him; some recent scholars have attempted to include both kinds of endings using parentheses or slashes, while Włast himself used mostly masculine endings after his transition.

2 Cf. Schreber's explanation: "human shapes set down for a short time by divine miracles only to be dissolved again," in Daniel Paul Schreber, *Memoirs of My Nervous Illness*, trans. Ida Macalpine and Richard A. Hunter (New York: NYRB New York Review Books, 2000), 43.

3 On the rapid development of institutions and clinics for the mentally ill in German-speaking countries, see e.g. *A Historical Dictionary of Psychiatry*, 3–16.

4 Even the word "psychoanalysis" did not appear often in Polish psychiatric literature starting in the 1960s. The perfect example is the work by Jan Malewski and Michał Łapiński entitled *Nerves and Psychotherapy* (*Nerwice i psychoterapia*), published in 1971, see: *Jak feniks z popiołów? Odradzanie się psychoanalizy w powojennej i dzisiejszej Polsce*, ed. Ewa Kobylińska-Dehe and Katarzyna Prot-Klinger, (Kraków: Universitas, 2021), 5. According to Ewa Kobylińska-Dehe and Katarzyna Prot-Klinger, apprehension concerning Sigmund Freud's discipline in countries of the Eastern Bloc stemmed from it being widely considered as a "bourgeois relic." Still, recent research on the reception of psychoanalysis in Polish lands has shown that Freud and his collaborators' thought, though officially absent, has left a mark on Polish culture.

5 Janion's critical opinion was supported by younger researchers: Izabela Filipiak and Brigitta Helbig-Mischewski. Filipiak assessed Pigoń's initiative as harmful to the poet, while Helbig-Mischewski attributed insincere intentions or even a need for cheap sensationalism to the editor. Meanwhile, Karolina Krasuska, the author of the most recent study on Włast, has not even mentioned Pigoń's document.

6 Pathographies, which were especially popular at that time, consisted in a combination of a biographical narrative with the author's contemporary psychiatric knowledge. Works by Sigmund Freud's close collaborator in Vienna Isidor Sadger (1867–1942) on people such as Friedrich Hebbel or Conrad Ferdinand Meyer were a good example of the continuation of pathographic writing in the twentieth century.

7 A partial attempt to reconstruct late-nineteenth-century sexological discourses was made by Izabela Filipiak, see I. Filipiak, *Obszary odmienności* (Gdańsk: Słowo/obraz terytoria, 2006); however, her discussion on theories of non-normative sexuality took only six pages out of her almost-six-hundred-page book (293–297). At the same time, her statement that "at the turn of century a female artist who desires to define her identity and believes she is not 'a real woman' is presented with the choice between 'the third sex' or 'degeneration.' Attempting to retain a bit

of respect for herself, she chooses 'the third sex' and accepts the idea that a male mind and soul live in her body" (297) is an extreme oversimplification and a failure to notice the multitude of identity models and gender expressions developed by nineteenth-century culture. For more on that, see Jack Halberstam's seminal book (whose first edition was published eight years before Filipiak's work) *Female Masculinity* (Durham: Duke University Press, 1998).

8 The poem *The Devils* (*Biesy*) was published in 1902 (*Chimera*, vol. 5, no. 13 and 14). Later, in 1903, it appeared as a separate book.

9 The beginnings of the biographical portraits of great artists which tied their general personality and life experiences to their works can be traced back to Giorgio Vasari's *The Lives of the Artists*, first published in 1550. An interest in the lives of famous figures was also expressed earlier by Plutarch in his *Parallel Lives* in the second century CE.

10 Nineteenth-century psychographic writing significantly contributed to the increasing psychologization of "cases" described by doctors which had previously been treated solely as evidence of illness and degeneration. As has been stressed by multiple scholars, the psychiatric institution in the nineteenth century worked closely with policing institutions, linking sexual "perversion" to criminality. However, the biographical narrative forced doctors to shift from the oversimplified image of "punishable" acts by "sick" individuals to the reconstruction of their protagonists' lives. In their attempts to create psychological portraits of their cases, psychiatrists readily relied on lifewriting, especially autobiographical essays which gave them unique insight into their patients' intimate experiences.

11 Krafft-Ebing explained his decision in these words: "I feel justified in calling this sexual anomaly 'Masochism,' because the author Sacher-Masoch frequently made this perversion, which up to his time was quite unknown to the scientific world as such, the substratum of his writings. I followed thereby the scientific formation of the term 'Daltonism,' from Dalton, the discoverer of colour-blindness. During recent years facts have been advanced which prove that Sacher-Masoch was not only the poet of Masochism, but that he himself was afflicted with this anomaly," R. Krafft-Ebing, *Psychopathia Sexualis* (New York: Arkade, 2011), 198; cf. the psychoanalysis of Sacher-Masoch's case by Gilles Deleuze, "Coldness and Cruelty," in *Masochism* (Princeton: Zone Books, 2011), 15–138.

12 Cf. Freud, "Group Psychology and the Analysis of Ego," in The St*andard Edition of the Complete Psychological Works of Sigmund Freud*, Vol. 18, ed. J. Strachey (London: The Hogarth Press, 1955), 72–81.

13 On the anti-feminism and homophobic discourse in the late nineteenth century, see Anne Fausto-Sterling, *Sexing the Body* (New York: Basic Books, 2020).

14 Franz Ludwig van Neugebauer (1856–1914) was a Polish-German physician and Freud's peer. He was born in Polish land and worked in the Evangelical hospital in Warsaw.

15 See: Chapter 2, 71–75.

16 On the shifting understanding of the relationship between physical and mental illness, and the body as a site where symptoms of mental conditions can reveal themselves, see Katja Guenther, *Localization and Its Discontents: A Genealogy of Psychoanalysis and the Neuro Disciplines* (Chicago-London: The University of Chicago Press, 2015), 5–8; 13–23.

17 On the close ties between fin-de-siècle culture and a crisis of gender, the masculine/feminine binary and an increasing fear of effeminacy, see Jacques Le Rider, *Le cas Otto Weininger. Racines de l'antiféminisme et de l'antisémitisme* (Paris: Presses Universitaires de France, 1982); Misha Kavka, "*The Alluring Abyss of Nothingness*: Misogyny and (Male) Hysteria in Otto Weininger," *New German Critique* 66 (1995): 123–145; Chandak Sengoopta, "The Unknown Weininger: Science, Philosophy, and Cultural Politics in Fin-de-Siècle Vienna," *Central European History*

vol. 29, no. 4 (1996): 453–493; Susan C. Anderson, "Otto Weininger's Masculine Utopia," *German Studies Review* vol. 19, no. 3 (1996): 433–453.

18 For comparison, it is worth noting that a publication of Włast's 1908–1914 correspondence edited by Edward Boniecki included twenty-six letters sent to Anna Komornicka from Obornik, Kraków, Opava, and Micin, while in the 1964 *Archiwum Literackie* Stanisław Pigoń was only able to print short passages from eight letters from that period with the permission of Aniela Komornicka.

References

Amenta, A., Kaliściak, T., & Warkocki, B. (Eds.) (2021). *Dezorientacje. Antologia polskiej literatury queer*, Warszawa: Wydawnictwo Krytyki Politycznej.

Anderson, S. C. (1996). Otto Weininger's Masculine Utopia, in *German Studies Review* 19 (3), 433–453.

Braslow, J. (1997). *Mental Ills and Bodily Cures: Psychiatric Treatment in the First Half of the Twentieth Century*, Berkeley: University of California Press.

Chmurski, M. (2015). Trans/figuracje nowoczesności? Spory o twórczość Marii Komornickiej-Piotra Odmieńca Własta, in *Poznańskie Studia Polonistyczne. Seria Literacka* 26 (46), 395–419.

Deleuze, G. (2011). *Masochism*, Princeton: Zone Books.

Dernałowicz, M. (1977). Piotr Odmieniec Włast, in *Twórczość* 3, 75–88.

Deutsch, H. (1932). Über die weibliche Homosexualität, in *Internationale Zeitschrift für Psychoanalyse* 18 (2), 219–241.

Fausto-Sterling, A. (2020). *Sexing the Body*, New York: Basic Books.

Filipiak, I. (2006). *Obszary odmienności*, Gdańsk: Słowo/obraz terytoria.

Freud, S. ([1905] 1953). Three Essays on the Theory of Sexuality, in J. Strachey (Ed.), *The Standard Edition of the Complete Psychological Works of Sigmund Freud.* Vol. 7, London: The Hogarth Press, 125–245.

Freud, S. ([1921] 1955c). Group Psychology and the Analysis of Ego, in J. Strachey (Ed.), *The Standard Edition of the Complete Psychological Works of Sigmund Freud*, Vol. 18, London: The Hogarth Press, 65–144.

Freud, S. ([1920] 1955c). The psychogenesis of a case of homosexuality in a woman, in J. Strachey (Ed.), *The Standard Edition of the Complete Psychological Works of Sigmund Freud.* Vol. 18, London: The Hogarth Press, 145–172.

Freud, S. ([1911] 1958). Psycho-Analytic Notes on an Autobiographical Account of a Case of Paranoia, in J. Strachey (Ed.), *The Standard Edition of the Complete Psychological Works of Sigmund Freud.* Vol. 12, London: The Hogarth Press, 1–82.

Freud, S. ([1908] 1959a). Hysterical Phantasies and their Relation to Bisexuality, in J. Strachey (Ed.), *The Standard Edition of the Complete Psychological Works of Sigmund Freud.* Vol. 9, London: The Hogarth Press, 155–156.

Freud, S. ([1908] 1959b). Creative Writers and Day-Dreaming, in J. Strachey (Ed.), *The Standard Edition of the Complete Psychological Works of Sigmund Freud.* Vol. 9, 141–154.

Freud, S. ([1931] 1961b). Female Sexuality, in J. Strachey (Ed.), *The Standard Edition of the Complete Psychological Works of Sigmund Freud.* Vol. 21, London: The Hogarth Press, 221–244.

Guenther, K. (2015). *Localization and Its Discontents: A Genealogy of Psychoanalysis and the Neuro Disciplines*, Chicago/London: The University of Chicago Press.

Halberstam, J. (1998). *Female Masculinity*, New York/London: Duke University Press.

Halperin, D. M. (2002). *How to Do the History of Homosexuality*, Chicago/London: The University of Chicago Press.
Helbig-Mischewski, B. (2010). *Strącona bogini*, Kraków: Universitas.
Horwitz, A. V. (2002). *Creating Mental Illness*, Chicago: University of Chicago Press.
Janion, M. (2006). *Kobiety i duch inności*, Warszawa: Sic!.
Kavka, M. (1995). The Alluring Abyss of Nothingness: Misogyny and (Male) Hysteria in Otto Weininger, in *New German Critique* 66, 123–145.
Kobylińska-Dehe, E. & Prot-Klinger, K. (Eds.) (2021). *Jak feniks z popiołów? O odradzaniu się psychoanalizy w powojennej i dzisiejszej Polsce*, Kraków: Universitas.
Komornicka, M. (1902). Biesy, in *Chimera* 5 (13–14).
Komornicka, M. (2011). *Listy*, Warszawa: Muzeum Historyczne Warszawy.
Krafft-Ebing, R. von (2011). *Psychopathia Sexualis*, New York: Arcade Publishing.
Krasuska, K. (2012). *Płeć i naród: Trans/lokacje. Maria Komornicka/Piotr Odmieniec Włast, Else Lasker-Schuler, Mina Loy*, Warszawa: Instytut Badań Literackich PAN.
Le Bon, G. (2001). *The Crowd: A Study in Popular Mind*, Kitchener: Batoche Books.
Le Rider, J. (1982). *Le cas Otto Weininger. Racines de l'antiféminisme et de l'antisémitisme*, Paris: Presses Universitaires de France.
Mak, G. (2013). *Doubting Sex: Inscriptions, Bodies and Selves in Nineteenth-century Hermaphrodite Case Histories*, Manchester: Manchester University Press.
Ochorowicz, J. (1877). *Twórczość poetycka ze stanowiska psychologii*, Lwów: Nakładem K. Wilda.
Ochorowicz, J. (1914). *Liryczna twórczość poetów. Szkic psychologiczny*, Warszawa: Biblioteka Dzieł Wyborowych.
Oszacki, A. (1925). *Choroby przemiany materii i energii u człowieka. Podstawy nauki o metabolizmie. Fizjopatologia tycia i chudnięcia, kliniczne postacie otyłości i chudości*, Kraków: Polska Akademia Umiejętności.
Oszacki, A. (1929). *Wymiana gazowa, jej teoria i zastosowanie kliniczne*, Kraków: Wydawnictwo Chirurgia Kliniczna.
Oszacki, A. (1930). *Über den Sauerstoffgehalt des Blutes bei Sarkomgeschwülsten*, Kraków: Polska Akademia Umiejętności.
Pigoń, S. (Ed.) (1964). Materiały dotyczące biografii i twórczości Marii Komornickiej, in *Archiwum Literackie* 8.
Przybyszewski, S. (1926). *Moi współcześni. Wśród obcych*, Warszawa: Instytut Wydawniczy Biblioteka Polska.
Przybyszewski, S. (1966). Z psychologii jednostki twórczej, in *Wybór pism*, Wrocław: Zakład Narodowy im. Ossolińskich.
Schreber, D. P. (2000). *Memoirs of My Nervous Illness*. Translated by Ida Macalpine & Richard A. Hunter, New York: NYRB New York Review Books.
Sengoopta, C. (1996). The Unknown Weininger: Science, Philosophy, and Cultural Politics in Fin-de-Siècle Vienna, in *Central European History* 29 (4), 453–493.
Shorter, E. (2005). *A Historical Dictionary of Psychiatry*, Oxford: Oxford University Press.
Weininger, O. (2005). *Sex and Character: An Investigation of Fundamental Principles*. Translated by Ladislaus Löb. Bloomington: Indiana University Press.

6

FREUD'S QUEER FELLOW

Georg Groddeck between psychoanalytic theory and literary modernism

German physician Georg Groddeck (1866–1934) was likely one of Sigmund Freud's most intriguing disciples.[1] Over the past four decades his writings have caught the attention of psychoanalysts and researchers involved in psychoanalytic circles. Apart from two biographies (Grossman & Grossman 1978; Martynkewicz 1997), a philosophical essay by Roger Lewinter (1974), two books: *Georg Groddeck. Psychanalyste de l'imaginaire* by Jacquy Chemouni (1984) and *Georg Groddeck. Präsentationsformen psychoanalytischen Wissens* by Galina Hristeva (2008), Groddeck's concept of the unconscious would become the subject of a significant number of studies on the genealogy and meaning of his concept of the unconscious (Grotjahn 1945: 9–24; Nitzschke 1983: 769–804; Will 1985: 150–169; Biancoli 1997: 117–125; Rudnytsky 2002: 141–206; Giefer 2008: 75–78; Poster, Hristeva & Giefer 2016: 161–182).[2] In this chapter, I propose an analysis of Groddeck's literary works, which would connect insights on the impact of his theoretical considerations on Freud with broader reflection on the relationship between Groddeck's writings and interwar literary trends at large.

Soon after the end of the First World War, Groddeck published two novels: *The Soul Seeker: A Psychoanalytical Novel* (*Der Seelensucher. Ein psychoanalytischer Roman*) (1921) and *The Book of the It* (*Das Buch vom Es*) (1923). The decision to present his theory in the literary form can be treated as a direct reaction to a paradigm shift in psychiatric writing (especially in classic case studies), which was brought about by psychoanalysis at the turn of the twentieth century. In their early-twentieth-century psychoanalytic case studies, Freud and his students created a new narrative framework for their patients' stories (Sealey 2011: 36–50; Makari 2008). While earlier psychiatrists – such as Richard von Krafft-Ebing and Havelock Ellis – took their patients' stories at face value, Freud was more inclined to believe that each statement had a

DOI: 10.4324/9781003441892-7

layer of hidden meaning. In his view, each confession concealed traces of unconscious processes (Lang & Sutton 2016: 421–422). Therefore, anything that patient said had to be treated with suspicion and vigilance of repressed wishes and fantasies.[3]

At the same time, psychoanalytic case studies – starting from the early *Studies on Hysteria*, and followed by lengthy descriptions of Dora, Little Hans, Daniel Paul Schreber, the Wolf Man, and the Rat Man – resembled literary texts (Forrester 2017). Thus, if Groddeck chose to elaborate on his theoretical ideas in books of fiction, he must have thought that literature was the right space for psychoanalytic reflection. His *Book of the It* converged the "double narrative" of psychoanalytic texts (which consisted of the patient's story and the doctor's interpretation) in the self-analytical voice of his protagonist Patrik Troll (Lang & Sutton 2016: 423).[4] Groddeck's theoretical concepts – which he developed in discussions with Freud and Freud's closest students – should be considered in the broader context of post-1918 experimental modernist writing.

In the first decades of the twentieth century, boundaries between fiction and life writing (the letter, the journal, the biography, and the autobiography)[5] were being deliberately blurred, while authors boldly created a space for images of non-normative sexuality and gender (Haralson 2004).[6] Groddeck's vision of an individual's subjectivity and sexuality both shaped and was shaped by modernist literature. His attitude towards psychoanalytic theory and practice was defined by his distinctive way of connecting the autobiographical with the fictional. This combination was also symptomatic of the importance that he ascribed to literary work in researching human psychology and sexuality.

Groddeck consciously remained on the margins of the psychoanalytic movement. However, this did not stop him from influencing Freud's most important associates as well as Freud himself. As we shall see, Groddeck's writings became a powerful alternative to the orthodox psychoanalytic thought after the Great War.[7] For Groddeck, psychoanalysis was a revolutionary language for speaking about human sexuality. At the same time, he noticed Freud's fear of heresy and openly criticized the psychoanalytic movement for its dogmatism. Groddeck wanted to understand psychoanalysis primarily as a form of self-analysis. Because it was an attempt to reveal the mechanisms of the unconscious, it was intimately related to literature and literary creation based on a free flow of associations. Freud was struck by the originality of Groddeck's theoretical ideas, but simultaneously intrigued by his ability to combine the role of a psychoanalyst and a writer. In fact, Groddeck was perfectly capable of doing both – developing a psycho-medical discourse and a literary one. In Groddeck's literary writings, Freud saw how psychoanalysis could transform into a space of literary creation.

The turn of the twentieth century saw an intensified flow of ideas between medical discourse and literature (Marcus 1994; 2014). Freud and his collaborators' perception of the psyche and sexuality as fundamental factors for shaping human identity significantly impacted the progressing psychologization of literature. At that time, there was a shift in understanding the essence of biographism (with the emergence of the so-called "new biography").[8] The portrayals of literary characters increasingly covered questions on the unconscious and the role of sexuality in the psychological life of the subject. Literature started to seem like the appropriate space to explore: non-normative desires and erotic fantasies (recall Wilhelm Jensen's *Gradiva*, Robert Musil's *The Confusions of Young Master Törless*, Marcel Proust's *In Search of Lost Time*, Arthur Schnitzler's *Eyes Wide Shut*), the idea of natural bisexuality in humans (Thomas Mann's *Buddenbrooks, Tonio Kröger*, and *The Magic Mountain*), or gender fluidity (Virginia Woolf's *Orlando*).

In the 1980s, Philippe Lejeune demonstrated that the process of unsealing the hermetic container of medical discourse started with doctors using life-writing genres, such as letters, diaries, and autobiographies. Importantly, the discourses on sexuality not only strengthened the oppressive system, but it could also work against the doctors' power. Therefore, the language of psychiatry at the turn of the century could also be seen as a speaking space for those who were considered "mad" and "degenerate." What was especially interesting was the gradual subversive process of lacing theoretical discourse with autobiographical narratives, which – paradoxically – were usually created at the doctor's suggestion. However, one must immediately distinguish between the autobiography as a genre and a text written in the autobiographical register (Saunders 2009: 1055–1056). While "the afflicted" continued to be a "medical case" even when their statements had been published, authors who revealed their intimate biographies to their readers could allow themselves to be sincere as long as they published the story as autobiographical fiction (Lejeune 2017: 19–23).[9]

As we will see, Groddeck wrote about himself by putting on the masks of his protagonists August Müller and Patrik Troll, and at the same time symbolically addressed these literary (self-)portraits to Freud. After establishing Groddeck's position in the psychoanalytic movement, this chapter will focus on the physician's literary strategies for writing about non-normative sexuality – for which he was labeled as a free thinker and an individualist on the one hand, and an instigator and an iconoclast on the other.

6.1 Freud's "queer" fellow: Groddeck in the psychoanalytic movement

In the spring of 1917, Freud received a long letter written by Georg Groddeck from the spa town of Baden-Baden in southern Germany. At that time, Freud could not have foreseen the extent to which his future collaboration with Groddeck would impact psychoanalytic theory and practice and open up new interpretive possibilities. In the letter, Groddeck showed Freud an outline of an intellectual autobiography which had led him from denying psychoanalysis any value to a fascination with its creator's thought. In 1913, he first familiarized himself with *The Interpretation of Dreams* and *The Psychopathology of Everyday Life* which – though he had not read them thoroughly – made a great impression on him. Groddeck explained that he had stopped reading because: "The effect of these books was so disturbing that I did not finish them, though I was aware of the fact that I deprived myself of an extraordinary enrichment of knowledge" (Groddeck 1917: 31). The reading experience shook him to his core. After several years of independent study and exploration, Groddeck decided to have his own ideas assessed by Freud. In order to anticipate any criticism, he wrote:

> Yet the wish to publish the results of many years of work in some form or other is still there. There is, however, one difficulty which I have not yet solved. After reading your papers on the history of psychoanalysis I began to doubt whether, according to your definition, I could count myself a psychoanalyst. I do not want to call myself the member of a movement if I am in danger of being rejected by the leaders of the movement as an intruder who does not belong to it, and this is why I want to ask you to give me a few more moments of your time and read this letter.
>
> *(Ibid.: 32)*

In his letter, Groddeck asked Freud for permission to call himself a psychoanalyst – but everything that he wrote from then on would stir extreme emotions in Freud's circle. On July 13, 1917, Freud reported to Sándor Ferenczi that he had received an "extremely interesting letter" from a German doctor, and he was looking forward to meeting the new student despite "his inclination toward sectarianism and mysticism" (Freud & Ferenczi 1993: 217–218). Then, several years later, in a December 12, 1928 letter from Ernest Jones, Ferenczi read the words:

> Groddeck is here lecturing and does not make a good impression on the sober English. He has very little knowledge on psychoanalysis and it is a pity he was admitted to the movement, *for he certainly does it more harm than good. It is plain to us that his philosophical id is little else than an Introjected God* [italics mine].
>
> *(Ferenczi & Jones [1928] 2013: 655)*

Jones was referring to Groddeck's category of the It (*das Es*), which he considered non-scientific. Since Groddeck's first letters to Freud, he had developed his concept of the unconscious which was divergent from the Freudian doctrine. He elaborated on his notion of the It in his 1923 epistolary novel *The Book of the It*, presenting a different model of the psyche from the one established the same year by Freud in *The Ego and the Id*. Between 1923 and 1924, a number of other works by Freud's close collaborators were published, including Otto Rank's *The Trauma of Birth*, and Ferenczi's *Thalassa*, as well as their co-authored *Development of Psychoanalysis*. Critics agree that the publication of *The Ego and the Id* was "a watershed in the psychoanalytic literature" (Grubrich-Simitis 1993: 138). However, as Peter L. Rudnytsky observed, Freud's treatise later proved to be not the only one, but one of many drivers of the shift which took place in psychoanalytic theory and practice of that time. After 1923, "psychoanalysis itself reached a crossroads: the choice between Freud's new model of ego psychology and what we can now recognize to be the relational turn" (Rudnytsky 2002: 142).

In *The Book of the It*, not only did Groddeck broaden the understanding of the unconscious, but he also cast doubt on the established relationship dynamic between the analyst and the analysand. Referring to "Miss G.'s" therapy, the narrator stresses: "I was confronted with the strange fact that I was not treating the patient, but the patient was treating me" (Groddeck [1923] 1949: 228).

Between 1917 and 1928, Groddeck's ideas were maturing, but the fundamental concept contained in his first letter to Freud remained unchanged. At that time, Groddeck had already written about the unlimited creative power of the It (*das Es*), which accounted for illness and health, and transcended all that is individual by permeating every person. In his first letter to Freud, Groddeck emphasized: "I am afraid that I have not made myself completely clear when I talk about my It as shaping the individual, causing it to think, act, and fall ill" (Groddeck 1917: 34). He perceived the human being holistically and rejected the divides between the body and the spirit, between the psychological and the corporeal, the healthy and the ill. Therefore, he wanted to draw Freud's attention to the possibility of using the technique of psychoanalytic therapy to treat physical illness.

His notion of the It contained a revolutionary proposal to abolish difference and the act of differentiation as basic human activity. It was this thought that Groddeck expounded upon in his essay "The It and Psychoanalysis" ("Das Es und die Psychoanalyse") published in 1925 in the magazine *Die Arche* which he edited. There, he made the provocative statement that "Every examination, especially the scientific examination, is a violation of the truth" (Groddeck 1925: 8), presupposing that descriptions of reality always distort the truth. In this sense, Groddeck perceived science as a fiction which relied on the arbitrary extraction of single elements from the wholeness of the universe. He explained that "We are constructing races, nations, families, and finally individuals, *all in an arbitrary way and against our knowledge* [italics mine]" (Ibid.: 6).

In a letter written on June 5, 1917, Freud commented favorably on the notion of the It, not seeing it as a threat to his own theory. However, several years later, he changed his mind. In April 1925, Ferenczi wrote a letter to the member of "the secret committee" (*Das Geheime Komitee*) in response to a growing dislike of the author of *The Book of the It* among analysts. In it, he addressed Karl Abraham in the following words:

> I think, dear Karl, that you are handling the case of Groddeck somewhat too rigidly, quite in contrast to your otherwise skillful diplomacy, which is praised by everyone. He is an original, whom one should allow to go his own way in side issues; the main thing is that he is a true adherent, and a respectable person to boot. He does not do pure psychoanalysis, but rather utilizes a not unskilled mixture of various therapeutic measures. It was perhaps not very tactful, even cocky, when he gave an example in public of his own free associations, but with him, *cockiness is really only an exaggeration of courage, which he does not lack.* He can be influenced by some criticism; threatening him with paragraphs would certainly only make him run wild [italics mine].
>
> *(Freud & Ferenczi [1925] 2000: 213)*

Ferenczi understood very well that Groddeck would never conform to top-down theoretical and practical solutions. If the psychoanalytic circle wanted him to remain a member, it had to allow him the freedom of thought and action.

Nevertheless, Freud accused Groddeck of imprecision and a proclivity towards metaphysics. In 1917, he wrote: "Why do you jump from your beautiful basis into mysticism, cancel the distinction between mental and somatic, commit yourself to philosophical theories which are not called for?" (Freud 1917: 37–38). Despite the criticism, Freud decided to use Groddeck's term of the It (*das Es*) in his 1923 description of the structure of the human psyche. While he had already written about the psychoanalytic understanding of the unconscious as early as 1915 (Freud [1915] 1964a: 159–215), Freud only introduced his famous terminology in 1923, which he explained as follows:

> Now I think we shall gain a great deal by following the suggestion of a writer who, from personal motives, vainly asserts that he has nothing to do with the rigours of pure science. I am speaking of Georg Groddeck, who is never tired of insisting that what we call our ego behaves essentially passively in life, and that, as he expresses it, we are "lived" by unknown and uncontrollable forces. We have all had impressions of the same kind, even though they may not have overwhelmed us to the exclusion of all others, and we need feel no hesitation in finding a place for Groddeck's discovery in the structure of science.
>
> *(Freud [1923] 1964b: 23)*

Freud believed that the conscious collided with the unconscious in each individual. When he wrote about "the I" as passive towards "the It," he drew nearer to Groddeck's idea that a person's life was lived by an unknown force. By stating in *The Book of the It* that "Man is lived by the It" (German: *Der Mensch wird vom Es gelebt*), Groddeck showed that the unconscious force was responsible for life and death, health and sickness, creation and impotence (Groddeck 1949: 11). "The It" referred to the entirety of human experience. In his 1920 article "On the It" ("Über das Es"), Groddeck wrote:

> The assumption that we are being lived by an It annihilates a number of concepts with which we are accustomed to do our thing. Thus I have already mentioned that the It knows neither body nor soul since they are both manifestation of the same unknown entity; that the Ego, individuality, becomes a doubtful concept since the It can be traced right back to the moment of fertilization and even beyond this to the chain of parents and ancestors. Thus the temporal limits are eliminated since the beginning and the end are lost in obscurity.
>
> *(Groddeck [1922] 1977: 135)*

For the German physician, the It not only shaped a person's life, but it was life itself, and it filled the person from the moment of conception until death. Because he assumed that it was impossible to study the unconscious in a rational way, Groddeck questioned whether scientific descriptions were indeed objective. In one of the final letters in *The Book of the It*, the narrator concludes:

> I must first impart to you the sad tidings that, in my own opinion, there is no such It as I have been presenting to you, that it is a fiction of my own imagination. Because I concern myself alone and entirely with the individual man, and shall continue to do so for the rest of my life, I must act in such a way as if there were, apart from the Universal Nature of God (German: *Ganzen Gottnaturs*), individual beings called men.
>
> *(Groddeck [1923] 1949: 221)*

For the author, the very possibility of uttering an objective statement was problematic because language created divides which were not present in extra-scientific reality. In order to clearly distance the It from Freud's theory, Groddeck purposefully blurred its definition and stressed that it did not reflect reality fully: "One can draw a distinction between conscious and unconscious, but never between the It and the conscious; one can confront Ego with unconscious, but never with the It" (Groddeck 1925: 8). In the unconscious, Groddeck saw a power which preceded language as well as all thought, and was therefore inexpressible through words ("I purposely use the expression stammering [...] because it is not possible to talk about the It") (Groddeck [1923] 1949: 133). Despite Freud's assurance in the letter from June 5, 1917 that whether one "gives the 'UCS' [unconscious] the name of 'Id' as well makes no difference" (Freud 1960: 317), a decade later, on March 25, 1927, he wrote to Ferenczi: "I gladly grant you and your friend Groddeck, but lately he has been doing all too much trickery and nonsense, the 'It' has gone to his head" (Freud & Ferenczi [1927] 2000: 304). Although Freud perceived him as "mad," Groddeck became his "queer" fellow. Freud continued the epistolary exchange and read all of Groddeck's papers, thus confronting himself with the unconscious implications of his own theory, mainly the unwanted truth of the psychoanalytic theory's potential for heresy.

Freud's dislike of Groddeck's writings could have resulted from the critique of the psychoanalytic movement that they featured. Groddeck had a very harsh opinion of the internal dynamic of the psychoanalytic milieu. In 1925, he wrote:

> Something else struck me at this congress [...]: the participants pretended that they do not know that there are also talented, well-trained, even excellent psychoanalysts outside the international association: in every one of the lectures that I had a pleasure of hearing, there was a talk of the wild analysis. As far as I know, not a single one of the leading psychoanalysts is trained in the sense that he can present himself otherwise than a wild analyst.
>
> *(Groddeck 1925: 3)*

He pointed to the psychoanalysts' conservatism, which – with time and the increasing internationalization of Freudianism – was expressed in efforts to solidify unbridgeable divisions between "real" and "false" psychoanalysis. He wrote not without irony that the group which was condemned for its unprofessionalism included most leading psychoanalysts, if only due to their education. Freud had written about "wild analysts" several years before, in his text "'Wild' Psycho-Analysis" ("Über Wilde Psychoanalyse"), sensing that as the popularity of psychoanalysis increased, it would be used contrary to his intentions (Freud [1910] 1957a: 219–228). Groddeck saw himself precisely as one of the "wild analysts." At the 1925 International Psychoanalytical Congress in Bad Homburg, he was mocked by members who jokingly congratulated him for joining the faculty of theology (Groddeck 1925: 5).

Accused of mysticism, Groddeck counterattacked Freud in *Die Arche* for doctrinairism. He compared the psychoanalytic movement to a church which excommunicates anyone it considers a heretic. In "The It and Psychoanalysis," Groddeck wrote:

> Psychoanalysis is a matter of the whole world [...]. If the psychoanalytic association wants to keep its importance, or one can say now that it wants to win it again, it must give up setting up doctrines in the manner of the Tridentine Council or the Augsburg Confession [...] That it selects its members it is its right, that it feels itself uniquely blest, is careless.
>
> *(Ibid.: 3)*

He was trying to demonstrate that the theory which had been created on the fringes of official science was beginning to repeat the same mistakes. By drawing lines and creating dogmas, the psychoanalytic environment limited the analysts' freedom of thought and therefore hindered the development of the theory. Groddeck challenged Freud's dogmatic approach to his invention. The German doctor wanted to treat psychoanalysis as a gift "for the whole world," a mode of thinking rather than a set of truths to be applied in an absolute manner.

When he asked Freud in his first letter whether he could call himself a psychoanalyst, Groddeck was alluding to the 1914 biographical essay *The History of the Psychoanalytic Movement*, and correctly reading it as an open letter to the "unfaithful" students: Alfred Adler, Wilhelm Stekel, and Carl Gustav Jung. Freud's narrative on the history of the psychoanalytic movement was intended to stabilize the "official message" of psychoanalysis. In 1914, Freud did not hesitate to assert that "psycho-analysis is my creation" (Freud [1914] 1957b: 7). He gave himself the exclusive right to judge the effects of his collaborators' work.[10] It is in this light that a letter from December 24, 1922 to Groddeck can be read. There, Freud confronted the German physician's unconventional attitude:

> I was very sorry that you find it necessary also to avoid a psychoanalytic career. This explanation of your indeed unsuccessful paper and your categorizing my person as a mother figure, a role which I quite obviously do not fit, show clearly that you are trying to evade the father transference.
>
> *(Freud 1922: 75)*

Freud did not think that Groddeck's ideas resulted from his boldness of interpretation. Rather, he suspected that Groddeck was obsessing over the mother figure – a role in which he wanted to cast his teacher. Although Freud did like Groddeck's book (on March 25, 1923 he wrote: "I like the little book very much") (Freud 1960: 342), he could not accept the mother being elevated over the father. On July 23, 1924, Freud directed a similar remark at Otto Rank, dismissing his ideas as a result of insufficient therapy (Rudnytsky 2002: 155). Another analyst who followed in Groddeck's footsteps was also one of Freud's closest students. In his *Clinical Diary*, Sándor Ferenczi wrote that he found a mother in his patient Elizabeth Severn ("R.N."): "namely the real one, who was hard and energetic and of whom I am afraid. R.N. knows this, and treats me with particular gentleness" (Ferenczi [1932] 1995: 44–45). The maternal dynamic of therapy can be identified in Groddeck's *The Book of the It* which consists of letters written by the protagonist and narrator Patrik Troll to his female friend. Groddeck purposefully made a woman the addressee and listener of the narrator's self-analysis, and called her his "judge beloved but stern" (Groddeck [1923] 1949: 47). In *The Book of the It*, she acts as an analyst-mother to whom Troll confesses his intimate history.[11]

6.2 Freud, Groddeck, and Nietzsche in a philosophical conundrum

When Groddeck wrote his 1917 letter to Freud, he had already authored several works which reflected his fascination with Romantic literature and its symbolism. Groddeck was born in 1866, and, like his father, he studied medicine at the Westphalian Wilhelm University of Münster, where he defended his doctoral thesis in 1889. In the years that followed, he managed a sanatorium in Baden-Baden with his teacher Ernst Schweniger. After 1899, Groddeck wrote short critical texts for the *Frankfurter Zeitung* and worked on his literary attempts. This was when he created the long poem *A Women Problem* (*Ein Frauenproblem*) (1903) inspired by Nietzsche's writings and the novel *A Child of the Earth* (*Ein Kind der Erde*) (1905). Less than a year later, he published *The Marriage of Dionysus* (*Die Hochzeit des Dionysos*), which was influenced by Nietzsche's early treatise *The Birth of Tragedy*. In his lifetime, Groddeck also completed *Towards God Nature* (*Hin zu Gottnatur*) and *Tragedy or Comedy: A Question for the Ibsen Readers* (*Tragödie oder Komödie. Eine Frage an die Ibsenleser*) (Martynkewicz 1997: 159–190).[12]

Freud emphasized Groddeck's debt to Nietzsche. In 1922, he wrote: "I think you got the It (in a literary, not an associative way) from Nietzsche. May I say that in my paper?" (Freud 1922: 76). He was convinced that Groddeck must have drawn on someone else's concept. By questioning its originality, Freud was trying to ascribe Groddeck's thought to Nietzsche's anti-Positivism. Moreover, he insisted that the German physician's considerations did not match the psychoanalytic approach (Freud [1923] 1964b: 23). Groddeck was thus symbolically excluded from the psychoanalytic movement, or in any case he was not welcomed by Freud as a representative. Freud returned to the problem of the split psyche in his 1933 *New Introductory Lectures on Psychoanalysis*, and again referred to Groddeck:

> We will no longer use the term "unconscious" in the systematic sense and we will give what we have hitherto so described a better name and one no longer open to misunderstanding. Following a verbal usage of Nietzsche's and taking up a suggestion by Georg Groddeck we will in future call it the "id".
>
> *(Freud [1933] 1971: 72)*

Compared to his 1923 remark previously mentioned, Freud diminished the physician's merit even further. He no longer mentioned the differences between his own notion of the it and the proposals put forward by Groddeck. In his lecture, he went on to consider the relationship between the conscious and the unconscious, and explained:

> The ego's relation to the id might be compared with that of a rider to his horse. The horse supplies the locomotive energy, while the rider has the

> privilege of deciding on the goal and of guiding the powerful animal's movement. But only too often there arises between the ego and the id the not precisely ideal situation of the rider being obliged to guide the horse along the path by which it itself wants to go.
>
> *(Ibid.: 77)*

The unconscious is a force which often rules over its "rider." Freud was evidently referring to Plato's *Phaedrus* where the human soul had been compared to a charioteer driving a pair of horses. One animal does not respond to desires while the other acts on every passion. The charioteer's role is to tame the impulsive animal. Freud's "id" was synonymous with repressed desires which were impossible to reconcile with commonly accepted social norms.

Crucially, the way that Groddeck's and Freud's understanding of the unconscious diverged translated directly into their understanding of culture. Freud ([1930] 1961b: 57–146), after Thomas Hobbes, perceived it as social consent to limitations on personal freedom, motivated by the need for security (as for Hobbes freedom was exercised outside the law). Conversely, Groddeck thought that culture was a direct result of the It's actions. In "The Compulsion to Use Symbols" ("Der Symbolisierungszwang"), Groddeck wrote that any artistic production (be it the visual arts, music, or literature) came from the unconscious. He thought that his stance was backed by the human mind's tendency towards associative thinking: finding references and connections in any image as they are inscribed in every cultural text. In this spirit, Groddeck read the biblical story of creation in *Genesis* and saw phallic symbolism in the tree of the knowledge of good and evil (Groddeck [1922] 1977: 158–159). "The unconscious expresses itself in them symbolically, [...] unconscious differences in age do not exist, or at least not in the sense in which they are registered by consciousness," he continued (Ibid.: 168). The unconscious knows no boundaries or divides as they result from man's social existence.

In his skeptical attitude towards the social order and scientific dogmatism, Groddeck resembled modernist philosophers. In the German philosophical tradition, from Schopenhauer to Nietzsche, freedom was understood as radical emancipation from existing schemes. Still, Nietzsche was the fiercest attacker of values and notions which had been taken for granted for centuries. He did not stop at criticizing conventional truths and the dogmatism of institutional religiosity, but he shook their very foundation: the idea of the objective truth.

Groddeck emulated Nietzsche – a critic of commonly accepted values, advocate for change and individual transformation, and author who designed new spaces of philosophical and literary expression – in his suspicious attitude towards truths discovered via reason and their resistance against academic conservatism. In *On Truth and Lies in a Nonmoral Sense*, Nietzsche asserted:

> As a means for the preserving of the individual, the intellect unfolds its principal powers in dissimulation, which is the means by which weaker, less robust individuals preserve themselves since they have been denied the chance to wage the battle for existence with horns or with the sharp teeth of beasts of prey. This art of dissimulation reaches its peak in man. Deception, flattering, lying, deluding, talking behind the back, putting up a false front, living in borrowed splendor, wearing a mask, hiding behind convention, playing a role for others and for oneself [...]. They are deeply immersed in illusions and in dream images; their eyes merely glide over the surface of things and see "forms." Their senses nowhere lead to truth; on the contrary, they are content to receive stimuli and, as it were, to engage in a groping game on the backs of things. [...] What does man actually know about himself? [...] Does nature not conceal most things from him – even concerning his own body – in order to confine and lock him in within a proud, deceptive consciousness, aloof from the coins of the bowels, the rapid flow of the blood stream, and the intricate quivering of the fibers!
>
> *(Nietzsche [1896] 2005: 14–15)*

Anything people considered certain proves to be a lie, a masquerade. The established normative order is revealed to be a mere illusion, while truth is nothing more than an ephemeral, oneiric flicker of light.[13] Nietzsche asks questions about man's self-awareness while simultaneously arguing that total self-understanding is impossible. Organic metaphors permeate his language in order to emphasize that the force of nature flows through people while concealing the truth about them. He closes the chasm between matter and spirit with an image of matter forming the spirit. Human consciousness is prone to turning a blind eye on this unconscious force and forgetting that "man is sustained in the indifference of his ignorance by that which is pitiless, greedy, insatiable, and murderous – as if hanging in dreams on the back of the tiger" (Nietzsche 2005: 15). By being unaware of it, man can be absorbed by "it" at any moment. In the same text, Nietzsche strengthens his claim about the impossibility of learning the truth by adding: "The various languages placed side by side show that with words it is never a question of truth, never a question of adequate expression" (Ibid.: 15–16). Language imminently demarcates the limits of human cognition, making it defective and imperfect. A similar belief can easily be found in *The Book of the It*. Groddeck argues in the Nietzschean spirit:

> On closer inspection, one finds that all concepts and names are inadequate and imprecise when applied to the It because they contain symbols and as a result of the compulsion to associate, they overlap with other conceptual areas thus expand more or less sharply defined complexes.
>
> *(Groddeck [1922] 1977: 133)*

The human being notices the presence and activity of the It, but he cannot put into words what the It is. The unconscious escapes all definition.

In this context, it is easy to see why psychoanalytic circles accused the German doctor of mysticism and of mixing the language of psychoanalysis with philosophy and theology. Groddeck's denunciation of dogmatism in academia was tinged with reluctance towards institutional science in general – which he shared with Nietzsche. In *Twilight of the Idols*, the philosopher wrote:

> As to learning how to think – our schools no longer have any notion of such a thing. Even at the universities, among the actual scholars in philosophy, logic as a theory, as a practical pursuit, and as a business, is beginning to die out. [...] What single German can still say he knows from experience that delicate shudder which *light footfalls* in matters intellectual cause to pervade his whole body and limbs!
>
> *(Nietzsche 1911: 59)*

He depicted thinking as a craft which must be learned like dance and continually practiced. Otherwise, it stops being alive and becomes an empty pattern. Groddeck also believed that the conservatism of psychoanalytic thought created a stiff interpretive framework for what had originally been a dynamic mode of thinking. In his eyes, reality was much richer than a person could imagine. Groddeck drew on Nietzsche's philosophy and enriched it with the psychoanalytic understanding of sexuality as a key dimension of every human life. By destabilizing the common truth of the established moral norms, the German psychoanalyst wanted to reveal the hidden truth of the plurality and complexity of human desire which manifested itself in different forms of sexual expression.

Despite these clear similarities between Nietzsche and Groddeck in their rebellious and iconoclastic attitude as well as their literary sensibility, it must be mentioned that Nietzsche did not use the category of the It in his writings in a systematic manner (Nitzschke 1983: 783–784; Will 1985: 151, 155–156, 158, 166–167; Rudnytsky 2002: 142–148; Martynkewicz 1997: 204–209). It is likely that Groddeck's other source of inspiration was a 1904 work *The Resurrection of Religion through Art* by Wilhelm Bölsche, who wrote about an unconscious, creative potentiality which stood behind any creative endeavor. Bölsche was inspired by Johan Wolfgang von Goethe's image of the spiritual, divine nature (German: *Gottnatur*). Indeed, similar ideas can be found it Groddeck's pre-psychoanalytic 1909 text *Towards God Nature*. In his pantheism and holistic approach to man (as part of all creation), Groddeck turned to Goethe. The protagonist of Groddeck's first psychoanalytic novel, August Müller, was modeled after Goethe. One day, Müller meets the poet's grandson, Wolf Goethe, who hands him an unusual gift as an expression of friendship. It is a small drawing on black paper which depicts a human figure sitting on top of planet Earth with a magnifying glass. Müller gives him a name: "der Seelensucher" (Groddeck 1921: 3, 100, 153, 201–202). Through the glass, the human is looking at a smaller female figure. Although the optical tool is clearly pointed at her pubic area, the little woman is turned towards the observer and exposes herself, unashamed, to his curious gaze. In his investigations, the "soul explorer" will be guided by psychoanalysis. For the protagonist of Groddeck's 1921 novel, sexuality was no more and no less than the unconscious: a constantly transforming force and a key to exploring the human soul.

6.3 Georg Groddeck's literary worlds

August Müller, the protagonist of *The Soul Seeker*, is a Quixotic dreamer and an ironist not unlike Simplicius Simplicissimus from the seventieth-century satirical novel by Hans von Grimmelshausen. One night, as a result of scarlet fever, Müller is transformed into Thomas Weltlein and declares himself to be the savior of man from bourgeois conventions. He becomes the embodiment of the unconscious. From that moment on, his life's purpose is to re-evaluate all values. He strives to reveal what has been socially repressed and culturally muted. In the novel, Thomas Weltlein draws an outline of a new anthropology whose main epistemological tool is intuition rather than reason. He understands education as a necessity to abandon the beaten paths of thinking about man and his role in the world.

Groddeck's work can be read as a critique of nineteenth-century scientism understood as a utopian pursuit of objective and total cognition. And thus, in the second part of the novel, Weltlein discovers psychoanalysis.[14] A key scene in the novel is Müller's "transfiguration night." Ill with scarlet fever, the protagonist sinks into obsessive thoughts about a bed bug infestation. He finds the first insect on a copy of Cervantes's *Don Quixote* placed beside the bed. After some time, he begins to differentiate between superior and inferior bed bugs. He develops a belief that bed bugs were created to call people to great, revolutionary accomplishments. Müller forms a mysterious bond with the insects, which is embodied in the scarlet fever consuming his mind and flesh. By Chapter 6, the bed bug has become a symbol of the fight against obscurantism, represented by clergymen among others. As August instructs his sister's friend, who is a seminarian: "You wear a black monk's habit because you feel pain of ecclesiastic fever […] a fever of humility" (Ibid.: 35). The blackness of the cassock contrasts with Müller's nudity. In the next scene, he jumps out of bed to tell his sister about the "divine" bed bug.

His illness culminates on the night of his death. In a letter left for his sister, August writes: "the human in me, August Müller, has died" (Ibid.: 45). Agatha also finds another letter, in which her brother writes about a new man, born out of doubt – the basis of all existence – whose "name shall be Thomas Weltlein" (Ibid.: 46). Like the biblical Adam, the new man Weltlein learns the truth about all creation. Adam-Weltlein discovers the world anew and notices that all categories (subject–object, alive–dead, man–animal) are mere figments of the human mind. In this spirit, he asks: "Why cannot a stone have an opinion? Why cannot there be something conscious in it?" (Ibid.: 48). The protagonist looks at his surroundings through the eyes of a child which does not separate itself from the perceived reality. Weltlein is an iteration of Nietzsche's Zarathustra ("When was thirty years old [...] his heart transformed") (Nietzsche 2006: 3). The transformation allowed Zarathustra to see more ("his eyes are pure"), freed him from human concerns ("no disgust is visible around his mouth"), and brought him closer to being a child rather than an adult ("Zarathustra has become a child") (Ibid.: 4). Like Zarathustra, who guides people to the truth about themselves ("I teach you the overman") (Ibid.: 6), in his fascinating adventures Weltlein discovers the truth about the human being's psychology and sexuality.

In several letters written between February and March 1921, Freud discussed Groddeck's novel with pastor Oskar Pfister. The analyst compared the author's language to the writings of François Rabelais, and thus defended Groddeck against the Swiss clergyman's critique. In his reply on March 14, 1921, Pfister accused Groddeck of using the blade of satire against science as well as switching back and forth between medicine and literature too casually. He concluded his letter by caustically referring to Groddeck's hybrid language:

> You say yourself that his trend is definitely scientific, but I dislike his spicing it with jokes. I like a clean sheet of paper, and I also like fresh butter, but butter-stains on a sheet of paper satisfy neither my eye nor my belly.[15]

The pastor doubtlessly supported clear divisions between science (understood as a tool of objective cognition) and creative endeavors (assumed to be subjective) – although Freud himself did not cultivate these divisions. Was Pfister, then, more bothered by the way Groddeck had decided to talk about psychoanalysis or rather by the criticism of the clergy and religiosity contained in *The Soul Seeker*? It is unlikely that the pastor would have missed the frequently recurring biblical themes in the German physician's writings. As we will see, apart from psychoanalytic theory, these references to the Old and New Testament were what connected *The Soul Seeker* to Groddeck's next work: *The Book of the It*.

6.4 *The Book of the It* as a self-portrait

The 1923 publication of *The Book of the It* – Groddeck's epistolary novel structured as the protagonist's thirty-three letters to a friend – marks the moment when he started forming a model of the unconscious and human desire which did not fit the narrow framework of the Oedipal triangle. In the book, Groddeck included long passages about the It (das Es), juxtaposing it against the bourgeois, civilized Freudian image of the unconscious. On June 18, 1925, Freud wrote in a letter:

> Thank you for your reports and enclosures. Everything from you is interesting to me, even if I may not follow you in detail. I do not, of course, recognize my civilized, bourgeois, demystified Id in your It. Yet you know that mine derived from yours.
>
> *(Freud 1925: 93)*

He rejected the mystical It, understood as a supernatural force, and adapted it to the limits of bourgeois imagination.

In Groddeck's novel, the narrator's thoughts are centered around three problem areas: the embodied metaphysics of the It, the philosophy of illness and psychoanalytic therapy, and the theory of sexuality. In the first letter, the protagonist addresses the readers:

> So I haven't been clear, after all; my letter was horribly muddled [...]. Well, dearest of friends, if you want to be instructed, let me advise you to consult a textbook, as they do at the universities. But for my letters you shall have herewith the key; *everything in them sounds reasonable, or perhaps only a little strange, is derived from Professor Freud of Vienna and his colleagues; whatever is quite mad, I claim as my own spiritual property* [italics mine].
>
> *(Groddeck [1923] 1949: 20)*

While the narrator associates Freud with reason, he maintains that psychoanalysis as a way of thinking has certain ties to madness. In the first part of the work, he criticizes medical discourse for creating artificial categorizations, and undermines the socially sanctioned divisions between the ill and the healthy, the normal and the deviant. For him, these terms are social constructs rather than neutral descriptors. In one of his letters, Patrik Troll contends:

> Natural laws are the creation of men [...]. Strike the word "unnatural" out of your vocabulary and there will be one stupidity less in your speech. [...] *We must abandon the accepted idea that there are unnatural lusts and adopt the view that what we are wont to call perversion, masturbation, homosexuality, sodomy, or whatever these things are named, are innate tendencies of man* [italics mine].
>
> *(Ibid.: 65)*

Clearly, the narrator does not believe that the categories of perversion and abnormality are functional in any way. Groddeck was sensing a paradigmatic shift in psycho-medical discourses, which transformed into spaces for negotiating and redefining what was "healthy" or "unhealthy" in the early twentieth century. Familiar with the psycho-medical literature of his time, he decided to pursue an unorthodox way of describing non-normative sexuality. This is why, after Wilhelm Stekel, Patrik Troll argues against Freud's idea of masturbation as a mere substitute for sexual satisfaction (Rudnytsky 2002: 148–150). Groddeck had likely read Stekel's *The Language of Dreams* (*Die Sprache des Traumes*) as well as his considerations on onanism printed in psychoanalytic journals (Stekel 1912: 557–566; 1913: 249–252; 1914a: 59–70; 1914b: 616–618). Groddeck disagreed with Freud's idea on the harmful effects on masturbation for two fundamental reasons: first, he considered it as a natural (and therefore legitimate) form of sexual gratification, and second, he deemed it a basic human sexual practice. In this view, sexuality escaped Freud's linear framework and evolutionary phases, proving to be a multi-layer amalgamate of diverse practices and expressions (Harris 2009: 25–47, 101–129). In *The Book of the It*, the body is a *desiring-machine* – to use Gilles Deleuze and Félix Guattari's term – whose actions elude the categories of medical discourse (Deleuze & Guattari 1983: 1–21).

Groddeck identifies the workings of the It in every text. In one letter, his protagonist Patrik Troll says: "For the It there exists no watertight ideas, it deals with whole structures of ideas, with complexes, which are formed under the influence of symbolization and association" (Groddeck [1923] 1949: 48). While reflecting on the unconscious, he points to the paradoxical nature of the symbol, which simultaneously reveals and conceals its meaning. In "The Compulsion to Use Symbols," Groddeck interpreted the story of the fall of Adam and Eve. As a text, *Genesis* was formative for the Western identity, and Groddeck viewed it through the lens of psychoanalysis. According to his protagonist: "The Fall of man is really the sex act between man and woman, and the expression *Erkenntnis* (knowledge) has the meaning it often has in the Bible of knowing, mating, cohabiting with the woman" (Groddeck [1922] 1977: 158). The sin of the first people consisted in the sex act: the carnal knowledge of another person's body (in this case: a woman's) which led to the discovery of man's own nudity. Tasting the forbidden fruit was synonymous with discovering the sexual difference.

Groddeck deliberately assumed a male-centric perspective in order to demonstrate that the fear of castration and the fear of knowing "the other" (the woman) is men's problem. Even though violating a taboo brings the man sexual satisfaction, its aftermath is the threat of castration. Troll writes about an "innate" fear of castration which is solidified in Western culture. As a "symbolizing creature" (Ibid.: 171), man learns about the world through images and tropes reproduced by culture. Meanwhile, Troll's Gospel assumes it is necessary to criticize the established imaginary-normative order and reject moral dogmatism.

In Chapter 28 of *The Book of the It*, Groddeck returns to the story of the creation of Adam. For Troll, "The Bible is a wise and entertaining book, with beautiful stories in it, which are doubly remarkable because people believed in them for thousands of years, [...] and for all of us were a part of our childhood" (Groddeck [1923] 1949: 207). It is a collection of stories which left a permanent trace in the human unconscious by being repeated over the centuries. Groddeck reads the Bible as a cultural text, discovering in it the source of human psyche. His narrator quotes the following passage from *Genesis*: "And the Lord God formed man of the dust of the ground, and breathed into his nostrils the breath of life; and man became a living soul."[16] Troll asks what that "breath of life" was. According to him, the story of Adam represents a vision of infantile sexuality. Troll argues that God formed man out of feces rather than dust. Like an uninhibited child, God played with his own waste (Groddeck [1923] 1949: 208). Thus, the first man is God's anal child. This image is then transposed by Troll onto his individual life story as he recounts his homosexual experiences. He insists that men want to feel physical pleasure the same way that women do. By the same token, the threat of castration is not only accompanied by fear, but it also awakens a desire to become a woman (Ibid.: 209).

Several years later, Groddeck wrote about "the new Adam": Jesus Christ. In the essay "The It and the Gospels" ("Das Es und die Evangelien"), which he published in *Die Arche* in 1926, he treated Jesus as the perfect personification of the It. At the same time, he interpreted the image of the humanized God in the Gospel as a sign that divinity (or the possibility of divinization) is latent in every human. Groddeck thought that Jesus had nothing to do with laws, including the moral law ("Christ and morality have nothing to do with each other") (Groddeck 1926: 4). This was because God's only law was love, and in Groddeck's view, love was naturally amoral ("Love has nothing to do with morality") (Ibid.: 4). Therefore, Christ's divine nature was best reflected in a child as the It could manifest itself most fully in a being who is unbridled by cultural norms and taboos. A child is closest to perfection because it is motivated by curiosity rather than law, shame, or guilt. An adult is unable to find his or her bearings in an environment without boundaries or clear divisions – the first of which is sexual difference. One key aspect of the gender binary in Western culture is the idea of an impotent (castrated) woman and the active, conquering man. Questioning the binary would mean giving men the right to experience their own femininity outside of the patriarchal order, and therefore to redefine the hegemonic model of masculinity.

The rejection of phallocentrism, which is evident in Groddeck's writings, did not go unnoticed in Freud's circle. Among the people inspired by the German physician's ideas was Karen Horney, who wrote "The Genesis of the Castration Complex in Women," "The Flight from Womanhood," and "The Dread of Woman" (Horney 1924: 50–65).[17] Her analysis of the problem of motherhood and the genesis of the castration complex in the woman echoes Patrik Troll's thoughts. In 1924, Horney wrote:

> My problem was the question whether that dissatisfaction with the female sexual role which results from "penis-envy" is really the alpha and omega of the castration complex in women. We have seen that the anatomical structure of the female genitals is indeed of great significance in the mental development of women. [...] But the deduction that therefore the repudiation of their womanhood is based on that envy seems inadmissible.
>
> *(Ibid.: 64)*

Horney did not quote Groddeck, but she similarly rejected the idea that "penis envy" was key to women's psychosexual development. In the fourteenth letter in *The Book of the It*, Troll mentions the biblical story of the creation of Eve, and argues: "the creation of woman, the cutting of the rib, which gives rise to the wound of woman – this castration is, in the end, punishment for masturbation" (Groddeck [1923] 1949: 105). When writing about punishment for masturbation, Groddeck again evokes Adam's sin which was the discovery of the sexual difference. The castration complex says more about men's psychology and sexuality rather than women's. For men, the history of the creation of Eve – the "founding myth of patriarchy" – functioned as a projection of autoerotic fantasies with the woman still absent. In one of his letters, Troll remarks with irony: "the woman comes into being through the castration of man" (Ibid.: 2007).[18]

He also talks about homosexuality, which he treats as a natural expression of human sexuality, rather than a "passing phase" of psychosexual development. He believes that determining a "proper" course of human sexuality is based on a rigid orientation of desire. Despite that, in the fourteenth letter, Troll walks Freud's beaten path by saying: "the life of man is governed by the Oedipus complex" (Ibid.: 104). Like his teacher, Troll limits desire to a reflection of infantile incestuous fantasies. The narrator tells the story of a patient called "M.D." who was obsessed by persecuting homosexual men. The patient could not help his thoughts about assaulting homosexuals he encountered in the street. This is how Troll identifies the source of M.D.'s desire: "The hatred with which D. [...] pursued the pederasts, was suppressed homosexuality" (Ibid.: 15). Groddeck perceived (latent) homosexuality as a result of an excessive love for one's mother – which was in accordance with Freud's disciple Isidor Sadger's intuitions (Sadger 1910: 59–133; 1914: 296–313).[19] Nevertheless, Groddeck did not pathologize that feeling (Lang & Sutton 2016: 419).[20]

Further in his argument, Groddeck crosses another boundary by asserting that a clear division between the feminine and the masculine is an illusion. In "On the It," he states:

> I shall make ample use of the fact that the individual is neither male nor female but both, that he is of no particular age but simultaneously one,

> ten, thirty years old, that everything that enters depends on the permission being given by the unconscious. [...] It follows from all this that it is useful to choose the child as the object of the It investigation. Sex distinction does not play a role yet, the apparent differences of age are irrelevant [...]. The result of an investigation of the child's It may teach us the saying "unless you be as children, you will not enter into the kingdom of heaven" is legitimate, that the aim in life is to become a child again and that we have only one choice – that of becoming childlike or childish.
>
> *(Groddeck [1922] 1977: 136)*

The human being is therefore neither a man nor a woman. Rather, they possess both feminine and masculine characteristics. Importantly, Troll is not thinking in mere metaphors of the feminine or masculine element, but he is really considering biological sex.

The figure of the polyamorous child returns as it experiences its body as an endless, paradisiac space of pleasure. Groddeck's emphasis on the problem of unity (the child) and difference (the adult) in experiencing one's own sexuality echoes the biblical description of creation. In *Genesis* 1, the human being is created as "male and female" (Bebe 2001: 115–117), and thus an androgynous entity. In their essence, the androgyne resembles a child which does not know the idea of the sexual difference yet. The human who was formed by God carries two elements within them (the feminine and the masculine) until the moment when God extracts the woman out of their body. From then on, they would be called man (Hebrew: *ish*) and woman (Hebrew: *ishah*). The tension which emerges between the feminine and the masculine element reflects the dichotomy of the sacred and the profane, the clean and the unclean, the light and the dark or the good or the evil, which are all fundamental to the religious imaginary. Thus, at its very origin, the gender binary is a symbolic opposition of two elements which are combined in every individual.

In the late nineteenth century, theories of natural human bisexuality – understood as innate "spiritual" androgyny – were gaining popularity among ideas on human sexuality. Inspired by these findings, in a letter on May 7, 1900 to Wilhelm Fliess, Freud wrote about the "feminine side" of his personality (Freud & Fliess [1900] 1985: 412). At that time, he was already convinced about the bisexual nature of every subject, which he later expressed in *Three Essays on the Theory of Sexuality.* There, he stressed the significance of the twofold psychological constitution of the subject: the feminine and the masculine (Freud [1905] 1953: 141–142).

In *Das Buch vom Es*, Groddeck assumes that – rather than being stable – both sex and gender are a spectrum between two qualities: the feminine and the masculine. This idea was repeated by Patrik Troll: "And so in the being we call a man, there lives also a woman, in the woman too a man" (Groddeck [1923] 1949: 14). Groddeck used the image of the androgyne in order to shed light on the oppressive workings of power which reproduced conservative patterns of gender (the gender binary) and sexuality (the rejection of all forms of sexual expression apart from the monogamous, officially registered relationship between two people of opposite sex). With its norms and taboos, culture defines every aspect of human life, influencing how the human being perceives themselves and others.

It seems that Patrik Troll successfully defies social conventions and rejects the resulting false morality. In this sense, he is far from the characters of Schnitzler's plays, Musil's short stories, or Mann's novels – who painfully experience the severity of moral principles. Rather than the modernizing city (as in Mihály Babits's first novel), the narrator's point of reference is the world of nature as the space where the unconscious really lives. The mysticism of the It thus relies on an animistic belief in the spirituality of all creation. In *The Book of the It*, Groddeck created a world out of blood, urine, and feces, and ascribed particular functions to these elements: blood-femininity-mother, urine-masculinity-father, feces-neutrality-child. The relationship between the mother and the child was especially important for him as a psycho-corporeal continuum which defined the subject's entire life. The image of the mother was an ideal which the child would follow throughout its life. In the sixth letter, Troll reiterates:

> Man's emotional life reaches after this mother imago as long as he lives, reaches so longingly, that the yearning for sleep, for rest, for protection, for death, may well be regarded as a yearning for the mother imago, and I shall take this view in my letters.
>
> *(Ibid.: 57)*

By giving importance to the psycho-corporeal bond with the mother, Groddeck explored new territories of unorthodox thought for Freud's rebellious students. Rank and Ferenczi, who focused on the mother-child relationship post-1924, were among the first readers of *The Book of the It*. Ferenczi surely could not have missed the thirtieth letter in which the narrator transposes the mother-child relationship onto the analyst-patient relationship. Troll tells one patient's story which shaped his therapy technique:

> In Fräulein G.'s case everything went on quite differently from the start. Her childlike attitude towards me – indeed, as I understood later, it was that of a child of three – compelled me to assume the mother's role. [...] Later on, when I came to look into my own medical activities more searchingly, I discovered that often before I had been forced by mysterious influences of this kind to adopt some other attitude than the parental one towards my patients, although consciously and theoretically I held the firm conviction that the doctor must be friend and father, must control his patients.
>
> *(Ibid.: 228)*

According to the narrator, transference understood as an emotional projection onto the analyst involves the mother figure rather than the father figure. Crucially, Troll discovers that therapy serves both his patient and him.[21]

The mother-child relationship also reveals the basic dynamic of the It, which – to Troll – is simultaneously a metaphor for the process of creation and artistic prolificness. *The Book of the It* describes a distinct vision of the creative process as a psycho-corporeal act. Troll refers to his own writing practice as a symbolic iteration of the sex act (Rudnytsky 2002: 165–166).[22] When discussing his writing technique, Troll discloses:

> In my right hand I hold a pen; with my left I am fondling my watch chain. [...] My mood is uneasy and I have cold fingerprints. Let me begin, my dear, at the end. My fingerprints are cold; that makes writing very difficult, and therefore means: "Be careful, or you'll write nonsense." [...] There is more to the story. From the pen flow out the ink which fertilizes the paper. When it is covered with writing, I fold it up, put it in an envelope, and send it to the post. You open the letter [...] what you are about to read deals with pregnancy and birth. And then you think of the many people who are scolded for writing so little, and you understand why they find it so hard to write.
>
> *(Groddeck [1923] 1949: 129–130)*

The writer's block is caused by an unconscious fear of giving birth to a child. The act of putting the pen to paper is compared to pregnancy and labor. Troll's idea of working on a book as being with child is more than metaphorical, as evidenced by these words:

> The most striking sign of pregnancy is the enlarged stomach. What do you think about my idea [...], that an enlarged stomach betokens the appearance of pregnancy even in the case of a man? Indisputably he carries no child in his body. But his It creates the swollen stomach by means of eating, drinking, [...], because it wishes to be pregnant, and accordingly believes itself to be so.
>
> *(Ibid.: 16)*

For the narrator, "male pregnancy" is a natural psycho-somatic phenomenon. This way, writing becomes part of the mother-child continuum in which the author "mothers" his work. Although the "pregnancy" happens at the psychological level and is physically visible as words on the page, its traces can sometimes be found in the male writer's body. The body becomes a space for the play of the unconscious which signals to the human being that it is necessary to fully participate in the mother-child continuum – to relive childhood and symbolically return to her womb. In *The Book of the It*, Groddeck forms an indissoluble connection between biological and symbolic motherhood, relating it to the bond between creators and their work.

6.5 Groddeck's self-analysis and literary experimentalism

The Book of the It appeared at a moment which was not only pivotal to psychoanalytic thought, but also to the development of modernist literature. In 1921, Robert Musil began working on *The Man Without Qualities*, James Joyce's *Ulysses* was published in 1922, Italo Svevo's *Zeno's Conscience* in 1923, Thomas Mann's *Magic Mountain* a year after that, and Virginia Woolf's *Orlando* in 1928. As Max Saunders observes, turn-of-the-century literature was characterized by a blurring of boundaries between literary genres and forms, culminating after 1918. In *Self-Impression: Life-writing, Autobiografiction, and the Forms of Modern Literature*, Saunders writes:

> the fact that a modernist author blurs generic boundaries does not invalidate the concept of genre. It may highlight the inevitable overlapping of genres, since genres are not pure entities. Saying an autobiography contains fiction is comparable to saying epics contain history, myth, or indeed fiction. So they do, but that does not mean epic isn't a genre. [...] Reading something as "autobiographical," then, is different from reading it as "autobiography"; its autobiographical dimension can be covert, unconscious, or implicit.
>
> *(Saunders 2010: 4)*

Thus, modernist writers need not choose the genre of autobiography to use the autobiographical register and reveal parts of their own biography (Ibid.: 5). If we acknowledge that "life-writing is fundamentally intertextual," almost every literary text will inevitably contain an element of the autobiographical (Ibid.: 5). Groddeck's work includes such polyphonous, hybrid fragments. Troll's letters to his friend echo Groddeck's arguments from his correspondence with Freud. It is no coincidence that Patrik Troll's life story resembles Groddeck's – who speaks his own words in the fictional analyst's voice. Moreover, Saunders stresses that not only had the early twentieth century softened the lines between biography and autobiography, but it had also introduced the dialogue of autobiography and fiction. At that time, literary autobiographies were treated as fictional texts, and fiction was increasingly being read as autobiographical (Ibid.: 7).

In the first letter, Groddeck described his own road to psychoanalysis in Troll's voice, mixing a personal story with fiction and psychoanalytic theory. His text counterbalanced Freud's *The Ego and the Id*, while simultaneously being a masterful literary iteration of his own self-analysis. In that first letter, Patrik Troll talks about why he became a physician and explains the origin of his skepticism toward science. Troll's story is thick with dark affects and repressed desires. They include a sadistic need to inflict suffering, which was revealed when he and his sister Lina played with dolls. One day Lina befriended a new girl by the name of Alma – which her brother took as the greatest betrayal. Patrick formed negative associations with the word "Alma." "Alma Mater" – the nourishing mother, the university he attended, and of course his sister's friend's name – would always fill him with dread. In *The Book of the It*, Troll covers both positive and negative aspects of motherhood, which he then translates into psychoanalytic therapy. By inscribing the relationship between the analyst and the analysand into the mother-child continuum, Troll exposes a desire dynamic which is directed at the mother's image. While working with his patient M.G., Troll abandons the active approach and attempts to attune to her instead. He believes that the success of the therapy relies on a positive reproduction of the roles of the mother and the child.

In one of his letters, Troll mentions his desire to meet Sigmund Freud in person, and quotes a fragment of a reply he received from the creator of psychoanalysis. By doing this, Groddeck started playing an intertextual game with his readers and with Freud himself, who would have recognized his own words from their private correspondence in the "wild analyst's" work: "If you have understood what transference and resistance are, you can undertake to give psychoanalytic treatment to the sick without any fear" (Ibid.: 125). When asking himself whether he understands what transference is, Troll replies: "the transference [...] is a reaction process in the patient" (Ibid.: 125). Here, he emphasizes the passivity of the analyst towards the patient, thus rejecting the therapy model in which only the analyst is entitled to interpret the patients' words.

Despite the differences between Groddeck's and Freud's theoretical concepts expressed in *The Book of the It*, Freud did not criticize the form of the work as fiction. In his writings, he repeatedly spoke about a number of writers – while insisting that the psychoanalyst was not a creator. However, in his text *Delusion and Dream in Jensen's* Gradiva, he argued that the author had successfully managed to present an insightful psychiatric study – hence the conclusion that both the psychoanalyst and the writer drew from the same source, namely: the unconscious. Still, while the psychoanalyst's work "consists in the conscious observation of abnormal mental processes in other people," the writer "directs his attention to the unconscious in his own mind, he listens to its possible developments and lends them artistic expression instead of suppressing them by conscious criticism" (Freud [1907] 1959a: 92). The artist translates the result of self-analysis into a text which does not meet scientific requirements. According to Freud, because the writer did not suppress his feelings with self-aware criticism, he gained an advantage over the analyst who was forced to choose between artistic creation and medical practice. In "Creative Writers and Day-Dreaming," Freud introduced an analogy between the writer's work and children's day dreams. The poet has an inner child, and the child has an inner poet. Therefore, an adult's day-dreaming is not far from child's play:

> The creative writer does the same as the child at play. He creates a world of phantasy which he takes very seriously – that is, which he invests with large amounts of emotion – while separating it sharply from reality. [...] The unreality of the writer's imaginative world, however, has very important consequences for the technique of his art; for many things which, if they were real, could give no enjoyment, can do so in the play of phantasy, and many excitements which, in themselves, are actually distressing, can become a source of pleasure for the hearers and spectators at the performance of a writer's work.
>
> *(Freud [1908] 1959a: 144)*

Reality clashes with the world of imagination. While the latter is dominated by fantasy, the former is organized by rationality. The adult is left with a choice between an ironic or distanced attitude, with humor remaining one of the last spaces of socially acceptable immaturity. Whereas in *The Book of the It* the child is depicted as a day-dreaming being with access to truths which are unavailable to adults, Freud considered fantasizing to be a result of disappointment in everyday life. People dreamt of what they were missing: "The motive forces of phantasies are unsatisfied wishes" (Ibid.: 146). In this view, literature was a substitutive formation, used to fulfill impossible desires by proxy. Whereas both Groddeck and Freud saw the unconscious as the origin of creation, Groddeck did not reduce the creative power of the It to the "zivilisiertes, bürgerliches Es." The It was at the very source of the essence of literature. For him, writing was not simply synonymous with creating parallel realities of fantastic images (as in *The Soul Seeker*), but it was also a way of creating a space for connecting to the unconscious more closely and creatively.

Groddeck encouraged his readers to rethink the relationship between literature and psychoanalysis, which he perceived as literature's legitimate child rather than a mere method of the analysis and interpretation of literary works.[23] For him, both literature and psychoanalysis served the exploration of an individual's psyche, which was motivated by the desire to know oneself. Both tried to reach the unconscious and uncontrollable forces which drove the internal life of the subject and created new meanings in the process of symbolization, while at the same time broadening the human's cognitive horizons. Knowing oneself relied on free association, while an unrestricted flow of thought allowed the individual to partially leave the claustrophobic space of the ego. However, the process required confrontation with internal affective flows, such as love-hate tensions, to which Groddeck devoted Troll's first two letters on the ambivalence of the mother-child relationship. The dichotomy between thoughts and feelings is untenable because they both transform thought into a symbolic medium. Real knowledge – Troll argues – consists of every creative thought which reshapes the psyche of the thinking and experiencing human from the inside.

Although Freud would not have called himself a creative writer, he was aware of the literary character of his works. The issue of scientific erudition arises when psychoanalytic discourse is opened up to the autobiographical register. In his works, Freud made room for subjective and personal stories, skillfully intertwining theoretical discourse with life writing. Tensions between biography, autobiography, and the classic case study are evident both in his analytical texts and his two essays on the history of psychoanalysis. Merging lifewriting genres with the language of psychiatry and psychoanalysis was popular among Freud's students especially in the first decade of the psychoanalytic movement. In *The Book of the It*, Groddeck showed that the biography of a fictional analyst could be a veiled autobiography as well as a fragment of self-analysis and a theoretical text.[24] In the twenty-eighth letter, Troll maintains that he only writes for pleasure and does not want to publish the letters because he is first and foremost a physician. His main task is to analyze and treat patients. However, as he is writing lengthy letters to a friend which contain the most intimate details of his private and emotional life, Groddeck-Troll casts her in the role of the analyst.

In the eighth letter, Troll returns to the category of nature and behaviors which are socially deemed "against nature." Incestuous fantasies, dreams of returning to the womb, masturbation, and homosexuality manifest fully in the multi-perverse child. To the narrator, this clearly indicates that they are part of human nature. For Groddeck, the real problem was not the human, but the norms and laws which humanity had imposed on itself. Troll is not ashamed to talk about his sadistic nature, homosexual adventures, the erotic longing for his mother, or the desire to become a woman. Through his protagonist, the author successfully painted a courageous (self-)portrait of sexual and gender transgression. Thus, he became part of a broader trend of using psychiatric and sexological knowledge as literary material – starting from Thomas Mann's early short stories where non-normative desires were inseparably bound up with art and illness, and concluding with mature modernist novels which revealed the psychological profiles of non-normative characters. By publishing *The Book of the It* in 1923, Groddeck joined the authors who explored queer identities by using both psychoanalytic discourse and the autobiographical register. This is exactly how Freud must have perceived Groddeck – not as a psychoanalyst, but rather as a psychoanalytic writer. For him, Groddeck must have possessed the secret of literary creation. In the end, Groddeck's ability to create a literary work enabled him to transcend the existing horizon of any psychoanalytic theorization of literary work.

At the same time, modernist experiments with lifewriting genres were informed by the key belief of psychoanalysis that the mind distorts memories. As Freud showed in *The Interpretation of Dreams*, the past is converted to a series of emotionally charged fantasies which mix fiction with reality. Rather than being a linear order of facts, the subject's life story is therefore woven out of a distorted, shifted images of actual events. Therefore, both a patient undergoing psychoanalytic therapy and the subject of an (auto)biography practice thinking in free associations, which reveals the non-linear, non-chronological dynamics of memory (Marcus 2018). Like psychoanalysts, modernist authors such as Woolf, Stein, or Svevo played with lifewriting genres. They understood that an overtly autobiographical work can be less personal than a text of theory or fiction (e.g. Freud's highly personal *Interpretation of Dreams* and the rather impersonal *Autobiographical Study*). In Groddeck's hands, psychoanalysis became a language of literary modernism. Moreover, the generic hybridity of his writings was intended to reflect the heterogenous nature of human desire.

In *The Book of the It*, Groddeck combined the genres of the biography (Patrik Troll's story), the memoir (the author's life described in Troll's words), and the letter (addressing thoughts to someone: the female friend, the reader, Freud himself). By choosing the convention of the epistolary novel, Groddeck was able to code fragments of his own self-analysis into it. For this reason, the non-linear narrative does not develop chronologically. Some images appear and disappear, others keep returning persistently. The book is organized through the dialogic form of correspondence with the friend who remains an active listener rather than a passive reader (though her replies are not published, Troll refers to them in each letter). She is both a mother-analyst and the child-writer's muse. She encourages him to write, inspires him, and sometimes intimidates or overwhelms him. By creating the space for Troll's expression, the analyst-muse initiates the process of self-analysis and the creative work of his thoughts. Groddeck gives both a social and a symbolic dimension to the desire to know oneself. Ultimately, *The Book of the It* depicts the pursuit of self-knowledge as a literary mapping of oneself-the-child and oneself-as-a-child – a journey through the landscape of childhood fantasies and images which converge in the mother's image.

6.6 Conclusion

Georg Groddeck's *Book of the It* was an experiment in modernist literature based on a creative combination of life writing with the language of psychoanalysis. In it, Groddeck created an alternative vision of the subject thereby exposing the limitations of Freud's thought. Although a number of key words in *The Book of the It* were drawn from the psychoanalytic dictionary, they were passed through a stream of free associations and lost the direction which the creator of psychoanalysis had imposed on them. By combining literary and psychoanalytic discourses, Groddeck's writings created a space for free interactions between psychology, medicine, philosophy, and literature. The case of the German doctor thus became the perfect example of an unstable dynamic between the literary and the theoretical.

Groddeck rejected Freud's idea of human psychosexual development as a fixed series of phases which culminated in a heterosexual choice of the object of desire. By choosing the multi-perverse child to be his ideal, Groddeck twisted Freud's evolutionary model and revealed to his readers that desire was multi-directional and escaped the bourgeois framework. *The Book of the It* can therefore be read as a critique of Freud's attempt to lock human desire in the tight cage of the Oedipal triangle. Troll's biography – which takes note of his non-binary gender (becoming-a-woman, becoming-a-man), his non-normative psychosexual orientation (the equal treatment of hetero- and homosexual relationships), and his recognition of masturbation as a legitimate sexual practice – provides a model for human sexuality which is freed from the necessity of renouncing the forms of desire which elude the heteronormative mold and are thus treated as socially unacceptable. It is no coincidence that Troll's vocabulary does not include words like "guilt" or "melancholy" as an effect of rejecting impossible love.[25]

Groddeck's *Book of the It* demonstrated that psychoanalytic theory and practice could be both revolutionary and reactionary. Whereas postulating that sexuality plays a dominant role in childhood development was a revolutionary step by psychoanalysts, the normativization of desire led to a loss of the restorative impetus which had been achieved by the discovery of unconsciousness in the psychological life of the subject. By putting the unconscious into the Oedipal normative frame, Freud merely proved the oppressive nature of the Western normative order, ultimately reproducing it in his own developmental model of sexuality.

Thus, it was not due to "mysticism" that Freud could not accept Groddeck's idea of the It. Rather, he disapproved of it because of the radical conclusions presented in *The Book of the It*. By persuading his female friend to bravely follow the voice of the unconscious and explore human nature, Troll openly takes a stance against any attempts at mediation between the social norm and the desires that escape it. Patrik Troll's letters are therefore an intimate account of self-examination which broadens the understanding of human nature as a creative and socially irrepressible emanation of the unconscious. As we will see in the final chapter, self-analysis, self-expression, and their relation to the mutual understanding of the therapeutic encounter, discussed by Groddeck and Ferenczi in their correspondence, foreshadowed the relational and emotional turn in the theories and practices of psychoanalysis of the early 1930s.

Notes

1 This chapter is a revised version of an article previously published in *Oxford German Studies*, see A. Sobolewska, *Freud's Queer Fellow: Georg Groddeck Between Psychoanalytic Theory and Literary Modernism*, Oxford German Studies 2022, vol. 51, no. 1, 45–76.

2 In 2016, the Georg Groddeck Gesellschaft held an international conference "Das Es in Zeiten von Unvernunft" (14–16 October in Berlin). Abstracts and full papers

presented during this event are available online: www.georg-groddeck.de/de/GGzum150DieVortraege, accessed April 1, 2020,

3 This particular model of psychoanalytic reading, where the focus is on the unconscious desires of the text itself, could also be destructive, as Eve Kosofsky Sedgwick argued in her seminal essay "Paranoid Reading and Reparative Reading, or, You're So Paranoid, You Probably Think This Essay Is About You," in *Touching Feeling: Affect, Pedagogy, Performativity* (Durham, London: Duke University Press, 2003): 23–151.

4 On the development of the confessional mode through the western history see Michel Foucault, *The History of Sexuality*, 3 vols., vol. 1: *The Will to Knowledge*, trans. Robert Hurley (New York: Pantheon Books, 1978), 61–66.

5 On generic blurring within the modernist literature see Max Saunders, "Autobiografiction: Experimental Life-Writing from the Turn of the Century to Modernism," *Literature Compass* vol. 6, no. 5 (2009): 1041–1059. The relation between biography and autobiography in the nineteenth and twentieth centuries has been thoroughly examined in the chapter "Biography and autobiography," in *The Cambridge History of Twentieth-Century English Literature*, ed. Laura Marcus and Peter Nicholls (Cambridge: Cambridge University Press, 2004), 286–303.

6 Using Eve Kosofsky Sedgwick's, Shoshana Felman's, and Eric Savoy's understanding of non-normative and homoerotic sexualities in the turn-of-the-century literature, Haralson examines works of James, Gertrude Stein, Willa Cather, and Ernest Hemingway and argues that their writings both intersected with social context of queer lives and framed the ways of imagining and writing about non-normative sexuality (see especially the chapter devoted to James's *The Turn of the Screw* interpreted in the light of Oscar Wilde's 1895 trials, 79–101).

7 In their *Anti-Oedipus*, Gilles Deleuze and Félix Guattari saw Groddeck as their precursor. The authors manifestly contrasted Freud's thought with Groddeck's. However, they also seemed to explicitly overlook the fact that between 1917 and 1934, Groddeck developed his own psychoanalytic system based on a non-Freudian approach to the unconscious and non-linear sexual development. Moreover, the manner in which Deleuze and Guattari criticized Freud, stressing his patriarchal and dogmatic mode of thinking, resembles Groddeck's. It is even more surprising that the authors of *Anti-Oedipus* mention Groddeck only once in their book, thus suppressing the (probably unwanted?) truth about the genealogy of their own thinking.

8 On the shift in modern biography-writing see Virginia Woolf's 1939 seminal essay "The Art of Biography" in her collected minor works *The Death of the Moth and Other Essays* (London: The Hogarth Press, 1942), 119–126. See also Elena Gualtieri, "The Impossible Art: Virginia Woolf on Modern Biography," *The Cambridge Quarterly* vol. 29, no. 4 (2000): 349–361.

9 Although Lejeune's argumentation is strong and convincing, he seems to overlook exceptional cases of using novels against its authors in courts, for example in the case of Wilde in 1895 or Radclyffe Hall after the publication of *The Well of Loneliness* in 1928.

10 It is interesting to note that Freud's disciples often compared him to Christ. In this context, Peter Rudnytsky mentions an interesting conversation Freud once had with Ludwik Binswanger: "Whereas, at his best, Freud could be as inspiring as Jesus, at his worst he arrogated to himself the infallibility of a Pope. Indeed, in April 1913, Freud quipped to Ludwig Binswanger that the reason Adler and Jung had broken away from him was 'precisely because they too wanted to be Popes,' implying that he wished to reserve the title of Supreme Pontiff for himself," Rudnytsky, "Inventing Freud," *The American Journal of Psychoanalysis* 68 (2008): 68.

11 The name of Groddeck's friend is unknown, yet Wolfgang Martynkewicz suggested that she was probably modeled after Hanneliese Schumann. Groddeck corresponded with Schumann between 1909 and 1919. See Groddeck, *The Book of the*

It, 198–199; W. Martynkewicz, *Georg Groddeck. Eine Biographie*, 211–212; Rudnytsky, *Reading Psychoanalysis*, 165–166. Peter L. Rudnytsky argued that Groddeck, while working on *The Book of the It*, could have thought of his future wife, Emmy von Voigt.

12 For more details concerning Groddeck's early writings see W. Martynkewicz, *Georg Groddeck. Eine Biographie*, 159–190. On Ibsen's influence on Groddeck's *The Book of the It* see: Rudnytsky, "Freud, Ferenczi, and Rosmersholm: Incestuous Triangles and Analytic Thirds," *American Journal of Psychoanalysis* vol. 73, no. 4 (2013): 335.

13 Even though in his early writings Nietzsche criticized the truth of the existing (religious, social, intellectual) order, he did not dismiss the category of truth as a whole. As Bernard Williams argued in his *Truth and Truthfulness*, truthfulness as a category "implies a respect for the truth." The Nietzschean "unconditional will to truth does not mean that we want to believe any and every truth. It does mean that we want to understand who we are, to correct error, to avoid deceiving ourselves, to get beyond comfortable falsehood." See Bernard Williams, *Truth and Truthfulness: An Essay in Genealogy* (Princeton: Princeton University Press, 2002), 11, 15.

14 See the whole chapter "Wie sich Frauen und wie sich Thomas die Hebung der Sittlichkeit denken."

15 Letter from Oskar Pfister to Sigmund Freud, March 14, *International Psycho-Analytical Library* 59 (1921), 81.

16 *King James Bible*, "Genesis 2:7." For feminist and queer reinterpretations of this fragment see: Delphine Horvilleur, *En tenue d'Eve. Féminin, Pudeur et Judaïsme* (Paris: Grasset, 2013): 171–177; Pauline Bebe, *Isha. Dictionnaire des femmes et du judaïsme* (Paris: Calmann-Lévy, 2001), 115–119; Abby Chava Stein, *Becoming Eve: My Journey from Ultra-Orthodox Rabbi to Transgender Woman* (New York: Seal Press, 2019).

17 Cf. Lou Andreas-Salomé, "Zum Typus Weib," *Psychoanalytische Bewegung* vol. 3, no. 2 (1931): 122–137; Marie Bonaparte, "Passivität, Masochismus und Weiblichkeit," *Internationale Zeitschrift für Psychoanalyse* vol. 21, no. 1 (1935): 23–29; Joan Riviere, "Womanliness as Masquerade," *The International Journal of Psychoanalysis* 10 (1939): 303–313. It is interesting to note that Helene Deutsch's theory of motherhood presents many similarities with the first three letters of *The Book of the It*, see: Deutsch, "The Psychology of Women in Relation to the Functions of Reproduction," *International Journal of Psycho-Analysis* 6 (1925): 405–418.

18 Cf. Rudnytsky, *Reading Psychoanalysis*, 168.

19 On Freud's understanding of homosexuality see Laurence A. Rickels, "Heil Homosexuality," *GLQ* vol. 2, no. 1–2 (1995): 37–83; Mary Jacobus, "Russian Tactics. Freud's *Case of Homosexuality in Women*," *GLQ* vol. 2, no. 1–2 (1995): 67–79; Ruth Menahem, "Désorientations sexuelles. Freud et l'homosexualité," *Revue française de psychanalyse* vol. 1, no. 67 (2003): 11–25.

20 The new understanding of "sexual inversion," developed within the early psychoanalytic movement, focused primarily on the excessive affective relation between mother and a (homosexual) man.

21 Ferenczi would reach similar conclusions several years later and write about "mutual analysis" (*Mutuelle Analyse*) based on a bilateral conversation between the doctor and the patient. Like Groddeck, Ferenczi argued that the analyst is cast by the patient in the role of the mother rather than father. He criticized Freud's psychoanalysis for a male-centric orientation (*die einseitig androphile Richtung seiner Sexualtheorie*) starting with his own relationship with Freud. Ferenczi had expected a full partnership and he received harsh fatherly judgement. As a result, he rejected the authoritarian model of the relationship between the analyst and the analysand, basing his appointments on a friendly rapport instead. He was largely indebted to Groddeck for this idea. The two men bonded over their fascination

with Freud coupled with a disappointment in their teacher's authoritative and conservative attitude. See: Ferenczi, *Clinical Diary*, 251; cf. Chapter 7.

22 Groddeck also wrote about it in his 1922 article "The Compulsion to Use Symbols," 168–169.

23 On psychoanalysis as an aesthetic and imaginative discipline, a true child of modern literature see Meg Harris Williams and Margot Waddell, *The Chamber Of Maiden Thought: Literary Origins of the Psychoanalytic Model of the Mind* (London-New York: Routledge, 2014).

24 Peter L. Rudnytsky, for example, interprets the relationship between Patrik Troll and his female friend as a metaphor of the psychoanalytic therapy, see *Reading Psychoanalysis*, 164–165.

25 I refer to Freud's 1917 essay "Mourning and Melancholia." See Freud, "Mourning and Melancholia," in *The Standard Edition of the Complete Psychological Works of Sigmund Freud.* Vol. 14 (1914–1916): *On the History of the Psycho-Analytic Movement, Papers on Metapsychology and Other Works*, ed. J. Strachey (London: The Hogarth Press, 1957c), 237–258, and Judith Butler's seminal analysis of psychoanalytic concept of "melancholia" in *Gender Trouble* (New York-London: Routledge, 1999), 73–83 (chapter "Freud and the Melancholia of Gender").

References

Andreas-Salomé, L. (1931). Zum Typus Weib, in *Psychoanalytische Bewegung* 3 (2), 122–137.

Bebe, P. (2001). *Isha. Dictionnaire des femmes et du judaïsme*, Paris: Calmann-Lévy.

Biancoli, R. (1997). Georg Groddeck, the Psychoanalyst of Symbols, *in International Forum of Psychoanalysis* 6 (2), 117–125.

Bonaparte, M. (1935). Passivität, Masochismus und Weiblichkeit, in *Internationale Zeitschrift für Psychoanalyse* 21 (1), 23–29.

Butler, J. (1999). *Gender Trouble*, New York/London: Routledge.

Chemouni, J. (1984). *Georg Groddeck. Psychanalyste de l'imaginaire*, Paris: Payot.

Deleuze, G. & Guattari, F. (1983). *Anti-Oedipus. Capitalism and Schizophrenia.* Translated by Robert Hurley, Mark Seem, & Helen R. Lane. Minneapolis: University of Minnesota Press.

Deutsch, H. (1925). The Psychology of Women in Relation to the Functions of Reproduction, in *International Journal of Psycho-Analysis* 6, 405–418.

Forrester, J. (2017). *Thinking in Cases*, Cambridge: Polity Press.

Ferenczi, S. (1995). *Clinical Diary.* Translated by Michael Balint & Nicola Zarday Jackson. Cambridge, Massachusetts: Harvard University Press.

Ferenczi, S. & Jones, E. (2013). *Sandor Ferenczi – Ernest Jones: Letters 1911–1933*, F. Eros, J. Szekacs-Weisz & K. Robinson (Eds.), London: Karnac.

Foucault, M. (1978). *The History of Sexuality, vol. 1: The Will to Knowledge.* Translated by Robert Hurley. New York: Penguin Random House.

Freud, E. L. (Ed.) (1960). *Letters of Sigmund Freud 1873–1939*. Translated by Tania & James Stern. New York: Basic Books.

Freud, S. (1917). Letter from Sigmund Freud to Georg Groddeck, June 5, 1917, in *International Psycho-Analytical Library* 105, 36–38.

Freud, S. (1922). Letter from Sigmund Freud to Georg Groddeck, Christmas, in *International Psycho-Analytical Library* 105, 75–76.

Freud, S. (1925). Letter from Sigmund Freud to Georg Groddeck, June 18, in *Int. Psycho-Anal. Lib.* 105, 93.

Freud, S. ([1905] 1953). Three Essays on the Theory of Sexuality, in J. Strachey (Ed.), *The Standard Edition of the Complete Psychological Works of Sigmund Freud.* Vol. 7, London: The Hogarth Press, 125–245.

Freud, S. ([1910] 1957a). Wild Psycho-Analysis, in J. Strachey (Ed.), *The Standard Edition of the Complete Psychological Works of Sigmund Freud.* Vol. 11, London: The Hogarth Press, 219–228.

Freud, S. ([1914] 1957b). On the History of Psycho-Analytic Movement, in J. Strachey (Ed.), *The Standard Edition of the Complete Psychological Works of Sigmund Freud*, Vol. 14, London: The Hogarth Press, 1–66.

Freud, S. ([1917] 1957c). Mourning and Melancholia, in J. Strachey (Ed.), *The Standard Edition of the Complete Psychological Works of Sigmund Freud.* Vol. 14, London: The Hogarth Press, 237–258.

Freud, S. ([1907] 1959a). Delusions and Dreams, in Jensen's Gradiva, in J. Strachey (Ed.), *The Standard Edition of the Complete Psychological Works of Sigmund Freud.* Vol. 9, London: The Hogarth Press, 7–96.

Freud, S. ([1908] 1959a). Creative Writers and Day-Dreaming, in J. Strachey (Ed.), *The Standard Edition of the Complete Psychological Works of Sigmund Freud.* Vol. 9, London: The Hogarth Press, 141–154.

Freud, S. ([1930] 1961b). Civilization and its Discontents, in J. Strachey (Ed.), *The Standard Edition of the Complete Psychological Works of Sigmund Freud.* Vol. 21, London: The Hogarth Press, 57–146.

Freud, S. ([1915] 1964a). The Unconscious, in J. Strachey (Ed.), *The Standard Edition of the Complete Psychological Works of Sigmund Freud.* Vol. 14, London: The Hogarth Press, 159–215.

Freud, S. ([1923] 1964b). The Ego and the Id, in J. Strachey (Ed.), *The Standard Edition of the Complete Psychological Works of Sigmund Freud.* Vol. 19, London: The Hogarth Press, 1–96.

Freud, S. ([1932] 1971). New Introductory Lectures On Psycho-Analysis, in J. Strachey (Ed.), *The Standard Edition of the Complete Psychological Works of Sigmund Freud.* Vol. 22, London: The Hogarth Press, 1–182.

Freud, S. & Groddeck, G. (1974). *Briefe über das Es*, Frankfurt am Main: S. Fischer Verlag.

Freud, S. & Fliess, W. ([1900] 1985). *The Complete Letters of Sigmund Freud to Wilhelm Fliess, 1887–1904*, Cambridge, Massachusetts: Harvard University Press.

Freud, S. & Ferenczi, S. (1993). *The Correspondence of Sigmund Freud and Sándor Ferenczi. Vol. 1: 1908–1914*, Cambridge, Massachusetts: Harvard University Press.

Freud, S. & Ferenczi, S. (2000). *The Correspondence of Sigmund Freud and Sándor Ferenczi. Vol. 3: 1920–1933*, Cambridge, Massachusetts: Harvard University Press.

Giefer, M. (2008). Max Eitingon und der "wilde" Analytiker Georg Groddeck, in *Luzifer-Amor* 21 (42), 75–78.

Grossman, C. & Grossman, S. (1978). *The Wild Analyst: The Life and Work of Georg Groddeck*, New York: Braziller.

Groddeck, G. (1917). Letter from Georg Groddeck to Sigmund Freud, May 27, *International Psycho-Analytical Library* 105, 31–35.

Groddeck, G. (1921). *Der Seelensucher*, Leipzig/Wien/Zürich: Internationaler Psychoanalytischer Verlag.

Groddeck, G. ([1923] 1949). *Das Buch vom Es. Psychoanalytische Briefe an eine Freundin*, Leipzig/Wien/Zürich: Internationaler Psychoanalytischer Verlag.

Groddeck, G. (1925). Das Es und die Psychoanalyse, in *Die Arche* 10, 1–15.

Groddeck, G. (1926). Das Es und Evangelien, in *Die Arche* 18, 1–17.

Groddeck, G. (1949). *The Book of the It*, New York: Vintage Books.
Groddeck, G. ([1922] 1977). *The Meaning of Illness: Selected Psychoanalytic Writings Including His Correspondence with Sigmund Freud*, London: International Universities Press.
Grotjahn, M. (1945). Georg Groddeck and his Teachings about Man's Innate Need for Symbolization. A Contribution to the History of Early Psychoanalytic Psychosomatic Medicine, in *Psychoanalytic Review* 32 (1), 9–24.
Gualtieri, E. (2000). The Impossible Art: Virginia Woolf on Modern Biography, in *The Cambridge Quarterly* 29 (4), 349–361.
Grubrich-Simitis, I. (1993). *Zurück zu Freuds Texten: Stumme Dokumente sprechen machen*, Frankfurt am Main: S. Fischer Verlag.
Grubrich-Simitis, I. (1993). *Back to Freud's Texts: Making Silent Documents Speak*. Translated by Philip Slotkin. New Haven: Yale University Press.
Haralson, E. (2004). *Henry James and the Queer Modernity*, Cambridge: Cambridge University Press.
Harris, A. (2009). *Gender as Soft Assembly*, New York: Routledge.
Harris Williams, M. & Waddell, M. (2014). *The Chamber of Maiden Thought: Literary Origins of the Psychoanalytic Model of the Mind*, London/New York: Routledge.
Horvilleur, D. (2013). *En tenue d'Eve. Féminin, Pudeur et Judaïsme*, Paris: Grasset.
Horney, K. (1924). On the Genesis of the Castration Complex in Women, in *International Journal of Psycho-Analysis* 5, 50–65.
Hristeva, G. (2008). *Georg Groddeck. Präsentationsformen psychoanalytischen Wissens*, Würzburg: Königshausen & Neumann.
Jacobus, M. (1995). Russian Tactics: Freud's Case of Homosexuality in Women, in *GLQ* 2 (1–2), 67–79.
King James Bible, available online: www.kingjamesbibleonline.org.
Kosofsky Sedgwick, E. (2003). *Touching Feeling: Affect, Pedagogy, Performativity*, Durham/London: Duke University Press.
Lang, B. & Sutton, K. (2016). The Queer Cases of Psychoanalysis: Rethinking the Scientific Study of Homosexuality, 1890s-1920s, in *German History* 34 (3), 419–444.
Lejeune, P. (2017). *Autobiographie et homosexualité en France au XIXe siècle*, Paris: Éditions de la Sorbonne.
Lewinter, R. (1974). *Groddeck et le royaume millénaire de Jérôme Bosch*, Paris: Ivrea.
Makari, G. (2008). *Revolution in Mind: The Creation of Psychoanalysis*, New York: Harper Perennial.
Marcus, L. (1994). *Auto/biographical Discourses: Theory, Criticism, Practice*, Manchester: Manchester University Press.
Marcus, L. (2014). *The Dreams of Modernity*, Cambridge: Cambridge University Press.
Marcus, L. (2018). *Autobiography: A Very Short Introduction*, Oxford: Oxford University Press.
Martynkewicz, W. (1997). *Georg Groddeck. Eine Biographie*, Frankfurt am Main: S. Fischer Verlag.
Menahem, R. (2003). Désorientations sexuelles. Freud et l'homosexualité, in *Revue française de psychanalyse* 1 (67), 11–25.
Nietzsche, F. (1911). *Twilight of the Idols*, New York: T. N. Foulis.
Nietzsche, F. ([1896] 2005). *Truth: Engagements Across Philosophical Traditions*, London: Wiley-Blackwell.
Nietzsche, F. (2006). *Thus Spoke Zarathustra*, Cambridge: Cambridge University Press.

Nitzschke, B. (1983). Zur Herkunft des "Es": Freud, Groddeck, Nietzsche – Schopenhauer und E. von Hartmann, in *Psyche – Zeitschrift für Psychoanalyse* 37 (9), 769–804.

Pfister, O. (1921). Letter from Oskar Pfister to Sigmund Freud, March 14, *International Psycho-Analytical Library* 59, 81.

Poster, M. F., Hristeva, G. & Giefer, M. (Eds.) (2016). Georg Groddeck: "The Pinch of Pepper" of Psychoanalysis, in *American Journal of Psychoanalysis* 76 (2), 161–182.

Rickels, L. A. (1995). Heil Homosexuality, in *GLQ* 2 (1), 37–83.

Riviere, J. (1939). Womanliness as Masquerade, in *The International Journal of Psychoanalysis* 10, 303–313.

Rudnytsky, P. L. (2002). *Reading Psychoanalysis: Freud, Rank, Ferenczi, Groddeck*, Ithaca: Cornell University Press.

Rudnytsky, P. L. (2008). Inventing Freud, in *The American Journal of Psychoanalysis* 68 (2008): 117–127.

Rudnytsky, P. L. (2013). Freud, Ferenczi, and Rosmersholm: Incestuous Triangles and Analytic Thirds, in *American Journal of Psychoanalysis* 73 (4), 323–338.

Sadger, I. (1910). Ein Fall von multipler Perversion mit hysterischen Absenzen, in *Jahrbuch für psychoanalytische und psychopathologische Forschung* 2 (1), 59–133.

Sadger, I. (1914). Sexuelle Perversionen, in *Jahrbuch für psychoanalytische und psychopathologische Forschung* 6 (1), 296–313.

Saunders, M. (2004). Biography and autobiography, in L. Marcus & P. Nicholls, *The Cambridge History of Twentieth-Century English Literature*, Cambridge: Cambridge University Press, 286–303.

Saunders, M. (2009). Autobiografiction: Experimental Life-Writing from the Turn of the Century to Modernism, in *Literature Compass* 6 (5), 1041–1059.

Saunders, M. (2010). *Self Impression: Life-Writing, Autobiografiction, and the Forms of Modern Literature*, Oxford: Oxford University Press.

Sealey, A. (2011). The Strange Case of the Freudian Case History: The Role of Long Case Histories in the Development of Psychoanalysis, in *History of the Human Sciences* 24, 36–50.

Sobolewska, A. (2022a). Freud's Queer Fellow: Georg Groddeck Between Psychoanalytic Theory and Literary Modernism, in *Oxford German Studies* 51 (1), 45–76.

Stekel, W. (1912). Uber ein Zeremoniell vor dem Schlafengehen, in *Zentralblatt für Psychoanalyse* 10 (11), 557–566.

Stekel, W. (1913). Die Onanie. Eine Gegenkritik der vorhergehenden Kritik von Otto Kaus, in *Zentralblatt für Psychoanalyse* 3 (4–5), 249–252.

Stekel, W. (1914a). Erotische Reizungen als Heilmittel, in *Zentralblatt für Psychoanalyse* 4 (1–2), 59–70.

Stekel, W. (1914b). Sadger: Die Psychoanalyse eines Autoerotikers, in *Zentralblatt für Psychoanalyse* 4 (11–12), 616–618.

Stein, A. Ch. (2019). *Becoming Eve: My Journey from Ultra-Orthodox Rabbi to Transgender Woman*, New York: Seal Press.

Will, H. (1985). Freud, Groddeck und die Geschichte des "Es", in *Psyche – Zeitschrift für Psychoanalyse* 39 (2), 150–169.

Woolf, V. (1942). *The Death of the Moth and Other Essays*, London: The Hogarth Press.

Williams, B. (2002). *Truth and Truthfulness: An Essay in Genealogy*, Princeton: Princeton University Press.

7

PRACTICING FRIENDSHIP – A NEW BEGINNING FOR PSYCHOANALYTIC THEORY AND PRACTICE

Ferenczi between Georg Groddeck and Elizabeth Severn

Shortly after the end of the Great War, while Georg Groddeck was experimenting with the languages of psychoanalysis and literature, Sándor Ferenczi was searching for the most effective methods of psychoanalytic therapy.[1] As many scholars pointed out, Ferenczi's friendship with Groddeck played a crucial role in the development of the idea of mutual analysis. As a friend and analyst, Groddeck made it possible for Ferenczi to work through his failed analysis with Freud. The therapeutic method of mutual analysis was rooted in the rejection of the strict boundary between analyst and patient, who were henceforth equally involved in the analytic process, both intellectually and emotionally.[2] As Peter L. Rudnytsky noted in this context: "There can be no doubt that Ferenczi's willingness to enter into a mutual analysis with [Elizabeth] Severn is one of the most controversial episodes in the history of psychoanalysis" (Rudnytsky 2022: 2). The development of mutual analysis is well documented in the *Clinical Diary*, which became Ferenczi's last major project before his death in 1933.

Written in its entirety in 1932, it comprises one hundred and thirty-two entries, in which Ferenczi addressed his ongoing patient analyses, the problems of psychoanalytic theory and his self-analysis. Michael Balint described the structure and character of the *Clinical Diary* as follows:

> It is entirely spontaneous, as a true diary should be. It is true that a large part of it, about 80%, is typed, which means that Ferenczi dictated those parts to his secretary whenever he could get away from his work for a few moments.
>
> *(Ferenczi 2014: 11–12)*

Occasionally Ferenczi would also record several remarks on the same day, which reflects the dynamics of his diary as being written during breaks from

DOI: 10.4324/9781003441892-8

his daily analytic routine. As Rudnytsky pointed out, Ferenczi's experiments with the methods of psychoanalytic treatment eventually paved the way for "the contemporary shift to a two-person conceptualization of clinical work, just as Freud's self-analysis was paradigmatic for the one-person perspective of classical theory" (Ibid.: 8). With mutual analysis emphasizing a reciprocal, intellectual, and affective relationship between analyst and patient, self-analysis gave way to an essentially relational and dialogical practice.

In this final chapter, I take a closer look at the paradigmatic turn in the field of psychoanalytic theory and practice based on the shift from (Freud's) one-person to (Ferenczi's) two-person model of approaching the therapeutic situation. In my analysis of this fundamental change in the history of psychoanalysis, I point to the significance of everyday writing practices developed by Ferenczi late in life. As the first chapter has demonstrated, a key element of Freud's early psychoanalytic theory was the necessity of expressing his love to and reworking his affection for Fliess. Their correspondence became the first step in establishing the language of psychoanalysis as a complex of hybrid discourses created at the intersection of psychology, medicine, personal writing, and literature. I will show that mutual analysis as an experimental therapeutic method, developed by Ferenczi together with Elizabeth Severn, led Ferenczi in a direction opposite to where Freud's self-analysis had gone more than three decades earlier.

Over the years, Ferenczi would write more and more sparsely, increasingly leaning toward short forms such as brief theoretical remarks, notes on his work with patients, and self-analytical reflections, which later were published as *Final Contributions* and the *Clinical Diary*. Significantly, though, the vast majority of Ferenczi's diary was dictated rather than written. Through an inquiry into how Ferenczi's diary was mediated by his voice, I consider it an oral-based tool for (self-)analytic practices. I argue that the spoken character of the diary made it possible for Ferenczi to directly extend the situation of analysis which is primarily an oral activity based on the practices of talking and listening. Before turning to this aspect, however, it is crucial to take a closer look at the origins of mutual analysis, which can be found in Ferenczi's and Groddeck's friendship on the one hand, and in his personal relationship with Freud on the other hand.

7.1 Discourse on psychoanalytic methods: Groddeck–Ferenczi letters from 1921–1922

In the mid-1920s, a new person appeared in the Freud–Ferenczi–Groddeck constellation – Elizabeth Severn, with whom Ferenczi successfully developed the framework of the new trauma theory, revisiting "seduction theory" that Freud had abandoned in 1897.[3] As Peter Rudnytsky argued:

> It has been long recognized that Ferenczi's friendship with Groddeck served as a catalyst for his emotional detachment from Freud. But what

> has gone unnoticed is the way this pattern was subsequently recreated when Ferenczi moved closer to Severn and away from Groddeck.
>
> *(Rudnytsky 2022: 197)*

Severn also succeeded Groddeck as Ferenczi's analyst with whom he was able to freely develop new ideas in the field of psychoanalytic theories and practices (Ibid.: 197–198). Although the friendship between Groddeck and Ferenczi has become the subject of numerous analyses (Fortune 2018: 78–84), what calls for deeper reflection is the impact that his personal relationship with Groddeck had on Ferenczi's late understanding of theoretical practice in the field of psychoanalysis.

Ferenczi and Groddeck's correspondence from the period 1921–1933 constitutes a material trace of their friendship. These letters, unlike Ferenczi's extensive correspondence with Freud, are occasional, written and sent irregularly. At the same time, the inconsistency of their correspondence may be misleading. In fact, the two friends would travel to talk in person. The self-analytic letter dated December 24, 1921, was sent by Ferenczi less than a year after the beginning of their correspondence (April 26, 1921). In September 1921, Ferenczi and his wife Gizella had visited Groddeck in Baden-Baden. They repeated the trip later in 1924. In 1925, Groddeck visited Ferenczi in Budapest. These scarce letters filled the gaps between these meetings – thus offering an invaluable record of their intimate exchange of experiences and thoughts.

In the intellectual-affective relationship between Groddeck and Ferenczi, two different sensibilities were juxtaposed: Groddeck's resistance to orthodoxy and his creative fantasy, and Ferenczi's rationalism and his search for the best methods of psychoanalytic therapy. In their discussions, differences in their views on the basic principles of psychoanalysis came to the fore relatively quickly. In 1922, Groddeck wrote:

> I think the difference between us is that you are driven to want to understand things, and I am driven not to want to understand. In other words, […] I feel comfortable in the imago of the maternal womb with its darkness, and you want to get away from it. With such differently oriented drives, there is no lack of entertainment, and this is a guarantee for the duration of [our] friendship. There will always be something to discuss. […] I like the indefinite, I prefer to doubt […]. That is why the invention of the It is so comforting to me. I have the feeling that you like to laugh, I love to do that too. *So why should we take what calls itself scientific so seriously* [italics mine]*?*
>
> *(Ferenczi & Groddeck [1922] 2006: 81)*

In accusing his friend of having a drive for definitive knowledge, Groddeck was referring to his own belief in the imperfection of all cognition. He thought that all knowledge – both in the empirical sciences and in literature – contained a kernel of the "unknown," a mystery impossible to grasp intellectually. As the previous chapter has demonstrated, in his experimental novels and writings Groddeck challenged the dogmatism he had observed in Freudian circles. He also opposed the view that psychoanalysis was a stable system of inflexible signifiers and categories that resisted any reshaping. In this spirit, in a letter to Ferenczi, Groddeck stressed: "That we project our own complexes onto scientific findings is self-evident. How else would we discover even the slightest thing?" (Ibid.: 82). In his eyes, every scientific theory included a subjective, self-analytic element, and was an extension of the person who created it. However, replying to his friend's words, Ferenczi came to the exact opposite conclusion:

> I think we wrongly strayed into this territory so foreign to psychoanalysis by attempting to convince each other with "arguments." […] I think I have proven that I am not a principle-rider [German: Prinzipienreiter] but someone who is always ready to learn. […] you also work with the same instrument as I do, namely with logic. Therefore, it is unfair of you to deny your own working method and to pretend that you work with some mystical, mysterious *daimonion* or, more precisely, with an instrument that has nothing to do with logic.
>
> *(Ibid.: 85–86)*

Unlike Groddeck, Ferenczi was referring to the rational (logical) dimension of every scientific inquiry. That is why he also invoked Groddeck's category of "the It" (das Es), which to Freud's closest associates seemed too obscure and closer to theology than psychoanalysis. In an effort to persuade Groddeck to agree with his point, Ferenczi addressed the parallels between the work of scientists and writers:

> Even if you guess something unconsciously, you cannot escape the logic […], the logic of the unconscious. I admit that every scientist works with the imagination […]. The poet also classifies – even if only with the help of symbolic (i.e. imprecise) units of measurement. But the poetic, intuitive desire to understand is also *a desire to understand* [italics mine].
>
> *(Ibid.: 87)*

Ferenczi pointed out that although they were based on the work of the unconscious, both artistic and scientific creative practices required a specified method. In a later letter (dated October 13, 1926), Ferenczi returned once more to the differences in the understanding of psychoanalytic theories and practices that had developed between him and Groddeck. As he noted:

> There are pronounced differences between the two of us concerning the scientific methodology we apply; however, with mutual good will, we have always managed to bridge these formal differences and bring our essential

> views into harmony. [...] However, it is also flattering to me to have had some influence on your development. In any case, psychoanalysis owes you significantly; the best in our profession know this very well, even if your priority rights are treated somewhat as secondary in the literature.
>
> *(Ibid.: 138–139)*

The above letter shows perfectly that Ferenczi spent several years trying to get to the heart of methodological differences between Groddeck and himself. What seems to be crucial is the fact that the differences in their theories and methods stemmed from their divergent understandings of psychoanalysis as a discursive tool. Since the beginning of his friendship with Groddeck, Ferenczi closely observed his friend's experiments with the language of psychoanalysis which resulted in the creation of Groddeck's two books of psychoanalytic fiction: *Der Seelensucher* (1921) and the self-analytic epistolary novel *The Book of the It* (1923). Groddeck's writings revealed not only how the language of psychoanalysis could intersect with the language of literature, but also how psychoanalysis could transform into literature.[4] In Groddeck's eyes, both literary and theoretical writing practices required the release of creative energy that was susceptible to unpredictable breakdowns and inhibitions. Therefore, it was no coincidence that Ferenczi sought answers to his questions about the psychology of theoretical practice and the inhibition of creative processes in his exchanges with Groddeck.

In the last years of his life, Ferenczi wrote relatively little, which can be interpreted as a symptom of his gradual shift away from the language of theory to the development of a new understanding of analysis as a mutually experienced oral event. On the one hand, unlike Freud, Ferenczi did not seek to create literary interpretations of his patients (his "cases"). Rather, he wanted to keep precise records of his impressions formed during the therapeutic encounters. Consequently, Ferenczi's patients did not become the subjects of great psychoanalytic case studies. On the other hand, unlike Groddeck, Ferenczi did not want to transform psychoanalysis into literature, although the experiments undertaken by his friend highlighted the infinite plasticity of the psychoanalytic language both as a tool for expressing the knowledge gained through analyses and as a creative practice of (re)interpreting patients' stories. Groddeck's writings shed new light on psychoanalysis as a literary and lifewriting enterprise, making the psychoanalyst someone who deliberately sculpts the matter of language. His work thus significantly disrupted the boundaries between theoretical, autobiographical, and literary discourses, at the same time reminding other psychoanalysts of the heterogeneous and plastic dimension of the psychoanalytic narrative – the basic tool for expressing knowledge about the human psyche.

7.2 Practicing friendship: Ferenczi and Groddeck

The surviving correspondence between Groddeck and Ferenczi – unlike that between Ferenczi and Freud – is rather one-sided. There are only three letters sent by Groddeck out of Ferenczi's fifty-two letters and postcards (Ibid.: 11–12). Over the years, the exchange of letters became increasingly rare. In this context, Michael Giefer notes:

> One can only speculate about why Ferenczi did not discuss his new ideas and experiments with his close friend Groddeck, at least not by letter. [...] *Possibly, he did not feel sufficiently understood by Groddeck, who could not or did not want to follow him on his way* [italics mine].
>
> *(Ibid.: 19)*

A close reading of selected letters from the first period of their correspondence (1921–1922) allows us to see why Groddeck and Ferenczi drifted away from each other over the following years. For one, Severn's appearance played a significant role in weakening their relationship. Not only was she eager to follow her analyst's intuitions, but living in Budapest, she was physically closer to Ferenczi, which naturally facilitated their communication. In a letter dated May 2, 1922, Ferenczi wrote to Groddeck about the inconveniences of exchanging correspondence: "We feared that the letter [...] was lost. But also the answer to a lengthy letter from me is very slow in coming" (Ibid.: 66). The long wait for a letter and the concern about missing correspondence significantly complicated the exchange of ideas between Ferenczi (in Budapest) and Groddeck, who remained in Baden-Baden. Thus, the two men only had the few brief moments of their meetings left for intensive discussions and analyses. It is also worth remembering that both Groddeck and Ferenczi became aware of the differences between them rather quickly. Indeed, two distinct portraits emerge from their early correspondence: one of Groddeck as an unorthodox psychoanalyst who used theory primarily as a tool for developing his philosophy of culture and bent language freely for autobiographical and literary expression; and the other of Ferenczi as a psychoanalyst who treated theory as an infinitely fertile tool for improving therapeutic methods.

After Herbert Will, Giefer systematically presented theoretical and methodological assumptions that Ferenczi took from Groddeck in the period following the end of the Great War (Will 1994: 728–732). He listed the principles that should guide every analyst according to Groddeck and Ferenczi:

> 1. Not to educate the patient, but to let him develop; 2. To allow and promote regression ("becoming a child again"), to emphasize the importance of emotionality; 3. To intensify the transference analysis; 4. To adopt a natural and sincere approach; 5. To allow relaxation and freedom; 6. To understand the language of the body in the symptom; 7. To create a maternal space, to encourage play as a form of relationship; 8. To share mutual analysis; 9. To perceive the unconscious connection

> between analyst and the analysand; and 10. To encourage the patient to express his criticism of the analyst.
>
> *(Ferenczi & Groddeck [1922] 2006: 28)*

Giefer assumed that all the critical aspects of Ferenczi's late thought had had their origins in his discussions with Groddeck. What should be noted, however, is the fact that the desire to move from one-sided analysis (with the analyst cast as a teacher who has the key to the patient's story) to mutual analysis was signaled by Ferenczi very early in his relationship with Groddeck (in the letter of December 24, 1921).

In Groddeck, Ferenczi sought to find a mother-analyst with whom he could establish a relationship that was open and free. Recreating the child–mother relationship in the process of analysis offered a chance to work through the experience of a lack of love for those patients who had not received it as children. In his reflection, Ferenczi was coming from his own experience – that of someone who "as a child experienced too little love and too much strictness from her [the mother]" (Ibid.: 52). In a parent–child relationship based on the caretaker's omnipotence, a bond of trust could not be formed. The result of such upbringing, Ferenczi argued, was hypocrisy ("What else can be the result of such education but hypocrisy?"), which forced the child to be insincere and left the adult insensitive and cold (Ibid.: 52).

Ferenczi pointed out that in the patient–analyst relationship – which develops analogously to the child–caretaker relationship – the free expression of emotions is necessary. To Groddeck, he wrote: "So, taken objectively, it is no small matter if [...] I declare myself defeated by your naturalness, your natural kindness, and friendliness. Never before have I expressed myself so openly to a man, not even to 'Sigmund' [Freud]" (Ibid.: 53). Openness, warmth, and trust were impossible to achieve with Freud in the role of an analyst. As Ferenczi admitted, "I could not open up to him completely freely" (Ibid.: 53). Under the circumstances of being unable to "open up freely" to the analyst, the analysis itself ceased to be possible. As Ferenczi recalls from his example, Freud was "too big, too much of a father" for him (Ibid.: 53).

In the same letter, Ferenczi revealed another important aspect of the patient–analyst relationship. Freud's lack of openness and his frigidity not only reduced the effectiveness of Ferenczi's analysis itself, but they also harmed the Hungarian's intellectual work and, as a result, his career in the psychoanalytic movement. Freud's authoritarian approach and his narcissism, diagnosed by Ferenczi in the *Clinical Diary*, had a destructive effect on the freedom of Ferenczi's thinking, preventing him from achieving something he could see in Groddeck: the unrestrained expression of creative fantasy liberated from Freud's orthodoxy. Ferenczi did not hesitate to posit that the affect and the intellect are inseparable in theoretical and analytical work, developed in daily writing practices based on logic, intuition, inspiration, and creative imagination. As Ferenczi added, recalling his close collaboration with Freud in the first years of their relationship:

> The consequence was that in Palermo, where he wanted to work on the famous paranoia case (Schreber) together with me, in a sudden outburst of rebellion, on the very first evening of our work, when he wanted to dictate something to me, I stood up and declared that this was not working together after all if he simply dictated to me.
>
> *(Ibid.: 53)*

Ferenczi identified Freud's failure to recognize an intellectual partner in him as the principal cause of his desire to rebel – to break with the Father's Law – and to gain freedom of thought. In describing the famous Palermo incident, Ferenczi addressed not only the sources of his future unsuccessful analysis but also diagnosed the destructive effect of casting Freud in the role of his master and teacher. Although in his text "Analysis Terminable and Interminable" (1937) Freud used Ferenczi's case as an example of successful analysis, the self-analytic letter to Groddeck from 1921, as well as his late correspondence with Freud, leave no illusions about Ferenczi's judgment. His own experience led him to criticize the accepted models of treatment in psychoanalysis. One problem was the length of analysis. While it seemed obvious that the therapy of neuroses required many years, the analysis of future psychoanalysts could have lasted only a few months. From this, Ferenczi deduced in his seminal paper "Confusion of Tongues Between the Adults and the Child – (The Language of Tenderness and of Passion)" that "our patients gradually become better analysed than we ourselves are" (Ferenczi [1933] 1949a: 226).

Ferenczi's December 1921 letter to Groddeck can be read as a reflection on and a supplement to a different self-analytic fragment he had sent to Freud nine years earlier (in 1912). In his letter to Freud, Ferenczi had attributed his psychosomatic problems (such as shallow breathing, shortness of breath, panic attacks, insomnia) to traumatic childhood experiences that involved sexual abuse. He had written: "It is possible that my mother's strict treatment (and my father's passiveness) had the result in me of a displacement of the Oedipus complex: (mother's death, father's love); i.e., a strengthening of homosexuality" (Freud & Ferenczi 1993: 452). The problem of recognizing homoerotic tension in Ferenczi's relationships with men had surfaced in this letter. In the following years, he would write about it to Groddeck in the context of his autobiographical novel *The Book of the It*. In a self-analytic letter from 1921, Ferenczi stressed: "Now I am noticing that I have echoed your 'Briefe zur Freundin' in the witty pieces I have inserted into this letter. Are you the female friend or is your friendship a homosexual substitute for me?" (Ferenczi & Groddeck [1922] 2006: 57). He recognized that he was literally imitating the poetics of Patrik Troll's narrative from Groddeck's epistolary novel. Thus, he was deliberately playing with the self-analytic discourse of *The Book of the It*, amusing himself by stepping into the role of the narrator-patient writing to a female friend-analyst. The very use of Groddeck's poetics – at once literary and theoretical – testifies to the creative openness with which Ferenczi addressed Groddeck. As he stated: "For a very, very long time I have been proudly reserved and have hidden my feelings, often even from my closest people. I don't need to tell you that this goes back to infantile feelings" (Ibid.: 52). The letter began with the warm phrase "Lieber Freund," and went into intimate detail about Ferenczi's affective life almost immediately.

An entirely different dynamic had governed the self-analytic letter sent to Freud on December 26, 1912. Whereas in his correspondence with Groddeck Ferenczi "bared his soul" while playing with his friend's literary language, the December letter to Freud had begun with an extensive paragraph in which Ferenczi assured him of his greatness and superiority over Jung:

> Mutual analysis is nonsense, also an impossibility [German: Die gegenseitige Analyse ist ein Unsinn, auch eine Unmöglichkeit]. Everyone must be able to tolerate an authority over himself from whom he accepts analytic correction. You are probably the only one who can permit himself to do without an analyst. [...]. Despite all the deficiencies of self-analysis (which is certainly lengthier and more difficult than being analyzed), we have to expect of you the ability to keep your symptoms in check. If you had the strength to overcome in yourself, without a leader (for the first time in the history of mankind), the resistances which all humanity brings to bear on the results of analysis, then we must expect of you the strength to dispense with your lesser symptoms. The facts speak decidedly in favor of this. *But what is valid for you is not valid for the rest of us. Jung has not achieved the same self-mastery as you* [German: Was aber für Sie gilt, nicht für uns andere] [italics mine].
>
> *(Freud & Ferenczi 1993: 449)*

In his *Clinical Diary* (written almost two decades later), in which the idea of a fully open, genuinely empathetic analyst was accompanied by a sharp critique of the basic premises of psychoanalytic theory, such as the understanding of trauma, the Oedipus complex, and self-analysis, Ferenczi challenged his very own words addressed to Freud in earnest in 1912. In his 1912 letter, Ferenczi had only moved on to his own self-analysis after he had reassured Freud of the validity of Freud's position in his conflict with Jung. This merits a detailed commentary. On the one hand, the fragment reveals Ferenczi's rivalry against Jung for Freud's fatherly favor. On the other hand, it highlights the inherent inequality in Freud's relationship to Ferenczi: in order to take care of his student-patient, the analyst-teacher demands emotional gratification.

Concerns related to self-analysis as an effective method of self-discovery and self-knowledge reappear in Ferenczi's letter to Groddeck dated October 11, 1922. He wrote:

> I do not believe in self-analysis. The unconscious is clever enough to mislead one just in the most important aspects. The analysis involves a degree of self-expression that is not possible if one allows a large part of one's psyche to act as a critical instance – and that is what one does in self-analysis if one wants to be both father and son. [...] That way, one does not arrive at essentially new insights about oneself. For this, the "boiling heat of the transference" is necessary, which is missing in the self-analysis.
>
> *(Ferenczi & Groddeck [1922] 2006: 73)*

Ferenczi's words echo both the arguments made against self-observation as an effective method of psychological expertise that were typical for the second half of the nineteenth century and the concerns about this technique formulated by Freud in his letters to Fliess. In Ferenczi's eyes, self-analysis as a method of reaching the unconscious was too prone to error. That was because the individual was unable to look at himself in a critical, purely objective way. The work of transference was also impossible in self-analysis (Ferenczi 1921a: 233–251). Therefore, Ferenczi concentrated on the effects that self-analysis had had on Freud:

> That self-analysis contradicts the rule of "sociality" is also proved by the following facts: can the mentally ill, who, as a result of the change of their mental structure, make themselves independent from society (become asocial), truly analyze themselves, i.e., discharge the content of their unconscious effortlessly, without the help of a midwife?
>
> *(Ferenczi & Groddeck [1922] 2006: 74)*

Ferenczi's explicit objection to self-analysis as a method was addressed to Groddeck, whose novel *The Book of the It* – like Freud's *The Interpretations of Dreams* – was situated at the intersection of autobiography, fiction, and psycho-medical discourse. However, the critique of self-analysis in this case was meant to serve as an encouragement to subject oneself to analysis understood as a relational (interpersonal) event.

As we read in the following part of Ferenczi's letter: "I am writing all this to invite you once again to *urgently* come to Budapest and *continue your analysis here* [italics mine]" (Ibid.: 75). Ferenczi was most likely referring to the attempts to mutually analyze each other that he and Groddeck had made during their stay in Baden-Baden in 1921 and 1922. Groddeck's response from October 12, 1922 made it clear that discussions around self-analysis had become a central aspect of their disagreement over methods in psychoanalytic inquiry. In his reply, Groddeck wrote: "I will pass over the self-analysis and its results [...]. In my opinion, the main analyzer is life itself, and what we doctors do in the process is mostly a miserable self-exaltation" (Ibid.: 79).

Characteristically, Groddeck regarded life – understood as synonymous with *élan vital* – as the greatest teacher, and considered every man a tool in the hands of the unconscious – "das Es." At the same time, the "life itself" described by Groddeck lay deep inside every individual. Therefore, in this case, self-analysis allowed one to see the mysterious workings of "das Es." As the excerpts from Ferenczi's and Groddeck's correspondence quoted above represent well, the main issue was their different evaluation of self-analysis as a method of psychological expertise. Nevertheless, Ferenczi's critical reflection on self-analysis as a method strengthened his conviction that analysis was first and foremost a social fact – an interpersonal event based on affective exchange and reciprocal, empathic engagement.

7.3 Around the inhibition of the creative process

In his self-analytic letter to Groddeck from Christmas 1921, Ferenczi raised another issue that had not appeared earlier in his discussion with Freud. He wrote about the inhibition of the creative process, commonly known as writer's block. Ferenczi turned directly to Groddeck, who, as a psychoanalyst and a writer, understood in the best possible way the difficulty Ferenczi was facing. In this context, he recalled the story of working on *Thalassa*:

> Let me list the symptoms for you: The first thing that comes to mind is the inhibition of my work. (*Ideas about this: You must not surpass the father*). In 1915/1916 […] I developed a great and "magnificent" theory of genital development as a reaction of animals to the danger of desiccation when adapting to terrestrial life. *I could never decide to put this valuable – so far the most important – work on paper.* When I […] want to write, I get a backache [italics mine].
>
> *(Ibid.: 55–56)*

Ferenczi considered writing as a practice that was at once intellectual, affective, and somatic – that is, equally involving logic, emotions, and the body. The inhibition of the creative process manifested itself at all three levels, leaving its traces in the dynamics of thought, in the emotional attitude toward one's work (creativity) and in one's body. In this context, Ferenczi stressed his psychosomatic symptoms: acute back pain that significantly interfered with writing, which required spending at least several hours at a desk. Transcending the state of inhibition was supposed to make it possible to write freely.

Inhibition could be triggered either by an upcoming lecture, publication, or by phenomena much more difficult to overcome, such as fear of criticism from one's closest circle (by a family member or collaborators). In Ferenczi's case, however, the role of the main inhibitor was played by Freud ("After all, I wanted to be loved by Freud") (Ibid.: 53).[5] Ferenczi shifted the problem of remaining in Freud's shadow to the plane of an emotional-erotic relationship.

As he stated: "The bad thing is that my eroticism does not seem to be satisfied with these explanations, I want an analytical interpretation, the 'It' does not; rather, it wants something real, a young woman, a child" (Ibid.: 57). In the letter, Ferenczi thus pointed to the "real" reasons behind the inhibition of the creative process. His desire for creative work was not blocked by some vague, quasi-metaphysical force, but precisely by the urge to leave behind a real child rather than a metaphorical one (like a theory or a book). Groddeck only replied months later – in May 1922. He wrote about the problem of inhibition in a self-analytical perspective, referring to his own experience:

> Some words then about the resistance to writing. In your last letter, you mentioned your stay in Vienna and your treatment by Freud. The letter came to me just at the moment when all kinds of difficulties with my new book [*The Book of the It*] had culminated in resentment on my part. […] a letter arrived from Rank, which was at the same time friendly and forceful, I dealt a little with this Freud complex and found the solution.
>
> *(Ibid.: 69)*

In his letter, Groddeck referred to the criticism he had received from Freud, which involved accusations of having copied the theories of Freud's "expelled" disciple – Wilhelm Stekel. The problem of the "father complex" highlighted by Groddeck had also appeared in the context of Ferenczi's inhibition of the creative process in his letter of February 27, 1922: "Pr[of]. Fr[eud] dealt with my conditions for 1–2 hours; he insists on his former opinion that the main problem with me is the hatred against him, who […] prevented my marriage with a younger bride (now stepdaughter)" (Ibid.: 62).[6] The problem of Freud-as-father-figure was at the center of Ferenczi's reflections on the issues with his own theoretical practice. The shadow of the "father complex" loomed over *Thalassa*, which Ferenczi had begun to write during the war, but did not publish until almost a decade later. Ferenczi regarded this work as his first independent achievement. The book was intended as a revelatory proposal that went beyond Freud's previous insights, thus opening new possibilities in the psychoanalytic theory. For Ferenczi, *Thalassa* had a similar significance as *The Book of the It* did for Groddeck.[7]

The influence Groddeck's novel had on Ferenczi is best evidenced by his adoption of Groddeck's imaginative language in his letters. In Groddeck's second novel, the protagonist mentioned difficulties in writing, which he linked to the activity of the unconscious. In one of the letters to a friend discussed in the previous chapter, Patrik Troll returned to the unpleasant experience of the ossification of his fingers that effectively prevented him from writing. In *Das Buch vom Es*, the practice of writing is shown to be a psychosomatic process through which writers immerse themselves in the unconscious. It is no coincidence that in the passages that follow Groddeck links the process of writing to pregnancy which is supposed to produce a child-masterpiece. Writing becomes a practice of making the imagination more dynamic (engaging in a free flow of thoughts); otherwise, it would be impossible to create any work (whether literary or theoretical). For Groddeck, writing and intellectual work were first and foremost exercises in the symbol, which, as a readable trace of the unconscious, penetrated the holistically conceived mind and body of the writer.

One of the central concepts of *The Book of the It* is prohibition, which refers to both the sphere of sexuality and the creative process. Every thought, idea, emotion, and desire leave a trace in the imagination and body of every person. This trace of the It becomes even greater if its source is repulsed. This, as Groddeck points out, inevitably shatters the prohibition and enforces the (at least partial) realization of the repressed wish. Ossifying fingers or a hurting back point to the constant activity of the It. The will to create manifests itself as its own distortion and even its opposite – the desire to create/give birth shifts into creative impotence. In his novel, Groddeck introduced a specific vision of the writer-psychoanalyst's work, in which periods of creative inhibitions are understood as moments of transformation and redirection of creative energy. A key role in this process is played by a mechanism that Groddeck referred to as the "compulsion to use symbols" (German: Symbolizierungszwang). As he explained:

> The unconscious expresses itself in symbols, sends them up to consciousness and gives the poet the material from which he builds his structures. He is not completely free while creating; he has to go the way the unconscious prescribes to him by sending up symbols.
>
> *(Groddeck [1922] 1977: 160)*

According to Groddeck, the dynamics of association as a free play of symbols lie at the root of all creative processes. In this context, the writer's work is not much different from the theoretical work of a psychoanalyst. They both operate in language (in the symbol), and must face the power of the It. In this light, the psychoanalyst can be seen as both a creator and a thinker – someone who, like the philosopher or the writer, works with the living matter of language. As Groddeck added:

> I have deliberately used the expression unconscious element of the poem rather than of the poet because I wanted to suggest that the work of art – like every action perhaps – has its own life, its own soul, and that, in other words, the symbol, as soon as it has emerged, throws up new symbols by means of the compulsion to associate which make up the body of the poem. The artist's conscious activity consists merely in the shaping of the form.
>
> *(Ibid.: 162)*

The work as an effect of the creative process is an extension of its author (his or her symbolic child) and has its own unconscious. In the self-analytic letter from 1921, referring to his work on *Thalassa*, Ferenczi adopted Groddeck's understanding of the work as a form of creative activity in the realm of spoken and written language.

Yet, after *Thalassa*, Ferenczi did not devote himself to writing another voluminous case study or treatise on psychoanalytic theory.[8] Toward the end of his life, he kept a diary (from January 7 to October 2, 1932) in which he noted fragmentary comments on the analyses of his patients. In his dated entries, he spoke of the progress of the analyses conducted at the time with Clara Thompson ("Dm."), Izette de Forest ("Ett."), Roberta Nederhoed ("N. D."), Alice Lowell ("B."), Angelika Frink ("G."), Elizabeth Severn ("R.N."), and others (Brennan 2015: 5–18; Rudnytsky 2022: 136).[9] The *Clinical Diary* is thus an indispensable source of knowledge about the transformations of psychoanalytic theories and practices. The most important element of Ferenczi's late theoretical system was the concept of mutual analysis – a revelatory therapeutic experiment that aimed to critically confront Freud's most important assumptions and improve the efficiency of the psychoanalytic methods of working with patients.

7.4 The morphology of the *Clinical Diary*: self-analysis and auto-genesis

Whereas contemporary readings of Ferenczi's diary have focused more on the content of the diary than on its form, reading the *Clinical Diary* for its genre has revealed that it is a "research diary."[10] In research diaries, readers are faced with a form determined by a combination of analysis and autobiographical reflection. Although the starting point is theoretical thought, in the end, the writer themself becomes the subject of analytic inquiry. As Béatrice Galtier has aptly pointed out, although research diaries fundamentally and inseparably combine the objective with the subjective, this does not at all take away from their scientific character (Galtier 1997).

The close reading of the *Clinical Diary* shows that, as a published work, it did not have one author. Rather, its content was based on conversations with patients, who influenced the nature and form of the different entries, most of which were dictated by Ferenczi and typed by his secretary. Therefore, unlike many intimate diaries and notebooks, the *Clinical Diary* did *not* emerge from daily writing practices (only one-fifth of the text was handwritten), but from the time Ferenczi spent with his patients and secretary, who typed the words spoken between patient appointments. Moreover, the diary was not a "secret" text: Ferenczi's closest colleagues and family members, such as Gizella Ferenczi, Michael and Alice Balint, and Vilma Kovács, knew of its existence (Ferenczi 2014: 7–10, 19–32).[11]

When analyzing the *Clinical Diary*, Galtier introduced "the chronographic method" (*la méthode chrono-graphique*) to identify the psychoanalyst's late writing practices (Galtier 1997: 241). She applied the method to the handwritten notes from 1930 to 1932 (including the closing October entry of the diary), which allowed her to look at Ferenczi's late work not in terms of the content, but in terms of the writing and recording techniques he used (Ferenczi 1949b: 231–242). Ferenczi's diary was his final and unfinished project, in which his many years of work on therapeutic techniques in psychoanalysis were supposed to culminate. Remarks by Michael Balint – its first editor – indicate that it was not a collection of unrelated notes, but rather a deliberately created diary devoted to psychoanalytic methods.

The key issue I would like to address in the final part of this chapter concerns the specificity of the *Clinical Diary* in terms of its genre and its oral dimension. I will concentrate on the fact that what is commonly called a "clinical diary" in its greater part was in fact dictated, not written. Therefore, it is crucial to think not only about reading Ferenczi's diary, but also about listening to it. As we will see, as a spoken journal, the *Clinical Diary* represents a special case of a lifewriting genre. First, it was private (not intended for publication at the time of its creation) and intimate (because of its content, especially the self-analytic passages), and yet, paradoxically, also non-secret (created with the participation of another person – the secretary). Second, it was spoken. The oral dynamics of Ferenczi's recorded notes bring them closer to the situation of a meeting between the analyst and the analysand. Therefore, the *Clinical Diary* can be read to a much greater extent in the speaking–listening perspective (the inner dynamics of therapeutic work) rather than the narrative–interpretative one (the psychoanalyst as a writer), which earns it a special location on the map of prewar psychoanalytic literature.

The *Clinical Diary* consisted of one hundred and thirty-two notes, all but one dated and titled by Ferenczi. Minor parts were handwritten, while most were typed. Ferenczi addressed many topics: self-analysis related to his relationship with Freud, paranoia, denial, schizophrenia, homosexuality, the Oedipus complex, the question of the effectiveness of current therapeutic methods, and the new trauma theory. The *Clinical Diary* was composed at a significant time for Ferenczi's personal and professional biography. By the time he started working on the diary, his friendship with Groddeck had already weakened, while his relationship with Freud had gone from cool to open conflict. The last remarks in the diary followed an unpleasant meeting with Freud in Vienna and a later congress in Wiesbaden. Due to its novelty, *Clinical Diary* had to wait a long time to be published. As Balint recalled:

> We thought it would be better to wait until the immediate repercussions of the disagreement between Freud and Ferenczi had subsided. This would allow time for the creation of a more favorable atmosphere for the objective evaluation of Ferenczi's ideas contained in the *Diary*.
>
> *(Ferenczi 2014: 8)*

The reception of Ferenczi's late reflections, which were published under the title *Final Contributions* (1955), was further worsened by Ernest Jones's (Ferenczi's former analysand's) harmful remarks in the third volume of his monumental biography of Freud (Ibid.: 8–9).

The table shown in the Appendix is an overview of the problems addressed by Ferenczi in his diary, including their frequency of appearance and annotations on whether the selected fragment was written by hand or dictated. The manuscript of the diary contains two hundred and ninety-two pages, of which fifty-six were handwritten by Ferenczi.[12] The indication which entries were written by his own hand and which were typed is particularly important, because it opens up the question of which notes remained in the private domain (written down privately, for oneself) and which entered the public sphere upon their conception (by being spoken out loud while dictated and typed). The significant quantitative discrepancy between the spoken word and the written text once again raises the principal question whether the *Clinical Diary* is more of an oral (intended for the ear) or written work (intended for the eye).[13]

In a famous lecture given in 1994 at the Freud Museum London, Jacques Derrida paid particular attention to the institutionalization of knowledge – in this case, through the Freudian archive (of the history of psychoanalysis) and Sigmund Freud's private archive (Derrida 2005a). The power of legislation, Derrida argued, is based on drawing boundaries between the public and the private, the personal and the scientific. Following this path, Derrida asked: "What comes under theory or under private correspondence, for example? What comes under system? under biography or autobiography? under personal or intellectual?" (Ibid.: 4–5). Revealing and deconstructing the boundaries between the subjective and the objective would thus serve as a creative method of reinterpreting archive politics. Because psychoanalytic practice and institutions reveal the inextricable knot between personal history and the "invention of psychoanalysis" as a project of knowledge, one can look at the *Clinical Diary* without distinguishing between what is intimate and what is analytical in the text. That way, the influence of Ferenczi's everyday experiences on the development of psychoanalytic theory comes to the fore. The key to such an understanding of the psychoanalyst's diary is the date placed above the entry. It introduces an element of everyday life into Ferenczi's research practice, acting as a floating boundary between work and everyday life, between the theoretical system and the one who creates it.

Using Friedrich Nietzsche's deeply personal philosophical treatise *Ecce Homo* as a prime example, Derrida showed the mechanism by which a theoretical-autobiographical text was pushed outside the framework of philosophy and placed in the field of personal writing. In lectures devoted to "otobiographies," Derrida emphasized the relationship between autobiography and listening (the ear) – the dynamics of constructing a story in relation to the one who listens (Derrida 2005b). In this light, the relationship between what is considered intimate (self-analytic), related to the presence of others (the ear – listening), and the institutionalization of what is at once intimate and scientific (theoretical) becomes crucial for the autobiographical genre. Like *Ecce Homo*, Ferenczi's *Clinical Diary* simultaneously belongs to the space of theory and life writing.

The proximity of the theoretical discourse of psychoanalysis to the various forms of autobiographical records can be observed in the quest to discover the origins of the self. In both autobiography and psychoanalysis, the way to gaining knowledge of the self leads through self-analysis. At the same time, in his diary, Ferenczi turned to a new kind of self-analysis – to *auto-genesis*, for which communication with others (speaking–listening) rather than writing is necessary. In contrast to self-analysis, mutual analysis was an event that was both intimate and interpersonal because it implied the presence of the other person. In this sense, analysis and self-analysis conducted in Ferenczi's (spoken) diary ceased to be a form of solipsistic monologue and instead turned into an oral tool of understanding oneself in relation to others. Moreover, the *Clinical Diary* found its other side in his late correspondence with Freud.

7.6 A revolution in psychoanalysis: toward the origins of a new trauma theory

Revolutions in science usually proceed imperceptibly, and yet they lead to breakthroughs in the prevailing order of knowledge. As Thomas Kuhn accurately observed:

> A revolution is for me a special sort of reconstruction of group commitments. But it need not to be a large change, nor need it seem revolutionary to those outside a single community, consisting perhaps of fewer than twenty-five people. It is just because this type of change, little recognized or discussed in the literature of the philosophy of science, occurs so regularly on this smaller scale that revolutionary, as against cumulative, change so badly needs to be understood.
>
> *(Kuhn 1996: 180–181)*

A shift can evolve in years of discussion, but it can also be brought about by one or two publications. Ferenczi's "Confusion of Tongues" – a text that can be regarded as a direct result of the mutual (self-)analytic practices by Ferenczi and Severn – turned out to be such a watershed moment in the pre-World War II history of the theories and practices of psychoanalysis. In this case, as in the entire history of psychoanalysis, personal ties intersected with the practices of self-analysis and analytic work with patients. A new way of thinking about the patient–analyst relationship emerged in a place where listening to the patients' stories met a reflection on therapeutic techniques.

Severn came to Budapest for her analysis with Ferenczi after unsuccessful experiences with other psychoanalysts: Smith Ely Jelliffe, Joseph Asch, and Otto Rank. She recalled Rank and Jelliffe as insensitive, one-sided, and even sadistic. These difficult experiences shaped her critical judgment of Freudian therapeutic methods. In *The Discovery of the Self*, Severn wrote: "The greatest objection to be made against psychoanalysis as such is, in my opinion, its *rigidity*. Being devised as a systemic and observational method, *it lacks in flexibility and humanness in its personal application to sick people* [italics mine]" (Severn 2017: 51–52; Rudnytsky 2022: 74). Severn's critical remarks against "mainstream" psychoanalysis brought her close to both Ferenczi and Groddeck.

In her reflection on trauma, Severn drew from her own experience, placing herself as one of the subjects of her study. As Peter Rudnytsky points out: "Severn was not only sexually, physically, and emotionally abused but as a result suffered from what would today be classified as a dissociative identity disorder" (Rudnytsky 2022: 15). Confronting her patients' traumatic experiences, Severn – alongside Ferenczi – criticized the Freudian account of trauma. On January 31, 1932, Ferenczi noted that even in cases of paranoia, the psychoanalyst must search for a grain of truth in his patients' stories (Ferenczi 1995: 130). The difference between Freud's, Ferenczi's, and Severn's views on infantile sexuality and the techniques of working with patients had been revealed earlier in a heated discussion about the "Kusstechnik" used by Ferenczi in therapy with one of his patients (Clara Thompson).[14] On December 13, 1931, Freud had written to Ferenczi, hoping that no one else would learn about this "method." For Freud, the image of a patient kissing the analyst was sexually explicit, while Ferenczi believed that he was thus enabling the analysand to reclaim the role of a child severely abused by her parents.

Ferenczi had documented the progress of his work with Severn and the difficulties related to mutual analysis since January 1932. After a prolonged interruption to his diary entries (June 1932 to October 1932), he recorded the following remark: "Once mutuality has been attempted, one-sided analysis then is no longer possible – not productive" (Ibid.: 213). This fragment marks the moment when mutual analysis went beyond the experimental stage and became a method of therapy. Importantly, Ferenczi did not "invent" it alone. Rudnytsky wrote about mutual analysis as Ferenczi and Severn's shared achievement: "Ferenczi and Severn jointly gave birth to trauma theory in psychoanalysis […]. This revolution on the plane of theory goes hand in hand with a shift to a fully two-person, intersubjective approach to clinical practice" (Rudnytsky 2022: 15). The shift in analytic practices was primarily related to the appreciation of the importance of the patient–analyst relationship and empathy as a key element of the psychoanalyst's approach. In psychoanalytic literature of the time, the revolution was foreshadowed by Ferenczi's and Severn's texts: "Confusion of Tongues" and *The Discovery of the Self* respectively. Traces of the practice of "mutual analysis" and a departure from the one-sided understanding of the psychoanalyst–patient interaction had appeared earlier and flourished in "clandestine circulation" – in Ferenczi's spoken journal and in his 1932–1933 correspondence with Freud. The tension between the published (revealed) works and the intimate (hidden) revolutionary reflections clearly speaks to the dynamics of knowledge formation between the private and the public.

In his diary, under the date of February 20, 1932, Ferenczi stated:

> In another case, in spite of months of repetition of the trauma, there is no conviction. The patient says, very pessimistically: it will never be possible for the doctor really to feel the events I am going through. Thus he cannot participate in experiencing the "psychophysical" intellectual motivation. I reply: Except if I sink down with her into her unconscious, namely with the help of my own traumatic complexes. The patient appreciates this, but has legitimate doubts about such a mystical procedure.
>
> *(Ferenczi 1995: 38)*

Mutual analysis was intended as a technique to shorten the distance between the analyst and the patient. The trust between them hinged on mutual honesty and openness. The psychoanalyst and the patient, having found themselves in an equal position, were thus able to look at their own experiences anew – through the eyes of the other. In this context, on February 24, 1932, Ferenczi emphasized:

> Mutual analysis may originally have been invented by patients as a symptom of their paranoid distrust: to obtain confirmation that they were right to uncover diverse resistances, caused by antipathies, in the analyst, and to compel him to admit to these impulses. [...] The methodical analytical intentions assumed a rather more complicated form in the case of R.N. [...] After years of analysis came the idea of mutual analysis.
>
> *(Ibid.: 42–44)*

The relational dimension in the formation of psychoanalytic theory was evident from its very beginnings. Like Josef Breuer was guided to talk therapy (the talking cure) by Anna O. (Bertha Pappenheim), Ferenczi could experiment with mutual analysis with Severn. On March 13, 1932, Ferenczi wrote:

> Certain phases of mutual analysis represent the complete renunciation of all compulsion and of all authority on both sides: they give the impression of two equally terrified children who compare their experiences, and because of their common fate understand each other completely and

> instinctively try to comfort each other. Awareness of this shared fate allows the partner to appear as completely harmless, therefore as someone whom one can trust with confidence.
>
> *(Ibid.: 56)*

The image of the frightened and lonely child became a model for Ferenczi's understanding of the relationship between the patient and the analyst. The relationship was to be free from any hierarchy and from the psychoanalyst's interpretative power.

Ferenczi's late letters to Freud can be read as a negative of his *Clinical Diary*. The two analysts' late correspondence documented a process of the disintegration of their intellectual and affective relationship (Haynal 2002). In one letter to Freud, Ferenczi reported that his intensive work with his patients had led him to self-criticism, and, at the same time, to a rethinking of the psychoanalytic method's fundamental assumptions. On August 13, 1932, he stated in his diary:

> Psychoanalysis lures patients into "transference." The profound understanding and the keen interest in the most minute details of their life history and of the impulses of their psyche are naturally interpreted by the patients as a sign of profound personal friendship, indeed tenderness. As most patients are psychic shipwrecks, who will clutch at any straw, they become blind and deaf to the facts that would indicate to them how little personal interest analysts have in their patients. Meanwhile the unconscious of the patients perceives all the negative feelings in the analyst (boredom, irritation, feelings of hate when the patient says something unpleasant or something that stirs up the doctor's complexes). The analysis provides a good opportunity to carry out unconscious, purely self-seeking, ruthless, immoral, indeed so to speak criminal actions and similar behavior guiltlessly [...], such as a sense of power over a succession of helplessly devoted patients, who admire him without reservation.
>
> *(Ferenczi 1995: 199)*

Despite the friendly attitude, the analyst found it hard to get rid of the sadistic pleasure (Sadistisches Vergnügen) taken at the patient's expense (Ibid.: 264). In such a situation, the only thing that could help was to give up the position of power and step into the path of mutual analysis. Such a model of therapy did not suit Freud. And this was how Ferenczi commented on his objections: the symbolic death of the teacher–father is necessary for the disciple–child to find their own way in research practices.

7.7 Disciples must murder their teachers

Correspondence with Freud from the final years of Ferenczi's life provides an intimate testimony to the disintegrating bonds of affection between the disciple and the teacher, while at the same time shedding light on the breakthrough in the history of psychoanalysis.[15] In the last days of August 1932, Ferenczi assured Freud that he had never wanted to establish his own analytic school, but had only strived for an open discussion on therapeutic techniques (Freud & Ferenczi 2000: 90–93). In September 1932, on his way to Baden-Baden, Ferenczi arrived in Vienna to meet Freud for the last time before the 12th International Psychoanalytic Congress in Wiesbaden. The course of the tempestuous conversation between them can be reconstructed through an epistolary exchange in the following days between Freud, Max Eitingon, Sándor Radó, and Ferenczi (Ibid.: 441–443). Eitingon convinced Freud of his disciple's poor health and unstable emotional state – as did Radó. They tried to explain away Ferenczi's "psychoanalytic disorientation." It was a smart strategy – cast as a hysteric, Ferenczi was no longer a worthy opponent in a debate or polemic. On September 27, 1932, Ferenczi wrote to Freud:

> The second bad surprise was your desire that I abstain from publication; even today I can't acknowledge that I would harm myself or the cause with my communications. I still hope you will drop this idea. You certainly know just as well as I do what a loss it means for both of us that my visit with you could transpire in such a way. You can be assured that I remember all the beautiful earlier visits, even though I also have to concede that more courage and more open talk on my part about practical and theoretical things would have been advantageous to me. But, unfortunately, there is usually a lack of such courage in those who are younger and weaker.
>
> *(Ibid.: 443–444)*

While Ferenczi aimed to deescalate the conflict, Freud remained unmoved and treated him as another "sheep going astray," similarly to Adler, Stekel, and Jung. In a letter dated October 2, 1932, Freud wrote:

> The request that you shouldn't publish for another year was predominantly in your interest. I didn't want to give up hope that in your continuing work you would still recognize yourself the technical impropriety of your procedure and the limited correctness of your results. You seemed to agree with me, but I naturally relieve you of your promise and, of necessity, forgo any influence, which I don't possess anyway. I don't any longer believe that you will rectify yourself, the way I rectified myself a generation earlier. […] The traumatic effect dissipates in me, I am prepared, and used to it. Objectively, I think I would be in a position to point out to you the theoretical error in your construction, but for what? I am convinced you would not be accessible to any doubts. So there is nothing left for me but to wish you the best, which would be very different from what is going on at present.
>
> *(Ibid.: 444–445)*

Ferenczi's intellectual disobedience was explained by Freud solely as the result of his "personal trauma." The controversy over the psychoanalytic method and technique was thus transferred to the emotional–affective dimension, leading Freud to disregard its "critical potential."

Despite growing resentment between Freud and Ferenczi, the article "Confusion of Tongues" appeared in print in 1933. It centered around two issues: the relationships between the child and the adult as well as the patient and the psychoanalyst. Ferenczi began with a critique of the existing view on the etiology and treatment of neuroses, emphasizing the need to listen to patients' stories, which should not be reduced to hysterical fantasies. He emphasized the realistic rather than the phantasmagorical dimension of childhood memories. Most significantly, however, Ferenczi posited that the analyst's task was no longer to interpret his patients' stories, but to interact emotionally with patients in working through their traumatic experiences.

Ferenczi pointed out that patients were sometimes aware of their superiority over psychoanalysts, and yet – because of the physician's authoritarian attitude – they could not express it openly. Ferenczi called it a "hypocrisy of professional activity" (Hypokrisie der Berufstätigkeit), which he claimed was based on an internalized compulsion to defend one's right to infallibility (Ferenczi 1949a: 226). The first step toward a positive change in psychoanalytic therapy methods was to have a sincere conversation with the patient about mutual negative emotions. Ferenczi emphasized: "I cannot see any other way out than to make the source of the disturbance in us fully conscious and to discuss it with the patient, admitting it perhaps not only as a possibility but as a fact" (Ibid.: 226). This was a pioneering suggestion of mutual analysis in which both the patient and the psychoanalyst would be encouraged to freely express their thoughts and feelings. It is striking how ardently Ferenczi argued that the psychoanalyst's frigid approach was not the result of professionalism, but of veiled resentment.

Such a statement was enough to arouse distaste in Freud and most of his closest colleagues. Ferenczi, however, was convinced that the analyst's authoritarian attitude to his patients in therapy led to the repetition of the relationships that the analysands had had with their caretakers. If someone had experienced harm in childhood, such a mode of contact with the psychoanalyst – cast as their guardian – would be unbearable. For that reason, Ferenczi set himself the task of establishing a close relationship with the patient rather than of sorting out his or her story. The care with which the psychoanalyst should approach his patients was supposed to make it possible to overcome the difficult patient–child relationship with former caretakers. In this context, Ferenczi added:

> If we keep up our cool, educational attitude even vis-à-vis an opisthotonic patient, we tear to shreds the last thread that connects him to us. The patient gone off into his trance is a child indeed who no longer reacts to intellectual explanations, only perhaps to maternal friendliness; without it he feels lonely and abandoned in his greatest need, i.e. in the same

> unbearable situation which at one time led to a splitting of his mind and eventually to his illness; thus it is no wonder that the patient cannot but repeat now the symptom-formation exactly as he did at the time when his illness started. I may remind you that patients do not react to theatrical phrases, but only to real sincere sympathy.
>
> (*Ibid.*: 227)

When the traumatic experience is recreated, linear temporality is disrupted – patients become children not in a symbolic, but in a real way. Although they remain an adult, during analysis their needs are the desires of a child awaiting help and care from a parent. Subsequently, Ferenczi juxtaposed intellectual explanations (*intelligente Aufklärung*) with warmth (*Freundlichkeit*) and tenderness. The notion of "*Sympathie*" that he used in his last paper can be understood both as a kind of sympathetic attitude and a call to empathize (*mitfühlen*) with the patient. For Ferenczi, the patient's actual suffering remained the central interest of psychoanalysis. He believed it should not be subjected to complex theoretical divagations, but met with friendly affection. The shift of attention from analysis to empathy was the first and most important aspect of Ferenczi's revolution. The second aspect concerned the adoption of a non-canonical image of the analyst as a mother rather than a strict father. These two crucial issues raised by Ferenczi converged in the question of the reality of childhood traumas:

> I obtained above all new corroborative evidence for my supposition that the trauma, especially the sexual trauma, as the pathogenic factor cannot be valued highly enough. Even children of very respectable, sincerely puritanical families, fall victim to real violence or rape much more often than one had dared to suppose. Either it is the parents who try to find a substitute gratification in this pathological way for their frustration, or it is people thought to be trustworthy such as relatives (uncles, aunts, grandparents), governesses or servants, who misuse the ignorance and the innocence of the child. The immediate explanation – that these are only sexual phantasies of the child, a kind of hysterical lying – is unfortunately made invalid by the number of such confessions, e.g. of assaults upon children, committed by patients actually in analysis.
>
> (*Ibid.*: 227)

Because he considered the family home as the main space for potential sexual violence, Ferenczi was convinced of the prevalence of child abuse. Against Freud, he also argued that a child's emotions and emotional needs do not extend beyond tender affection. As he emphasized:

> It is not so, however, with pathological adults, especially if they have been disturbed in their balance and self-control by some misfortune or by the use of intoxicating drugs. They mistake the play of children for the desires

> of a sexually mature person or even allow themselves – irrespective of any consequences – to be carried away. The real rape of girls who have hardly grown out of the age of infants, similar sexual acts of mature women with boys, and also enforced homosexual acts, are more frequent occurrences than has hitherto been assumed. […] It is difficult to imagine the behaviour and the emotions of children after such violence.
>
> *(Ibid.: 227–228)*

Ferenczi ascribed sexual desire exclusively to the adult. Freud, however, could not accept the image of the child as an asexual being (Rudnytsky 2022: 245–263; 264–285). As Larry Wolff aptly stated, the fact that seduction theory was abandoned by Freud was extremely problematic in the face of so much evidence of child abuse within middle- and working-class families (Wolff 1988: 201). Thus, at a time when the Viennese press was reporting almost daily on cases of domestic violence against minors, Freud insisted that the "parent–child relation was one of sexual desire and mortal hatred" (Ibid.: 198). Therefore, in *The Interpretation of Dreams*, he turned the child victim into a "creature of murderous wishes" (Ibid.: 206).

The phantom of the repressed seduction theory returned with the publication of the "Confusion of Tongues" and Severn's *The Discovery of the Self.* Ferenczi merged the problem of the reality of childhood traumas with his attempt to reform psychoanalytic therapeutic methods, for which mutual analysis with Severn was the first step. Ferenczi devoted thirty dated entries in his diary to mutual analysis. They illustrate the transition from an experiment to the constitution of a new psychoanalytic method. For both Ferenczi and Severn, this partnership – as oriented around trauma and dissociation – had not only a theoretical dimension but also an autobiographical one. In his first note dedicated to Severn, Ferenczi wrote:

> The last great shock struck this person, who was already split into three parts, at the age of eleven and a half. In spite of the precariousness of that *tripartitum*, a form of adaptation to the apparently unbearable situation had set in over the years.
>
> *(Ferenczi 1995: 9)*

Following earlier findings by Pierre Janet and Morton Prince, he recognized the mechanism of dissociation in Severn and interpreted it as an effect of a series of traumatic experiences.

The result of the trauma was the loss of contact with one's feelings, which resembles the concept of "als ob" described by Helena Deutsch in 1934. In the *Clinical Diary* Ferenczi noted:

> After the second shock, we therefore have to deal with a third, soulless part of the personality, that is to say, with a body progressively divested

> of its souk, whose disintegration is not perceived at all or is regarded as an event happening to another person, being watched from the outside.
>
> *(Ibid.: 9)*

As a victim of childhood sexual abuse himself, Ferenczi could not help but see fragments of his own experience in Severn's account. References to her case were not only part of his work strategy but could also function as a catalyst for renewing his own self-analysis.

In *The Discovery of the Self*, Severn referred to Ferenczi's case as an illustration of the exact same mechanism that Ferenczi registered in his diary (Rudnytsky 2022: 94–100). Severn noted:

> The patient I have just referred to is one in point. He was a boy of six, his nurse the offender. She was a comely young woman of voluptuous type who, for the satisfaction of her own urgencies, seduced the child, i.e., used him forcibly as best she could in lieu of an adult partner. The effect on the child was twofold: he was, on the one hand, horrified, frightened, and emotionally shocked by coming in contact with such emotional violence. On the other hand, he was in a real sense "seduced" in that he was made suddenly and unduly precocious, a *desire* was aroused in him that was beyond his years.
>
> *(Severn [1933] 2017: 98)*[16]

The description of the seduced child as a victim of the confrontation with uncontrollable desire is further reflected in Ferenczi's "Confusion of Tongues." A comparative reading of the *Clinical Diary* and *The Discovery of the Self* shows that mutual analysis was primarily an interpersonal practice of working through a series of traumatic events from childhood that emotionally bound the analyst and patient together. The reciprocal self-analytic dimension of mutual analysis resonates in Ferenczi's diary and in *The Discovery of the Self*. As Rudnytsky emphasizes in this context:

> because Severn also includes her own case history, and that of her daughter, in *The Discovery of the Self*, her book takes its place in the venerable analytic tradition – extending from Freud and Ferenczi to Horney and Kohut – of covert autobiography, while at the same time employing material from the analyses of both a colleague and a family member.
>
> *(Rudnytsky 2022: 16)*

While Ferenczi's spoken diary consisted of brief and precise notes, comments and explanations that did not develop into a theoretical treatise due to their fragmentary form, Severn returned to the tradition of the psychoanalytic case study, bringing together her patients' heterogeneous voices in a polyphonic *quasi*-literary and -autobiographical narrative shaped by the psychoanalyst in the role of a writer.

7.8 Conclusion

Alongside the *Clinical Diary* and *The Discovery of the Self*, the "Confusion of Tongues" initiated a new order of thinking about and practicing psychoanalysis. The belief in the ineffectiveness of the interpretive methods of Freudian therapy, which had placed patients in the position of passive recipients of their own stories, was replaced by Ferenczi with a demand to democratize the patient–analyst relationship. After all, if one has experienced the inability to communicate with their caretakers (who were always in a position of domination), a successful analysis must not reproduce past situations and replicate the "confusion of tongues." Ferenczi paid particular attention to the lack of understanding between the psychoanalyst and the patient in most analysis, where each was forced to speak with a different voice – the analyst's was cold and insensitive, while the patient's was humble and stifled.

Ferenczi's considerations recovered the real dimension of trauma (in contrast to Freud and others' view of the patients' stories as mere wish-formations) and articulated a demand for a complete equalization of the positions of patient and psychoanalyst in therapy. Most importantly, however, Ferenczi questioned the fundamental characteristic of Freudian psychoanalysis – the drive for interpretation, which at the dawn of the twentieth century was increasingly replacing the descriptive model. In this final chapter, I have argued that mutual analysis was intended much more as a psychosomatic than an intellectual-analytic concept. Ferenczi's late considerations thus opened up another area of reflection on psychoanalysis not just as a method of therapy, but also as a certain ethical imperative.

As this chapter has shown, Ferenczi and Groddeck's discussions that preceded Ferenczi's mutual analysis with Severn centered largely around psychoanalysis as a narrative strategy. As exemplified by the *Clinical Diary* – a research document and an oral journal – Ferenczi recognized two central drives in psychoanalytic discourses. There was the "interpretive drive" which carried the danger of inserting the patient's story into the psychoanalyst's self-imposed frame (rather than listening to it). There was also the drive to create a universal theory – an ideal concept with which one would be able to explain any phenomenon related to the human psyche. I read Ferenczi's 1932 diary as a turn away from the psychoanalytic narrative toward oral commentary as a direct extension of the analytic encounter – an attempt to remain as close as possible to the spoken dimension of patients' stories. The emphasis on logic (rationalism) and the critique of vague concepts that became apparent in the Ferenczi–Groddeck debate on the method posed the risk of transforming the patients' words into a case study. Mutual analysis can thus be viewed not only as an experiment in the field of analytic practices but also as a break with previous practices of psychoanalytic writing.

Ferenczi's diary marks a shift in psychoanalytic literature – from the model of theorizing the patients' experiences to the relational model of empathizing with the analysand. At the same time, careful listening to the analysands' stories constituted a path toward a constantly renewed self-analytic confrontation with one's own emotional biography. In the last years of his life, in contrast to Freud and Groddeck, Ferenczi wanted to show that psychoanalysis was more of a relational practice based on mutual listening than a method of creating a narrative. That is why Ferenczi considered the continuously affected mind and, above all, the ear – rather than a pen and paper for the next great case study to be written – as the most important tools for the psychoanalyst's work and the proper centers of the psychoanalyst's intellectual fertility.

Notes

1 The problem of therapeutic techniques had troubled Ferenczi since early years of his career in the psychoanalytic movement. Among the most important texts in this field are: Sándor Ferenczi and Otto Rank, *The Development of Psycho-Analysis* (1924), trans. Caroline Newton (New York: Dover, 1956); Ferenczi, *Further Contributions to the Theory and Technique of Psycho-analysis*, ed. John Rickman, trans. Jane Isabel Suttie et al. (New York: Boni and Liveright Publishers, 1961). Cf. André Haynal, "Ferenczi and the Origins of the Psychoanalytic Technique," in *The Legacy of Sándor Ferenczi*, ed. Lewis Aron and Adrienne Harris (London: The Analytic Press, 1993); Thierry Bokanowsky, "The technical innovations (1918–1933)," in *The Modernity of Sándor Ferenczi: His Historical and Contemporary Importance in Psychoanalysis* (New York-London: Routledge, 2018), 45–58; Endre Koritar, "Ferenczi's experiments with technique," in *Ferenczi's Influence on Contemporary Psychoanalytic Traditions: Lines of Development – Evolution of Theory and Practice Over the Decades*, ed. Aleksandar Dimitrijevic, Gabriele Cassullo, and Jay Frankel (New York-London: Routledge, 2018), 153–158.

2 On mutual analysis, see: Therese Ragen and Lewis Aron, "Abandoned Workings: Ferenczi's Mutual Analysis," in *The Legacy of Sándor Ferenczi*, 217–226; Christopher Fortune, "Mutual Analysis: A Logical Outcome of Sándor Ferenczi's Experiments in Psychoanalysis," in *Ferenczi's Turn in Psychoanalysis*, ed. Peter L. Rudnytsky, Antal Bókay, and Patrizia Giampieri-Deutsch (New York: New York University Press, 1996), 170–186; Peter L. Rudnytsky, *Mutual Analysis: Ferenczi, Severn, and the Origins of Trauma Theory* (New York-London: Routledge, 2022).

3 Freud's propagation of the somewhat misleadingly named "seduction theory" – the idea that caretakers project their own sexual desires on children to then sexually abuse, or "seduce" them – ended with the publication of *The Interpretation of Dreams*. From then on, Freud claimed that neurotic patients' stories of sexual abuse represented fantasies rather than facts. For more on seduction theory, see: Larry Wolff, *Child Abuse in Freud's Vienna* (New York: Atheneum, 1988), 197–217; Jeffrey Moussaieff Masson, *The Assault on Truth: Freud's Suppression the Seduction Theory* (New York: Ballantine Books, 2003).

4 It is clear in the Groddeck–Ferenczi correspondence that Ferenczi knew Groddeck's literary works. See also Ferenczi's review of Groddeck's novel: Ferenczi, "Georg Groddeck: Der *Seelensucher. Ein psychoanalytischer Roman,*" *Imago* 7 (1921b): 356–359.

5 In *Clinical Diary* (2.10.1932) Ferenczi stated: "I was brave (and productive) only as long as I (unconsciously) relied for support on another power, that is, I had never really become 'grown up.' Scientific achievements, marriage, battles with formidable colleagues – all this was possible only under the protection of the idea that *in all circumstances* I can count on the father-surrogate," 212 (English translation).
6 Freud had dissuaded Ferenczi from pursuing Elma Pálos and convinced him to marry her mother Gizella, making Elma his stepdaughter. For more on that, see Emanuel Berman, "Sándor, Gizella, Elma: A biographical journey," *The International Journal of Psychoanalysis* vol. 85, no. 2 (2004): 489–520.
7 In *Thalassa* Ferenczi emphasized: "I too must confess that the ideas which I should now like to communicate, at least in their broad outlines, have lain buried in my desk for more than nine years, and I suspect that my hesitancy in making them known – *in giving birth to them, if you like* – was attributed not alone to external causes *but to my own resistances as well* (italics mine)," Ferenczi, *Thalassa: A Theory of Genitality*, trans. Henry Alden Bunker (New York: The Norton Library, 1968), 5.
8 In the *Clinical Diary* (August 4, 1932), Ferenczi returns to his treatise and asserts: "My theory of genitality may have many good points, yet in its mode of presentation and its historical reconstruction it clings too closely to the words of the master; a new edition would mean complete rewriting," 187.
9 Ferenczi's handwritten notes in the *Clinical Diary* include either his patients' initials or full names (e.g. "C. Thomson," *Clinical Diary*, manuscript, June 30, 1932, 179). My analysis is based on the manuscript of the *Clinical Diary* kept in the Freud Museum London (section: S. Ferenczi Archives). Page numbers are provided here according to the manuscript.
10 On the genre of the research journal, see René Lourau, *Le journal de recherche. Matériaux d'une théorie de l'implication* (Paris: Méridiens Klincksieck, 1988).
11 After Ferenczi's death, his manuscripts (the future *Clinical Diary* included) were given to Michael Balint by Gizella Ferenczi. Balint undertook their editing and was responsible for decoding the handwritten parts. The publication of Ferenczi's diary was not possible until the late 1960s because of his conflict with Freud as well as Jones's subsequent unjustified allegations about Ferenczi's mental illness.
12 It means that 19 percent of the diary was written by hand.
13 A perfect example of this is the (dictated) entry from January 19, 1932. Ferenczi spoke about himself in the third person: "Similarly, her [Severn's] partner of the mutual analysis [Ferenczi] had compensated in his youth by endless masturbatory activity […]," S. Ferenczi, *Clinical Diary*, 15; cf. his entry from August 4, 1932 (184–186). Notably, such a masking-strategy was no longer needed in his handwritten notes. At the same time, in another (dictated) entry (from March 17, 1932), Ferenczi speaks openly (in the first person) about the sexual trauma he had experienced in the early childhood, see: *Clinical Diary*, 61.
14 Cf. Ferenczi, *Clinical Diary*, 2–4 (January 7, 1932).
15 On Ferenczi's and Freud's letters, see for example Sharon R. Kahn, "Intolerance, Ambivalence, and Oedipus: The Reversal of Roles Between Sigmund Freud and Sándor Ferenczi," *Psychoanalytic Inquiry* vol. 17, no. 4 (1997): 559–569.
16 Cf. Rudnytsky, *Mutual Analysis*, 95.

References

Berman, E. (2004). Sándor, Gizella, Elma: A biographical journey, *in The International Journal of Psychoanalysis* 85 (2), 489–520.

Bokanowsky, T. (2018). *The Modernity of Sándor Ferenczi: His Historical and Contemporary Importance in Psychoanalysis*, New York/London: Routledge.

Brennan, B. W. (2015). Decoding Ferenczi's Clinical Diary: Bibliographical Notes, in *American Journal of Psychoanalysis* 75, 5–18.
Derrida, J. (2005a). *Archive Fever: A Freudian Impression*. Translated by Eric Prenowitz. Chicago/London: The University of Chicago Press.
Derrida, J. (2005b). *Otobiographies: L'enseignement de Nietzsche et la politique du nom propre*, Paris: Editions Galilée.
Ferenczi, S. (1921a). Weiterer Ausbau der aktiven Technik in der Psychoanalyse, in *Internationale Zeitschrift für Psychoanalyse* 7, 233–251.
Ferenczi, S. (1921b). Georg Groddeck: Der Seelensucher. Ein psychoanalytischer Roman, in *Imago* 7, 356–359.
Ferenczi S. & Rank, O. (1924). *The Development of Psycho-Analysis* (1924). Translated by Caroline Newton. New York: Dover.
Ferenczi, S. (1932). *Clinical Diary* (manuscript), Freud Museum London. Section: S. Ferenczi Archives.
Ferenczi, S. ([1933] 1949a). Confusion of Tongues Between the Adults and the Child – (The Language of Tenderness and of Passion), in *International Journal of Psychoanalysis* 30, 225–230.
Ferenczi, S. (1949b). Notes and Fragments (1930–1932), in *International Journal of Psychoanalysis* 30, 231–242.
Ferenczi, S. (1961). *Further Contributions to the Theory and Technique of Psycho-analysis.* Translated by Jane Isabel Suttie *et al.* New York: Boni and Liveright Publishers.
Ferenczi, S. ([1924] 1968). *Thalassa: A Theory of Genitality.* Translated by Henry Alden Bunker, New York: The Norton Library.
Freud, S. & Ferenczi, S. (1993). *The Correspondence of Sigmund Freud and Sándor Ferenczi. Vol. 1: 1908–1914*, Cambridge, Massachusetts: Harvard University Press.
Ferenczi, S. (1995). *Clinical Diary.* Translated by Michael Balint & Nicola Zarday Jackson. Cambridge, Massachusetts: Harvard University Press.
Freud, S. & Ferenczi, S. (2000). *The Correspondence of Sigmund Freud and Sándor Ferenczi. Vol. 3: 1920–1933*, Cambridge, Massachusetts: Harvard University Press.
Ferenczi, S. & Groddeck, G. ([1922] 2006). *Briefwechsel Ferenczi/Groddeck*, Frankfurt am Main/Basel: Stroemfeld Verlag.
Ferenczi, S. (2014). *Journal clinique*, Paris: Payot.
Fortune, C. (1996). Mutual Analysis: A Logical Outcome of Sándor Ferenczi's Experiments in Psychoanalysis, in P. L. Rudnytsky, A. Bókay, & P. Giampieri-Deutsch (Eds.), *Ferenczi's Turn in Psychoanalysis*, New York: New York University Press, 170–186.
Fortune, C. (2018). Georg Groddeck's influential friendship with Sándor Ferenczi, in A. Dimitrijevic, G. Cassullo & J. Frankel (Eds.), *Ferenczi's Influence on Contemporary Psychoanalytic Traditions: Lines of Development – Evolution of Theory and Practice Over the Decades*, New York/London: Routledge, 78–84.
Galtier, B. (1997). *L'écrit des jours. Lire les journaux personnels – Eugène Dabit, Alice James, Sandor Ferenczi*, Paris: H. Champion.
Groddeck, G. (1921). *Der Seelensucher*, Leipzig/Wien/Zurich: Internationaler Psychoanalytischer Verlag.
Groddeck, G. ([1923] 1949). *The Book of the It*, New York: Vintage Books.
Groddeck, G. ([1922] 1977). *The Meaning of Illness: Selected Psychoanalytic Writings Including his Correspondence with Sigmund Freud*, London: International Universities Press.

Haynal, A. (1993). Ferenczi and the Origins of the Psychoanalytic Technique, in L. Aron & A. Harris (Eds.), *The Legacy of Sándor Ferenczi*, London: The Analytic Press, 53–74.
Haynal, A. (2002). *Disappearing and Reviving: Sándor Ferenczi in the History of Psychoanalysis*, London: Karnac.
Kahn, S. R. (1997). Intolerance, Ambivalence, and Oedipus: The Reversal of Roles Between Sigmund Freud and Sándor Ferenczi, in *Psychoanalytic Inquiry* 17 (4), 559–569.
Koritar, E. (2018). Ferenczi's experiments with technique, in A. Dimitrijevic, G. Cassullo & J. Frankel (Eds.), *Ferenczi's Influence on Contemporary Psychoanalytic Traditions*, New York/London: Routledge, 153–158.
Kuhn, T. S. (1996). *The Structure of Scientific Revolutions*, Chicago/London: Chicago University Press.
Lourau, R. (1988). *Le journal de recherche. Matériaux d'une théorie de l'implication*, Paris: Méridiens Klincksieck.
Masson, J. M. (2003). *The Assault on Truth: Freud's Suppression the Seduction Theory*, New York: Ballantine Books.
Ragen, T. & Aron, L. (1993). Abandoned Workings: Ferenczi's Mutual Analysis, in L. Aron & A. Harris (Eds.), *The Legacy of Sándor Ferenczi*, London: The Analytic Press, 217–226.
Rudnytsky, P. L. (2022). *Mutual Analysis: Ferenczi, Severn, and the Origins of Trauma Theory*, New York/London: Routledge.
Severn, E. (2017). *The Discovery of the Self*, New York/London: Routledge.
Will, H. (1994). Ferenczi und Groddeck. Eine Freundschaft, in *Psyche* 48, 728–732.
Wolff, L. (1988). *Child Abuse in Freud's Vienna*, New York: Atheneum.

8

CONCLUSION

This book was intended as a contribution to the study of the history of psychoanalysis and psychoanalytic literature with special emphasis on the daily writing practices of the early Freudians. In the past seven chapters, I explored the close relationship between psychoanalysis, psycho-medical discourses, literature, and the visual arts of the late 1800s and early 1900s in Central Europe. I reflected on the specificity of psychoanalytic literary genres and the pivotal role of lifewriting genres in the psychoanalytic movement. My analysis started with a demonstration of how the origins of Freud's self-analysis developed in his epistolary practices. In the chapters that followed, I focused on the role of autobiography and (psycho)biography in psycho-medical discourses. I also wanted to take a closer look at the importance of diaries for the crucial transformations of psychoanalytic theories and practices in the early 1930s.

The relational dimension of theoretical and therapeutic practices in prewar psychoanalysis also became a focal point of my book. The first chapter ("Reading Sigmund Freud's Correspondence with Wilhelm Fliess: Between A Lover's Discourse and Self-Analysis") revealed how Freud's early psychoanalytic thought was entangled with affect and love. Chapter 2 ("The Sexological Discourse on Non-Normative Sexuality: Sándor Ferenczi, Richard von Krafft-Ebing, and Magnus Hirschfeld") demonstrated the linguistic polyphony of the psycho-medical discourses of the final decades of the nineteenth century, which emerged at the intersection of patients' autobiographical narrative strategies and physicians' descriptive methods. By highlighting the polyphonic nature of early sexological literature, I intended to break with the prevailing image of psychiatric practices viewed solely as a form of mistreating patients and turning them into psycho-medical "cases."

Examining the poetics of selected writings by Richard von Krafft-Ebing, Magnus Hirschfeld, and Sándor Ferenczi allowed me to discuss a paradigm

DOI: 10.4324/9781003441892-9

shift in the history of psycho-medical literature in Central Europe. I argued that it involved a move from the descriptive method (Krafft-Ebing) to the development of an empathetic approach toward the patient (Ferenczi). Most importantly, examples of narrative strategies developed by Hirschfeld and Ferenczi allowed me to uncover the roots of the image of the engaged physician, who was committed to fighting for social change and the improvement of his patients' fates. I also stressed that the modernist turn, which introduced a new way of seeing the human body as liberated from the chains of cultural and religious norms, played a critical role in the transition from descriptive case study writing to psycho-medical portraiture – a writing strategy of exploring the patients' personal histories and evoking empathy in readers.

In this book, I analyzed the relational dimension of psychoanalytic knowledge through selected examples of the dynamics of its circulation in Central Europe. As I have shown, psychoanalytic thought flourished simultaneously in literature, the visual arts, and science. Chapter 3 ("The Interpretation of Literary Dreams: Psychoanalysis, Trauma, and Painful Modernity – The Case of Mihály Babits"), which dealt with the diffusion of psychoanalytic and psycho-medical thought into modernist Hungarian literature, allowed me to take a closer look at the dynamics of what is usually referred to as knowledge "reception" and "transmission." Using newly emerging theories from psychiatry, psychology, and psychoanalysis, Mihály Babits created his literary take on daydreaming, trauma, and the mechanism of dissociation. The motifs drawn from the psycho-medical literature of his time allowed him to introduce a new understanding of split personality, which provided him with an opportunity to diagnose the painful experience of violent modernization processes. As I tried to show using the example of Babits's novel *Caliph Stork* (*The Nightmare*) and further in Chapters 4 and 5, the circulation of psychoanalytic knowledge progressed in irregular temporal and spatial shifts rather than linearly. I have emphasized that the reception of psychoanalysis in Hungarian and Czech contexts consisted in the adoption of established psychoanalytic theories and practices as much as in a creative rethinking and reinterpretation.

Chapter 4 ("The Specters of Psychoanalysis in Interwar Prague: Bohuslav Brouk and Jindřich Štyrský") dealt with the plasticity of the language of psychoanalysis as a set of diverse theoretical concepts and narrative strategies that inspired Czech surrealists to undertake far-reaching experiments with the genres of autobiography and diary. I have stressed that psychoanalysis found its way into groups of different specialties – the avant-garde, the university, and medical circles – influencing the thinking of entire communities. Tracing the circulation of psychoanalytic theories in the Czech context allowed me to highlight the collective dimension of theoretical and analytical practices. In Chapter 5 ("The Queer Case of Piotr Odmieniec Włast: (Psycho)biography, Psychoanalysis, and the Origins of Anti-Psychiatric Discourse in Poland"), I addressed the issue of the influence of fin-de-siècle psycho-medical discourses on non-normative sexuality in reinforcing the gender binary, which reduced gender or sexual transgression solely to "diseased nerves." The chapter focused on the clash between discourses of non-normative sexuality and Piotr Odmieniec Włast's self-analytical manifesto of gender transgression in an epistolary exchange. As was the case with Freud's letters to Fliess and the correspondence between Ferenczi and Groddeck, in Włast's personal history, the letter proved to be a dialogical genre *par excellence* and an ideal space for practicing self-analysis. Through a close reading of Aleksander Oszacki's essay on Włast, I was able to underscore the non-linearity of knowledge transmission as well as to situate this forgotten psycho-medical document in the long tradition of psychoanalytic psychographic writing that began in the early 1900s.

Georg Groddeck also referred to the genre of the psychoanalytic biography in his work. In his two psychoanalytic novels, he created the psychographic studies of Thomas Weltlein (*The Soul Seeker*) and Patrik Troll (*The Book of the It*). In *The Book of the It*, Groddeck combined the two key lifewriting genres for psychoanalytic literature – the letter and the autobiography, revealing them as the most suitable forms for expressing thoughts on the philosophy of the unconscious and the theory of sexuality. As Chapter 6 ("Freud's Queer Fellow: Georg Groddeck Between Psychoanalytic Theory and Literary Modernism") demonstrated, Groddeck's literary-psychoanalytic works were based on a combination of theory, life writing, and fiction. His psychoanalytic–literary work marked the "literary turn" in the psychoanalytic literature, in which psychoanalysis – after a long approach – became literature itself.

Groddeck's writings pointed to the creative dimension of literary work and theoretical practice. The theme of the psychology of theoretical practice and the inhibition of the creative process returned in Chapter 7 ("Practicing Friendship – A New Beginning for Psychoanalytic Theory and Practice: Ferenczi Between Georg Groddeck and Elizabeth Severn") in the context of Ferenczi and Groddeck's correspondence. Having examined their discussion on psychoanalytic methods, I suggested two portraits of the psychoanalyst developed before the outbreak of World War II: the cultural theorist and writer on the one hand, and the analyst and therapist on the other hand. Furthermore, in-depth reflection on Ferenczi's late writing and research practices enabled me to rethink the paradigmatic shift in the history of psychoanalysis linked to mutual analysis. In that final chapter, I argued that Ferenczi's introduction of an essentially relational therapeutic method (mutual analysis) involved a shift away from the primarily interpretive and narrative work of psychoanalysis to psychoanalytic practice as an exercise in empathy and emotional engagement with the personal history of the analyzed.

By rethinking the role of lifewriting genres in the history of psychoanalysis, I was able to stress the relational dimension of theoretical and analytical practice. For Freud, the letter served as a space for expressing and comprehending his emotional life. For Ferenczi and Groddeck, it was a space for practicing friendship and discussing psychoanalytic methods. For Piotr Odmieniec Włast, correspondence provided a chance to manifest the truth about themself in contradiction to their family and doctors. I presented the case of the self-analytic letters of this prominent Polish modernist poet as a particular manifestation of gender transgression in Central Europe in the early twentieth century that echoed the story of Daniel Paul Schreber. However, while Schreber's *Memoirs of My Nervous Illness* can be read today as a public manifesto of transgenderism, Włast's letters were intimate documents of self-discovery, made public only after the poet's death. Importantly, both Schreber and Włast resorted to religious discourse in order to liberate themselves from the chains of the normalizing poetics of descriptive psycho-medical discourse. Meanwhile, the story of (Róbert) Róza K. analyzed in Chapter 2 illustrated the practice of embedding patients' autobiographical stories in a medical narrative by the physician, which was common in fin-de-siècle psycho-medical discourses. As I have argued, Ferenczi's early text on (Róbert) Róza was a particularly important document in the development of Hungarian psychiatry and psychology, and was closely linked to the modernist breakthrough in Hungary. Typically for modernist cultures, it combined openness and progressiveness with evolutionism, which, in this case, manifested in the form of a pathologizing gaze on the body of a non-normative patient.

The series of paradigmatic shifts in the history of psychoanalysis that I have described in this book – which led from the descriptive model, through interpretive strategies, to an emotional engagement in the relational model – was closely related to the transformations of psycho-medical, lifewriting, and literary genres in the late 1800s and early 1900s. I have posited that writing about the theories and practices of psychoanalysis in Central Europe must be based on a thorough analysis of the genres of psychoanalytic literature which reveals its polyphonic nature. At the same time, my analyses of selected cases from the history of psychoanalysis, psycho-medical sciences, modernist literature, and the visual arts in Central Europe before the outbreak of the World War II highlighted the great variety of the lifewriting genres in psychoanalytic literature – from the love letter and the self-analytic letter, through the masked autobiography in the form of an epistolary novel, to the dictated (spoken) diary. Through the interdisciplinary character of this work, I was able to accentuate the inherent heterogeneity of psychoanalytic literature, which I have treated as a central element of the modernist turn in Central Europe.

Another problem addressed here was the relational and interpersonal dimension of the formation and transmission of psychoanalytic knowledge, which I described as the result of collective thinking, writing, and interpreting. A relational and emotional perspective on the history of psychoanalytic theories and practices reframed psychoanalysis as a collective invention developed on a local and transnational level. In this perspective, concepts such as "authorship" or "text" gained a relational dimension in a retelling of the history of psychoanalysis as one of cooperation and personal ties. I aimed to delineate new and still unexplored areas of the history of psychoanalytic theories and practices in the cultural contexts of knowledge circulation. Such areas included, for example, reflection on practicing friendships and the importance of personal and emotional ties for the formation of psychoanalytic theories and practices before the outbreak of World War II. The relational dimension of knowledge formation found itself at the very heart of the comparative cultural history of psychoanalysis in Central Europe which I have proposed in this book.

It is interesting that psychoanalytic reflection on the history of art and science has attached special value to solitude in the creative practices of artists, writers, and scientists. In his reflection on the importance of solitude in the creative process, British analyst Anthony Storr wrote:

> It is widely believed that interpersonal relationship of an intimate kind are the chief, if not the only, source of human happiness. Yet the lives of creative individuals often seem to run counter to this assumption. For example, many of the world's greatest thinkers have not reared families or formed close personal ties. This is true of Descartes, Newton, Locke, Pascal, Spinoza, Kant, Leibniz, Schopenhauer, Nietzsche, Kierkegaard and Wittgenstein. Some of these men of genius had transient affairs with other men or women: others, like Newton, remained celibate. But none of them married, and most lived alone for the greater part of their lives.
>
> *(Storr 1988: ix)*

Storr contrasted solitude with intimate personal ties: friendships, love affairs, and marriages. Yet, in Freud's biography, close professional and familial ties played a crucial role. I argued that psychoanalysis, as a set of theories and practices, developed within a wide network of relationships between Freud and his closest colleagues. Interpersonal ties ensured the psychoanalytic movement's rapid growth, first locally and post-1910 (with the establishment of the International Psychoanalytical Association) also internationally.

In this book, I tried to demonstrate that the dynamics of artistic fertility and scientific creativity in the psychoanalytic movement were fueled by relationships with other people, in which lifewriting genres played a particularly important role – rather than by solitude. In contrast to such a view, Storr emphasized:

> Modern insistence that true happiness can only be found in intimate attachments, more especially in sexual fulfilment, does not allow a place for characters like Gibbon. It is clear that, although his friendships were many, his chief source of self-esteem and of pleasure was his work.
>
> *(Ibid.: xi)*

Storr saw the professional world as disconnected from affective relationships. Nevertheless, my close reading of Freud's letters to Fliess (Chapter 1) as well as the correspondence between Ferenczi and Groddeck (Chapter 7) demonstrated that friendship, trust, and an emotional-intellectual exchange were crucial for their theoretical creativity. Moreover, the development of therapeutic techniques in the history of psychoanalysis would not have been possible without the participation of the patients, as proven by Ferenczi's experiments with Severn (in mutual analysis), described in the final chapter.

In my examination of personal and emotional ties between the people involved in the history of psychoanalysis, I wanted to reiterate that the development of *any* theory is also achieved through community, informal collective thinking, and writing practices. Historians and anthropologists of knowledge – from Peter Burke to Raymond Collins and Françoise Waquet – have written extensively about the collective dimension of scientific productivity. The history of sciences does not support Storr's conviction that the "men and women of science [...] may find their chief value in the impersonal rather than in the personal" (Ibid.: xii). My rejection of the individualist model in thinking about knowledge production is directly related to the discovery of the primary role of life writing in the history of psychoanalysis. In this book, I did not stop at saying that the theories and practices of psychoanalysis involved human relationships. Rather, I suggested that the authentic source of creativity of the first psychoanalysts lay in intellectual-emotional symbioses as well as mutual trust and fascinations (both erotic and intellectual).

The importance of practicing friendship and companionship in the history of psychoanalysis before 1939 stands in yet starker contrast to Storr's following statement:

> The creative person is constantly seeking to discover himself, to remodel his own identity, and to find meaning in the universe through what he creates. He finds this a valuable integrating process, which, like meditation or prayer, has little to do with other people, but which has its own separate validity. His most significant moments are those in which he attains some new insight, or makes some new discovery; and these moments are chiefly, if not invariably, those in which he is alone.
>
> *(Ibid.: xiv)*

In his book, Storr argued that creative work requires solitude. However, the study of theories and practices of psychoanalysis undertaken here allows us to abandon such a vision of solitary artistic and scientific productivity. When Storr asserted that: "Many ordinary interests, and the majority of creative pursuits involving real originality, continue without involving relationships" (Ibid.: xiv), he promoted an individualistic vision of artistic and scientific productivity. The examples of modernist literary and artistic groups provided in this book as well as their connections with medical and psychoanalytic communities contradict his vision of creative work as solitary and alienated.

It is worth noting that the emotional and communal dimension of research and writing practices had another, darker side. Sometimes, as Chapter 5 has demonstrated, personal relationships (in this case, family ties) may have had a destructive impact on an individual, especially if they were not accepted either in his family or in the surrounding community – as was the experience of Piotr Odmieniec Włast. Nevertheless, the example of Włast's biography can be seen as a different representation of the genius's solitude from the one suggested by Storr. Despite the isolation and harm he suffered at the hands of his family, Włast's letters became a way to manifest his identity.

In this book, I operated on the assumption that any intellectual work – whether artistic, literary, or psychoanalytic – in fact engages imagination, constitutes a more or less masked record of personal experience, and serves as a form of communication with others. As a result, any boundaries between artistic and scientific production remained blurred. This understanding of literary, artistic, and psychoanalytic creation also led me to question the very practice of work in the Humanities, for which writing is one of the core elements. In my view, our work as scholars in the Humanities involves establishing intimate relationships with the objects of our research, which gives it transformative power: a new view on the research subject transforms the researcher. Our reflections on the past bring better ways of understanding our present. This statement seems to be all the more valid in the history of psychoanalysis, which is unfinished and still developing. Therefore, a more profound knowledge about the advent of psychoanalysis – which ended with Freud's death in 1939 and the emigration of the most important representatives of Freudianism to Western Europe and the United States during World War II – helps to situate it as part of the modernist turn in Central Europe.

The intertwining of psychoanalytic discourses with the languages of psychiatry, psychology, philosophy, literature, and the visual arts birthed a new poetics of psycho-medical and psychoanalytic expression. My work aimed to identify the heterogeneity of psychoanalytic language, which – as a theoretical and therapeutic practice – involved lifewriting genres. Tracing the transformations that letters, diaries, psychographies, biographies, and autobiographies underwent in the writing practices of the first psychoanalysts brought to light the features of psychoanalytic literary genres that emerged as part of the modernist turn in Central Europe. As a narrative assemblage, psychoanalysis turns out to be a set of various poetics of thought and praxis, the heterogeneity of which I have shown in detail, primarily by investigating the writing practices of three prominent personalities: Freud, Ferenczi, and Groddeck. The examples of Freud's early love discourse, Ferenczi's early narrative strategies and his late writing practices, and Groddeck's experimental literary work provided an opportunity to treat psychoanalysis itself as a set of various forms of thinking and acting with words.

To conclude, in this book, I have traced the transformation of psychoanalytic theories and practices from two intersecting perspectives – a horizontal and a vertical one. The horizontal one consisted in following the transformations that occurred in psycho-medical discourses during the development of the early psychoanalytic thought, which I considered to be a transition from the descriptive model that was typical of the psychiatric language in the second half of the nineteenth century, through Freud's interpretive model (psychoanalysis as a hermeneutic method and narrative strategy), to Ferenczi's dialogical model. Meanwhile, the vertical perspective allowed me to highlight two crucial turns in the history of psychoanalytic literature: the "lifewriting turn" and the "literary turn." The former concerned a very early stage in the history of psychoanalysis, when personal writing gradually took a central place in psychoanalytic work (the autobiographical and biographical records of patients; life writing as a starting point for psychographies, autobiographies, and memoirs of Freud and his disciples). The latter was related to the transformation of psychoanalysis into literature (Groddeck).

I have tried to portray psychoanalysis as a dynamic and diverse poetics of thought – a narrative assemblage formed at the intersection of personal writing, psycho-medical discourses, philosophy, and literature. On this, I agree with George Steiner, who wrote:

> All philosophic acts, every attempt to think thought, with the possible exception of formal (mathematical) and symbolic logic, are irremediably linguistic. They are realized and held hostage by one motion or another of discourse, of encoding in words and in grammar. Be it oral or written, the philosophic proposition, the articulation and communication of argument are subject to the executive dynamics and limitations of human speech.
>
> *(Steiner 2011: 9)*

In the case of both philosophy and psychoanalysis, language and human speech determine the dynamics and limitations of the expression of thoughts. I paid particular attention to the fact that what always limits or mediates our thinking does not necessarily constitute an obstacle, but can also act as the source for creative transformations. Experiments in the field of the modernist discourses of philosophy, psychoanalysis, and literature prove this very successfully.

Ultimately, to paraphrase Steiner, my book has been an "attempt to listen more closely" (Ibid.: 13) to the polyphonic voices of psychoanalysis. In my view, psychoanalysis is a "poetry of thought," to use a beautiful phrase introduced by the philosopher. I aimed to show that the theories and practices of psychoanalysis, as diverse "poetries of thought," emerged from a tight tangle between self-analysis and autobiographical forms. In this sense, Freud and his early associates strove to capture in theoretical and literary forms the totality of the psycho-somatic, subjective experience of the inner and outer reality.

References

Steiner, G. (2011). *The Poetry of Thought: From Hellenism to Celan*, New York: New Directions Books.
Storr, A. (1988). *Solitude: A Return to the Self*, New York: Ballantine Books.

9

APPENDIX

Clinical Diary	*Handwritten notes*	*Typed notes*
mutual analysis / 30	19.07.32 (195–197); 13.08.32 (239–242); Undated/Mutuality – sine qua non (260)	17.01.32 (12–14); 19.01.32 (16–19); 31.01.32 (29–33); 2.02.32 (34–36); 16.02.32 (43–46); 20.02.32 (47–48); 24.02.32 (54–57); 3.03.32 (59–60); 6.03.32 (62–63); 10.03.32 (69–71); 13.03.32 (72–73); 17.03.32 (77–79); 20.03.32 (81–83); 29.03.32 (90–92); 31.03.32 (93–95); 12.04.32–14.04.32 (106–109); 1.05.32 (117–120); 3.05.32 (121–122); 5.05.32 (123–126); 12.05.32 (134–136); 19.05.32 (140); 18.06.32 (152–154); 19.06.32 (155); 6.07.32 (188–190); 23.07.32 (203–206); 30.07.32 (221–224); 8.08.32 (228–231)

Clinical Diary	*Handwritten notes*	*Typed notes*
therapeutic techniques / 63	3.06.32 (140i); 12.06.32 (140n/); 30.06.32 (179–180); 30.06.32 (184–187); 19.07.32 (194); 19.07.32 (195–197); Undated/What is “trauma” (224a–f); 13.08.32 (239–242); Undated/Mutuality – sine qua non (260); Undated/Progression (261)	07.01.32 (1–4); 17.01.32 (12–14); 19.01.32 (16–19); 28.01.32 (26–28); 31.01.32 (29–33); 2.02.32 (34–36); 4.02.32 (37–38); 14.02.32 (39–42); 16.02.32 (43–46); 20.02.32 (47–48); 21.02.32 (49–51); 24.02.32 (54–57); 3.03.32 (59–60); 6.03.32 (62–63); 8.03.32 (65–68); 10.03.32 (69–71); 13.03.32 (72–73); 15.03.32 (74–76); 17.03.32 (77–79); [Difficulties that arise from not accepting as real the splitting of personality] (80); 20.03.32 (81–83); 22.03.32 (84–86); 29.03.32 (90–92); 31.03.32 (93–95); 7.04.32 (102–104); 12.04.32–14.04.32 (106–109); 26.04.32 [Contribution to the phallus cult] (115–116); 1.05.32 (117–120); 3.05.32 (121–122); 5.05.32 (123–126); 8.05.32 (127–129); 12.05.32 (134–136); 19.05.32 (140); 12.06.32 (141–143); 16.06.32 (147–151); 19.06.32 (155); 21.06.32 (157–158); 23.06.32 (161–163); 28.06.32 [Utopia] (175); Undated/Influence of the passions of adults… (184–187); 6.07.32 (188–190); 23.07.32 (203–206); 24.07.32 (207–209); 27.07.32 (217–220); 30.07.32 (221–224); 4.08.32 (I.–IV.); 8.08.32 (228–231); 11.08.32 (232–234); 14.08.32 (243–245); 17.08.32 (246–248); 17.08.32 [Addendum to fragmentation] (249–250); 22.08.32 (251–252); 24.08.32 (253–255)
self-analysis / 13	29.05.32 (140b); 3.06.32 (140l); 19.07.32 (194); 19.07.32 (195–197); Undated/Identification versus hatred (210–213); 2(*12).10.32 (257–259); Undated/Progression (261)	19.01.32(16–19); 17.03.32 (77–79); 12.04.32–14.04.32 (106–109); 1.05.32 (117–120); 12.06.32 (141–143); 4.08.32 (I.–IV.)

Clinical Diary	*Handwritten notes*	*Typed notes*
trauma theory / 65	1.06.32 (140f); 30.06.32 (179–180); 19.07.32 (194); 19.07.32 (195–197); 19.07.32 (198); Undated/Identification versus hatred (210–213); Undated/What is "trauma" (224a–f); 13.08.32 (239–242); Undated/Terrorism of Suffering (256); 2(*12).10.32 (257–259)	10.01.32 (4–8); 12.01.32 (8–11); 17.01.32 (12–14); 19.01.32 (16–19); 24.01.32 (20–23); 28.01.32 (26–28); 31.01.32 (29–33); 2.02.32 (34–36); 4.02.32 (37–38); 14.02.32 (39–42); 20.02.32 (47–48); 21.02.32 (49–51); 23.02.32 (52–53); 24.02.32 [Trauma in an unconscious state] (58); 3.03.32 [On the terrorism of suffering] (61); 6.03.32 (62–63); 15.03.32 (74–76); [Difficulties that arise from not accepting as real the splitting of personality] (80); 20.03.32 (81–83); 22.03.32 (84–86); 25.03.32 (87–89); 3.04.32 (96–98); 5.04.32 (99–101); 7.04.32 (102–104); 10.04.32 (105); 24.04.32 (110–112); 26.04.32 (113–114); 1.05.32 (117–120); 3.05.32 (121–122); 5.05.32 (123–126); 8.05.32 (127–129); 10.05.32 (130–133); 12.05.32 (134–136); 17.05.32 (137–139); 12.06.32 (141–143); 14.06.32 (144–146); 16.06.32 (147–151); 18.06.32 (152–154); 21.06.32 (157–158); 23.06.32 (161–163); 26.06.32 (164–165); 30.06.32 (176–178); 7.07.32 (191–193); 24.07.32 (207–209); 26.07.32 [Clitoris and vagina] (214–216); 26.07.32 [A revision of the Oedipus complex] (215–216); 27.07.32 (217–220); 30.07.32 (221–224); 4.08.32 (I.–IV.); 7.08.32 (224–227); 8.08.32 (228–231); 12.08.32 (235–237); 14.08.32 (243–245); 17.08.32 (246–248); 17.08.32 [Addendum to fragmentation] (249–250); 24.08.32 (253–255)

Clinical Diary	*Handwritten notes*	*Typed notes*
gender and (homo)sexuality / 31	3.06.32 (140g); 10.06.32 (140/m); 14.06.32 (146b/a); 20.06.32 (156); 22.06.32 (158a–160); 19.07.32 (195–197); Undated/Identification versus hatred (210–213); 13.08.32 (239–242)	23.02.32 (52–53); 31.03.32 (93–95); 5.04.32 (99–101); 10.04.32 (105); 26.04.32 (113–114); 26.04.32 [Contribution to the phallus cult] (115–116); 8.05.32 (127–129); 10.05.32 (130–133); 17.05.32 (137–139); 19.05.32 (140); 14.06.32 (144–146); 16.06.32 (147–151); 19.06.32 (155); 21.06.32 (157–158); 26.06.32 [On the compulsion to alleviate others' pain…] (166–169); 28.06.32 (173–174); 21.07.32 (199–202); 23.07.32 (203–206); 26.07.32 [Clitoris and vagina] (214–216); 27.07.32 (217–220); 4.08.32 (I.–IV.); 7.08.32 (224–227); 22.08.32 (251–252)
R.N. (Elizabeth Severn) / 28	9.06.32(140m/a); 19.07.32 (195–197); Undated/What is "trauma" (224a–f); Undated/Mutuality – sine qua non (260)	12.01.32 (8–11); 17.01.32 (12–14); 19.01.32 (16–19); 24.01.32 (20–23); 31.01.32 (29–33); 24.02.32 (54–57); 24.02.32 [Trauma in an unconscious state] (58); 6.03.32 (62–63); 10.03.32 (69–71); 17.03.32 (77–79); 17.03.32 [Difficulties that arise from not accepting as real the splitting of personality] (80); 5.05.32 (123–126); 12.05.32 (134–136); 12.06.32 (141–143); 18.06.32 (152–154); 23.06.32 (161–163); 26.06.32 (164–165); 6.07.32 (188–190); 7.07.32 (191–193); 23.07.32 (203–206); 24.07.32 (207–209); 30.07.32 (221–224); 8.08.32 (228–231); 17.08.32 [Addendum to fragmentation] (249–250)

Clinical Diary	*Handwritten notes*	*Typed notes*
D.M. (Clara Thompson) / 16	3.06.32 (140j); 03.06.32 (140/k); 3.06.32 (140l); 14.06.32 (146b/a); 20.06.32 (156); 24.06.32 (170–172); 30.06.32 (179–180); 19.07.32 (195–197); Undated/Identification versus hatred (210–213); Undated/ Mutuality – sine qua non (260)	19.01.32(16–19); 13.03.32 (72–73); 24.04.32 (110–112); 12.06.32 (141–143); 19.06.32 (155); 6.07.32 (188–190);
Ett. (Izette de Forest) / 2	14.06.32(146b/a)	17.05.32(137–139);
N.D. (Roberta Nederhoed) / 1	-	23.06.32(161–163)
B. (Alice Lowell) / 25	3.06.32(140l); 10.06.32 (140/m); 14.06.32 (146b/a); 19.07.32 (195–197); 19.07.32 (198)	24.01.32 (20–23); 28.01.32 (26–28); 4.02.32 (37–38); 24.02.32 (54–57); 3.03.32 [On the terrorism of suffering] (61); 6.03.32 (62–63); 8.03.32 (65–68); 22.03.32 (84–86); 25.03.32 (87–89); 26.04.32 [Contribution to the phallus cult] (115–116); 19.05.32 (140); 12.06.32 (141–143); 6.07.32 (188–190); 21.07.32 (199–202); 23.07.32 (203–206); 27.07.32 (217–220); 30.07.32 (221–224); 8.08.32 (228–231); 12.08.32 (235–237); 17.08.32 (246–248)
G. (Angelika Frink) / 8	Undated/Identification versus hatred (210–213); Undated/What is "trauma" (224a–f)	26.07.32[A revision of the Oedipus complex] (215–216); 27.07.32 (217–220); 30.07.32 (221–224); 14.08.32 (243–245); 17.08.32 (246–248); 24.08.32 (253–255)

Clinical Diary	*Handwritten notes*	*Typed notes*
S.I. (Harriot Sigray) / 19	19.07.32(195–197)	24.02.32 (54–57); 24.02.32 [Trauma in an unconscious state] (58); 3.03.32 [On the terrorism of suffering] (61); 10.03.32 (69–71); 15.03.32 (74–76); 3.04.32 (96–98); 26.04.32 [Contribution to the phallus cult] (115–116); 12.05.32 (134–136); 19.05.32 (140); 12.06.32 (141–143); 16.06.32 (147–151); 18.06.32 (152–154); 23.06.32 (161–163); 26.06.32 (164–165); 28.06.32 (173–174); 6.07.32 (188–190); 7.07.32 (191–193); 12.08.32 (235–237)
U. (Teddy Miller) / 4	Undated/Mutuality – sine qua non (260)	14.06.32(144–146); 22.08.32 (251–252); 24.08.32 (253–255)
O.S./[R./R.S. in the manuscript] / 9	-	21.02.32 (49–51); 24.02.32 [Trauma in an unconscious state] (58); 8.05.32 (127–129); 14.06.32 (144–146); 23.06.32 (161–163); 26.06.32 [On the compulsion to alleviate others' pain…] (166–169); 30.06.32 (176–178); 21.07.32 (199–202); 12.08.32 (235–237)
F./[F.] / 1	-	7.08.32(224–227)

INDEX

Abraham, Karl 87n4, 133, 177
Abraham, Nicolas 22
An Autobiographical Study (Freud) 7, 41, 45–46
Anti-Oedipus 200n7
anti-Semitism 46, 119–120n13
Autobiografiction (Saunders) 194
autobiography, memoirs 7–9, 10, 15–16, 24–25, 27, 35; *An Autobiographical Study* (Freud) 7, 41, 45–46; autobiografiction 15–16, 194; *The Caliph Stork* as autobiographical case study 98–101; defining 41; Freud on 6–7, 8–9; *The Interpretation of Dreams* (Freud) 6, 16, 45–46, 51, 96, 123, 175, 197, 229; as masked self-revelations, non-normative sexuality 16, 19; patients' 68, 78, 80–81, 173–174, 210; as psychoanalytical genre 5–10; as psycho-medical document (Elemér Tábory) 98–101, 112, 117; as self-analysis 6
Autoeroticism and Psychoeroticism (Brouk) 124, 145
auto-genesis 41–47, 219–222

Babits, Mihály 25, 93–120; literary and academic career 93; *see also The Caliph Stork (A gólyakalifa)* (Babits)
Balint, Michael 206, 220, 220–223, 233n11
Barthes, Roland 23, 35, 35–36, 36, 37, 37–38, 48
Bates, David 141
Bernays, Martha 7
Bernays, Minna 61n18
Bernfeld, Siegfried 6, 10, 40, 58–59n1
Between Men (Sedgwick) 44
Beyond the Pleasure Principle (Freud) 136–137
biographies 6–7, 200n5; "The Art of Biography" (Woolf) 200n8; *The Book of the It* (Groddeck) 197, 198, 199; "A Defense of Biography" (Bonaparte) 9–10; *Freud: A Life for Our Time* (Gay) 6, 62n32; Freud on 7, 9; "new biography" 7–8, 174; as psychoanalytic genre 7; psychoanalytic psychography, (*see* psychography);
bisexuality: *Androgyne* (Przybyszewski) 83, 84; Fliess about 54–57; Freud about (auto-genesis, theory) 16, 24, 41–47, 54, 55, 61n18, 73, 78, 164–165, 191; Freud–Fliess relationship 41–47, 55–58, 61n18, 62n29, 62n33; natural human (innateness) 83, 174, 191; *Psychopathia Sexualis* (Krafft-Ebing) 78–81, 100, 158–159, 163–164; "The Sex" (Przybyszewski) 83; *Sex and Character* (Weininger) 83–84, 152; third sex (Hirschfeld) 81–82; *Three Essays on the Theory of Sexuality* (Freud) 55, 73, 78, 164–165, 191
Bölsche, Wilhelm 184
Bonaparte, Marie 9–10, 41, 56
The Book of the It (Groddeck) 11, 27; Adam and Eve, fall of man 188–189,

190; analyst–analysand relationship 176; gender, sexuality, sexual difference 184, 188, 189–191, 197, 198–199; genre experimentation, double narrative 173–174; illness/health, philosophy of 176, 187–188; main themes 187; self-analysis and literary experimentalism 194–198; as self-portrait 186–193; structure 186
Borgos, Anna 79
Bortnyik, Sándor 70, 72
Breuer, Josef 13, 61n19
Brome, Vincent 57
Brouk, Bohuslav 122–123; *Autoeroticism and Psychoeroticism* 144–145; Freudianism critique 124–125; libido/sexuality and creative process 126, 131; pornophilic art, concept 26, 126, 128, 129, 131, 137; sexuality (Eros) and human liberation 124, 126–129; Štyrský collaboration 124; as "wild psychoanalyst", psychoanalytical theories 124–125
Bruckner, Anton 3
Budapest: *Budapest 1900* (Lukacs) 69, 70, 71; as city of psychoanalysis 4; modernist culture 69–71; Budapest Psychoanalytic School 4, 72
Butler, Judith 46–47
The Caliph Stork (A gólyakalifa) (Babits) 25, 93–118, 119nn3–4; automated writing 117; context: Anglo-American literature 97–98; context: Hauff fairytale 97; dissociation as modernity response 101–104; dream theories/understanding 94, 95, 96–97, 99, 101, 113–116; dream-death similarities 99; genre: as autobiographical case study 98–101; genre: as polyphonic (self-) narrative 105–111; genre: as psychoanalytical reading 111–116; genre: as psycho-medical reader 94–98; hallucination 96–97, 115–116, 117; literary source: Hauff fairytale 93–94; neurosis, psychosis, reality-loss 111–115; split personalities / dissociative identities 25, 94–95, 98, 99–100, 106, 115, 117; the unconscious 97, 99, 115

Chandler, Daniel 12
child: play and creative sensibilities 161, 195–198; mother-child relationship/continuum 101, 132–135, 192–194, 195, 197, 212; natural uninhibition 189; psycho-sexual development 29n5, 109–111, 144–145, 189, 191, 197, 199, 222–223, 229–230; seduction theory (Freud) 207, 229, 232n3; trauma 212, 213, 228–230; world perception 186
Chimera 158
Chmurski, Mateusz 150
Christine "Sally" Beauchamp 94–95
Clinical Diary (Ferenczi) 233nn5–13; Freud analysis 212; morphology 219–222; mother analyst, maternal therapy aspects 180; patient-therapist relationship 225, 229–230, 231; publication 233n11; as research diary 219–222; structure, character 206–207, 220–221; written-oral genre 245–250, 28, 207, 220, 233nn11–12
Collins, Randall 38, 39
"Confusion of Tongues between the Adults and the Child" (Ferenczi) 117, 213, 222–224, 227, 229–231
creative inhibition 216–219
creative process and libido 125–126, 131
creative process/creative sensibility, universality 10–11, 27, 138–139, 160–161, 216–219
"Creative Writers and Day-Dreaming" (Freud) 10–11, 160–161, 195–197
cultural paralaxis 4–5
cultural parataxis 4–5
culture: comparative cultural history 1, 5, 20, 28, 240; defining 5; history 5; as local, everyday practice 5; low vs high distinction, loss 15; psychoanalysis as cultural practice 1, 4–5, 10, 20, 242
Czechoslovakia, Czech Surrealism: class struggle and sexual revolution 131; dream poetic 130–137; *Edice 69* (Edition 69) series 26, 125–126, 128; Freudianism 123–125; humor and suffering 142–143; pornophiles, pornophilic art 26, 126, 128, 129, 131, 137; psychonalysis, pre-1939 knowledge transmission 122, 124–125, 145; sexuality (Eros) and human liberation 124, 126–129, 131, 145–146; Štyrský, dream diaries 137–141; Štyrský, erotic works 25, 125–126; "synthetism," artistic 137

Das Buch vom Es (*The Book of the It*, Groddeck); *see The Book of the It* (Groddeck)
"A Defense of Biography" (Bonaparte) 9–10

Deleuze, Gilles 17–19, 188, 200n7
"Delusion and Dream in Jensen's *Gradiva*" (Freud) 10–11, 195
Der Doppelgänger (Rank) 98
Der Seelensucher (The Soul Seeker, Groddeck) 27, 185–186, 210
Derrida, Jacques 221–222
destruction as symbol 108–111
Deutsch, Helena 165, 229
The Devils (Włast) 158–159, 162, 169n8
diaries, journals 10, 28, 29n5; *Clinical Diary* (Ferenczi) 245–250, 28, 180, 206–207, 212, 214, 219–222, 225, 229–230, 231, 233nn5–13; *The Discovery of the Self* (Severn) 230, 231; dream diary (Štyrský) 139–141; "Relics and Diaries" (Bernfeld) 10; research diary 219; spoken/oral journal 220, 224, 231
Die Don Juan Gestalt (Rank) 98
Discomfort in Culture (Freud) 229
The Discovery of the Self (Severn) 115, 229–231
The Dissociation of Personality (Prince) 92, 94–95
dissociative personality disorder / dissociative identity 25, 94–95, 98, 99–100, 106, 115, 117, 223, 229, 237
dreams: day-dreaming and creativity 160–161, 165, 195–197; dream diary (Štyrský) 25, 139–145; "dream" life (*The Caliph Stork*) 99, 100, 101, 106, 107, 110–112; *The Interpretation of Dreams* (Freud) 6, 16, 45–46, 51, 96, 123, 175, 197, 229; as knowledge source 115–116, 117, 145; nightmares 94, 101, 113–114, 115–117, 137; as source for autobiografiction 16; as source of psychobiographies 10–11; surrealism and 130–137; theories, interpretation (*The Caliph Stork*) 93, 94–98, 99

Edice 69 (Edition 69) series 26, 125–126, 128
The Ego and the Id (Freud) 176–177, 194
ego-psychology / egocentrism (Freud) 46, 176, 178–179, 181–182, 194
Ellis, Havelock 73, 172
Emilie Comes to Me in a Dream (Štyrský) 126, 130, 134–136, 143–145
epistolography; *see* letters, correspondences
Eros and Civilization (Marcuse) 126–128
experimental writing 5, 25, 173–174, 197–198, 200n5, 209–210, 242

Falzeder, Ernst 34
Fenichel, Otto 123–124, 147n5
Ferenczi, Sándor 68–88, 71–73, 112–113, 206–233; adult-child relationship 117, 213, 222–224, 227, 229–231; *Clinical Diary* (*see under own heading*); creative process, inhibition 216–219; dream theory 96; Groddeck–Ferenczi friendship 210–216; homosexuality, non-normative sexuality 24, 69, 72–74, 76–78, 85, 86, 112–115; lifewriting practices 28, 207; psychoanalysis popularization 72–73, 92–93; psycho-medical portraiture 73–78; relational model, psychoanalysis 22, 28, 176, 199, 207, 224–225, 232, 236–239; scientific methodology 208–210, 211–212; trauma theory 207, 222–230
Ferenczi, Sándor (psychoanalytic methods, discourse/development): *Clinical Diary* as documentation (1933) 206; Freud–Ferenczi relationship, correspondence/critique 38–39, 208–209, 212–217, 220–221, 223, 225–229; Groddeck–Ferenczi letters/visits (1921–1922) 207–210; mutual analysis as relational therapeutic method, developing 22, 229, 231, 233n13, 241 (*see also* mutual analysis); Severn–Ferenczi collaboration 206–208, 211, 222–225, 229–230, 238
fetish, fetishization 132–133, 136
Fetishism (Freud) 132
fiction 10
Filipiak, Izabela 168–169n7, 168n5
Fliess, Ida 41, 56, 61nn18–19, 62n27
Fliess, Wilhelm 23–24, 34–62, 191, 207, 238; bisexuality 54–57; *In eigener Sache* (*On My Own Account)* 56–57, 62n29; Freud: plagiarism affair 55–58; Freud: relationship, correspondence (*see* Freud-Fliess letters);
Foucault, Michel 17, 68, 119n12
Freud, Ernst L. 36
Freud, Sigmund 8; authoritarian style, Ferenczi critique 38–39, 212–213; auto-genesis (Fliess correspondence) 41–47; castration anxiety 142–143; creativity / creative sensibility 10–11, 160–161, 195–197; *The Ego and the Id* 176–177, 194; ego-psychology / egocentrism 46, 176, 178–179, 181–182, 194; humor and the

unconscious 142–143; seduction theory (Freud) 207, 229, 232n3; self-analysis (Fliess correspondence) 51–55; sexuality 16, 24, 41–47, 54, 55, 61n18, 73, 78, 164–167, 191; unconscious, concept 173, 174–185
Freud, Sigmund (correspondences): Fliess, Wilhelm 23–24, 34–62, 191, 207, 238 (*see also* Freud-Fliess letters); publication: censorship 34–35; publication: history 35, 60n10
Freud, Sigmund (texts): *Autobiographical Study* 7, 41, 45–46; *Beyond the Pleasure Principle* 136–137; "Creative Writers and Day-Dreaming" 10–11, 160–161, 195–197; "Delusion and Dream in Jensen's *Gradiva*" 10–11, 195; Discomfort in Culture 229; *Fetishism* 132; *The Interpretation of Dreams* 6, 16, 45–46, 51, 96, 123, 175, 197, 229; *The Interpretation of Dreams* (Freud) 6, 16, 45–46, 51, 96, 123, 175, 197, 229; "Screen Memories" 6, 16; *Studies on Hysteria* 13; *Three Essays on the Theory of Sexuality* 55, 73, 78, 164–168, 191
Freud: A Life for Our Time (Gay) 6
Freud-Fliess letters 23–24, 34–62, 191, 207, 238; bi-/homosexuality (auto-genesis, self-analysis, Freud) 41–47, 50, 54, 55, 61n18; bi-/homosexuality, theory (Freud); bisexuality, theory (Fliess) 54–57; friendship 23, 41, 44–45, 56–57, 62n32; as lover's discourse 22, 37–38, 41; plagiarism affair 55–58, 62n29; as psychoanalytical discourse 41; publication 34–35, 41; as relationship reflection (bisexuality, friendship) 41–47, 55–58, 61n18, 62n29, 62n33; self-analysis as writing practice (Freud) 51–55
friendship, concept 23; Ferenczi-Groddeck *see under their own names*, 206–233; Freud-Fliess (*see* Freud-Fliess letters); male, Western culture 42, 43–44; male platonic vs homoerotic love 44, 45, 48–50; Montaigne about 48–50, 51; scientific authority and 39; solitude vs friendship 240–241
Fuss, Diane 16–17, 19

Galtier, Béatrice 219–220
Garner, Shirley Nelson 43, 45
Gay, Peter 6, 62n32
gender, sexuality, bisexuality (Freud-Fliess) 42
gender, sexuality/non-normative sexuality 16–17; autobiografiction as masked self-revelations 16, 19; bisexuality (*see under own heading*); gender as universal moving principle 83; infantile sexuality 29n5, 109–111, 189, 222–223; non-normative sexuality, sexological discourse (*see under own heading*); psychoanalytic theory, emancipatory influence 16, 19; psychoanalytic theory, Oedipal triangle critique 16–18; queer sexuality 30n9; *scientia sexualis* 19, 92, 142; *Three Essays on the Theory of Sexuality* (Freud) 55, 73, 78, 164–165, 191; transgender identity 78–81, 150–170
"generalized Oedipus" concept 17–19
Generation 1900 71, 92–93
Giefer, Michael 211, 212
Goethe, Johan Wolfgang von 7–8, 184
Gradiva (Jensen) 10–11, 195
Graf, Max 8, 40
Groddeck, Georg 172–202, 206–233; *The Book of the It* (*see under own heading*); creative process, inhibition 216–219; cultural understanding 182; *Der Seelensucher* (The Soul Seeker) 27, 185–186, 210; Goethe's divine nature, influence 184–185; illness/health, philosophy of 176, 187–188; Nietzsche influence 181, 182–184, 186, 201n13; psychoanalysis as self-analysis 173, 214–216; scientific methodology 183–184, 208–210, 211–212; sexuality, model 184, 188, 189–191, 197, 198–199; unconscious (It/Es), concept 173, 174–185
Groddeck–Ferenczi psychoanalytic method discourse 206–216
Groddeck–Freud collaboration and controversies 174–185, 187–188, 190, 191, 194–199
Gross, Otto 109–110, 111, 112, 118
Guattari, Félix 17–19, 188, 200n7
Gyógyászat (Therapy) 71–72, 84, 87n7
Gyöngyi, Izsó 77

hallucination 96–97, 115–116, 117
Harris, Roy 14
Hauff, Wilhelm 93, 97, 106
Hermann, Imre 133–134
hermaphroditism 78, 82–84, 163–165, 164
Hirschfeld, Magnus 68–88

history, comparative cultural 1, 5, 20, 28, 240
Hobbes, Thomas 182
Hofmannsthal, Hugo von 3, 104
"Homosexualitas Feminina" ("Female homosexuality," Ferenczi) 24, 72–74, 76–78, 86
homosexuality: cultural tabu 46–47; as degeneration (spiritual, bodily) 76–77; desire, repression 112–115; Freud (auto-genesis, theory) 43–47; *Psychopathia Sexualis* (Krafft-Ebing) 78–81, 100, 158–159, 163–164; *Symposium* (Plato) 61n16, 84; *see also* bisexuality
homosocial desire 43–44
Horney, Karen 189–190
Hungary / Hungarian psychiatry and psychology: anti-Semitism 119–120n13; Babits, Mihály, *The Caliph Stork* 25, 93–94, 94–117; Ferenczi, Sándor, "Homosexualitas Feminina" 69, 73–78, 85; Ferenczi, Sándor, psychoanalysis popularization 72–73, 92–93; Ferenczi–Groddeck friendship/correspondence 206–233; Hermann, Imre 133–134; modernist breakthrough 69–71, 72, 92–94, 95, 102–103, 117; sexological discourses 24–25; Vay, Sarolta/Sándor 77–78, 79, 164

Ibsen, Henrik 104, 159
In eigener Sache (*On My Own Account*, Fliess) 56–57, 62n29
inhibition, creative processes 193, 210, 216–219, 238
International Psychoanalytic Association 4
The Interpretation of Dreams (Freud) 6, 16, 45–46, 51, 96, 123, 175, 197, 229

James, David 21–22
Janet, Pierre 25, 95, 117, 229
Jensen, Wilhelm 10–11, 195
Jolles, André 73
Jones, Ernest 7, 57, 175, 221, 233n11
journals, psychoanalytic genre; *see* diaries, journals
The Judgement (Kafka) 105

Kafka, Franz 104–105
Katharina C., case 13–14
Kernstok, Károly 3, 70
Kertbeny, Karl-Maria 72–73
Kincses 112, 114
knowledge (formation, transmission) 12, 20, 81–82, 145, 157, 208–209, 224, 237; (re)interpreting patients' cases 210; dreams as source 115–116, 117, 145; personal dimension 38–39; self-knowledge, self-analysis 51–55, 155, 191, 214–219, 222; support, restriction 85
knowledge transmission, personal dimension 38–39
Komornicka, Aniela 151, 152, 156, 170n18
Komornicka, Maria (Włast, Piotr Odmieniec)); *see* Włast, Piotr Odmieniec
Kosofsky Sedgwick, Eve 43–44, 60n12, 200n3, 200n6
Kósztolányi, Dezső 72, 93
Krafft-Ebing, Richard von 78–81, 85–86, 100, 158–159, 163–164, 169n11
Kramnick, J. 21
Kraus, Karl 11, 83
Krúdy, Gyula 69, 70, 72
Kuhn, Thomas 222

La Boétie, Étienne de 48
Langerová, Marie 122
Le Bon, Gustave 159
Lejeune, Philippe 41, 99, 119n12, 174, 200n9
letters, correspondences 34–35; as auto-genesis, self-analysis 41–47, 219–222; as cultural practice 35, 48; epistolary practice, nature, dynamic 36–37; Freud, Sigmund 36; Freud to Fliess 23–24, 34, 34–62, 191, 207, 238; Groddeck and Ferenczi 27, 207–210, 210–216; knowledge transmission 38–39; as "lover's discourse" 35–38, 58, 59n5; psychoanalytic community, historical significance 12, 37; as psychoanalytic genre 12; self-analysis in written correspondence 51–55; static and narrative genres 48; text–spoken word tension 35–36, 59n2; Włast to his family 26
life writing 6, 8–10, 151, 156, 173, 194, 197, 198, 241; *see also individual genres*
Literary Archive (Archiwum Literackie) 151
literary modernism and psychoanalytic theory 172–174; *see also* experimental writing
lover's discourse (*Le discours amoureux*, Barthes) 35–36, 37, 58, 59n5
Lukacs, John 69, 70, 71, 87n4

Mahler, Gustav 3
The Man Moses and the Monotheist Religion (Freud) 3
Marcus, Laura 2
Marcuse, Herbert 26, 123, 126–128
Maria Komornicka/Piotr Odmieniec Włast; *see* Włast, Piotr Odmieniec
"Materials on the Life and Work of Maria Komornicka" 151
Medusa 139–140, 141
memoirs; *see* autobiography, memoirs
Mészáros, Judit 72, 87n6
modernism 2, 92, 101–105, 173–174; Central and Eastern Europe 2–5, 19–20, 118; dissociation as modernity response 101–105; literary 14–18, 15, 173; low-vs-high culture, distinction loss 15; plurality (cultural parataxis, paralaxis) 4–5; private–public sphere inseparability 15; psychoanalysis and 2–3; Viennese 2, 3–4
Moebius, Paul Julius 83, 158
Moll, Albert 81
Montaigne, Michel de 48–50, 51
Moravian spirit 124–125
Moreau-Ricaud, Michelle 72
mother analyst, mother-child continuum 180, 192–193, 195, 196, 198, 201–202n21, 212, 212–213, 228
mother figure, phallic mother 110, 133–134, 139–140
Müller, August 174, 184, 185
Muñoz, José Esteban 128
Musil, Robert 194
mutual analysis: concept 219; framework, development (Ferenczi, Severn) 22, 229, 231, 233n13, 241; vs one-person therapeutic approach (Freud) 207; origins: Freud–Ferenczi relationship 207–216; origins: Groddeck–Ferenczi discourse 207–216; patient-therapist relationship 28, 201n21, 210, 212, 224–225, 227, 230; as relational therapeutic method 207–208, 223–225, 230, 231; vs self-analysis 222

Näcke, Paul Adolf 81
narrative assemblage 1, 4–5, 10, 20, 242
neurosis, neurotic conflicts 52, 53, 54, 96, 112–113, 115–116, 125–126, 144
Nezval, Vítězslav 130
Nietzsche, Friedrich 27, 119nn3–4, 182–185, 186, 201n13, 221–222
nightmares 94, 101, 113–114, 115–117, 137
non-normative sexuality, sexological discourse 17, 68–88; autobiographic manifesto 19; bi-sexuality as innate human disposition (Weininger, Przybyszewski) 82–83; emancipation 81–82; empathetic turn: normative gaze vs engagement/naturalization 75, 76, 82, 84, 88n11, 169n10; Ferenczi 24, 69, 72–74, 76–78, 85, 86, 112–115; Freud-Fliess relationship, correspondence 23–24, 43, 44–46, 58; generation 1900 71; Hirschfeld, Magnus 72–73, 80–82, 84–85; Krafft-Ebing, Richard von 73, 78–81, 85; life writing, literary (Sándor (Sarolta) Vay) 77–78, 79, 156; modernist society as framework 68–71; patients' autobiographical, self-analytical description 77, 79–81; polyphonic writing as genre and source diversity 78; polyphonic writing in *Psychopathia Sexualis* (Krafft-Ebing) 78–81; third sex (Hirschfeld) 81–82; Włast, Piotr Odmieniec 150
Nyugat (West) 72, 93, 96, 104, 118–119n2

Ochorowicz, Julian 160–161
Oedipus / Oedipus complex 17–19, 53, 190, 213, 214, 220
"On the Part Played by Homosexuality in the Pathogenesis of Paranoia" (Ferenczi) 112–116
"On the Symbolism of Destruction" (Gross) 108–111
On Truth and Lies in a Nonmoral Sense (Nietzsche) 182–183
one-person psychology 53, 207; *see also* self-analysis
oral journal 220, 224, 231, 239
Oszacki, Aleksander 26, 156–160, 161–163; modernity as aggregates of subjectivism 159; psychological hermaphroditism (Freud vs Oszacki) 164–167; Włast psychographic essay 158–167

pathography 7–8
patients' narratives 68, 78, 80–81, 173–174, 210; as objective, face value 173; as unconscious processing 173–174
Pfister, Oskar 186
phallic mother 110, 133–134, 139–140
Picture of Dorian Gray (Wilde) 97, 98
Pigoń, Stanisław 156–160, 167, 168n5, 170n18

Plato 37, 61n16, 84, 182
Polish literary history 150–151, 160
Polish psychoanalysis tradition 26, 59n2, 168n4; anti-psychiatric discourse 26, 167, 168, 169n10; *see also* Oszacki, Aleksander
Pór, Bertalan 70, 76
pornophiles, pornophilic art 26, 126, 128, 129, 131, 137
Prince, Morton 94–95, 119n6, 229
Przybyszewski, Stanisław 83–84, 160–161
psychoanalysis, literary dimension: autobiografiction 15–16, 98, 194–199; case study as literary genre 73; dialogical nature 14–15; Freud about 10–11, 13–14; literary modernism 14–18, 20, 21, 24–26, 172–174, 185–186, 194–197, 198, 238 (*see also* Groddeck, Georg); Włast "materials" 151, 156–157, 158, 160, 167; psychoanalysis and literature/fiction, commonalities 10–11; Wittels, Fritz 11; *see also The Caliph Stork (A gólyakalifa)* (Babits)
psychoanalysis / psychoanalytic movement, development: cities of 3–4; diversification, decentralization 4–5; Freud, contribution, authority 38–41; knowledge transmission, personal dimension 38–39; modernist break / modernism and 1–3; plurality 4–5; as universal theory 2–3
psychoanalysis: as cultural practice / narrative assemblage 1, 10, 20, 242; as self-analysis 173, 214–216; relational model of 22, 28, 176, 199, 207, 224–225, 232, 236–239; set of therapeutic techniques 19; text–spoken word relationship 12–15, 35–36, 59n2, transmission, pre-1939 Czechoslovakia 122, 124–125, 145;
"Psychoanalysis of the dream and its pathological significance" (Ferenczi) 96
Psycho-Analytic Notes on an Autobiographical Account of a Case of Paranoia (Freud) 8, 26, 166
psychoanalytic theory and literary modernism 172–174
psychoanalytic writings, languages genres: genre experimentation, blurring 5, 15–16, 25, 173–174, 197–198, 200n5, 209–210, 237, 242; language dimensions (subjective–scientific parallelism) 6–10, 220–222; language plasticity 237; life writing 6, 8–10, 151, 156, 173, 194, 197, 198, 241; literary, fiction 2, 10–12; narrative assemblage 1, 4–5, 10, 20, 242; psycho-medical (*see* psycho-medical discourse); scientific, theoretical 2, 5
psychoanalytic discourse 41
psychography 7–8, 26, 28–29n3, 169n10, 237–238; *The Book of the It* (Groddeck) 27, 197; *The Caliph Stork* (*A gólykalifa*, Babits) 25, 118; concept 8; Freud on 7–8, 28–29n3; "From Pathography to Psychography" (Sadger) 7; as psychoanalytic genre 7, 8; self-psychography 118; Włast, Piotr (Maria Komornicka) 26, 156–157, 161–167, 237–238
The Psychological Automatism (Janet) 117
The Psychology of a Creative Individual (Przybyszewski) 138–139
psychological hermaphroditism 78, 82–84, 163–165, 164
psycho-medical literature/discourses 6, 68–69; case study 73; fin-de-siècle modernist turn 14, 19, 24; homosexuality 44, 45–46; non-normative sexuality 23, 66–88 (*see also under own heading*); polyphonic writing (*Psychopathia Sexualis*, Krafft-Ebing) 78–81; portraiture (Róza K, "Homosexualitas Feminina," Ferenczi) 73–78; psycho-medical portrait, "Homosexualitas Feminina" (Ferenczi) 73–76, 77, 78–79, 239
Psychopathia Sexualis (Krafft-Ebing), homosexuality 78–81, 100, 158–159, 163–164
psychosis 96, 113, 115–116, 144

Rabelais, François 186
Rank, Otto 98, 140–141, 147n8, 180, 192, 223
relational model, psychoanalysis 22, 28, 176, 199, 207, 224–225, 232, 236–239
relational writings 51
"Relics and Diaries" (Bernfeld) 10
Reynolds, Stephen 15–16
R.N. (Severn, Elizabeth); *see* Severn, Elizabeth (R.N.)
Roazen, Paul 57
Róza (Róbert) K., psycho-medical portraiture (Ferenczi) 73–76, 77, 78–79, 239
Rudnytsky, Peter L. 61n18, 87n5, 176, 200n10
Ruhs, August 13

Sacher-Masoch, Leopold von 158, 158–159, 169n11
Sadger, Isidor 7–8, 168n6, 190
Sándor (Sarolta) Vay 77–78, 79, 156
Saunders, Max 15–16, 194
Schächter, Miksa 72, 85
Schopenhauer, Arthur 83, 182
Schorske, Carl E. 1–3, 5
Schreber, Daniel Paul 26, 112, 152, 166–167, 168n2, 239
Schröter, Michael 57–58, 62nn32–34
scientia sexualis 19, 92, 142, 146
Sedgwick, Eve Kosofsky 43–44, 60n12, 200n3, 200n6
seduction theory (Freud) 207, 229, 232n3
self-analysis 10, 158; *Clinical Diary* as research diary 219–222; epistolary practice and theory formation (Freud) 18, 23–24, 41–47, 58, 62, 205–206, 213–214; inhibitions and 216–217; letters (Ferenczi, Groddeck) 213–215; and literary experimentalism (Groddeck) 194–198, 199; objections (Ferenczi, Groddeck) 213–216; patients' descriptions 80–81; Surrealist experiments 118, 122–123, 138; as writing practice (Freud) 51–55
Self-Impression: Life-writing, Autobiografiction, and the Forms of Modern Literature (Saunders) 194
Severn, Elizabeth 14, 28, 180, 206–208, 211, 222–225, 229–230, 238
"The Sex" (Przybyszewski) 83
Sex and Character (Weininger) 83–84, 152
sexuality; *see* gender, sexuality/non-normative sexuality
Shakespeare, William 45
Słowacki, Juliusz 159
The Soul Seeker (Groddeck) 27, 185–186, 210
"The Spider as a Dream Symbol" (Abraham) 133–134
Spielrein, Sabina 109, 118, 137
split personality; *see* dissociative personality disorder / dissociative identity
Spohr, Max 73
spoken journal 220, 224, 231, 239
Steiner, George 243
Stekel, Wilhelm 188, 217
Steuer, Daniel 83
Stevenson, Robert Louis 97–98
Storr, Anthony 240–242
The Story of the Caliph Stork (Hauff) 93–94, 97
Strindberg, August 104, 159
Štyrský, Jindřich: autoeroticism 144–145; Brouk collaboration 124; destruction and desire, linking 136–137; dream as self-analysis 138; dream diaries 25, 137–141, 141–142; *Emilie Comes to Me in a Dream* 126, 130, 134–136, 143–145; erotic works, Edition 69 series 25, 125–126; fetishization 136; humor and suffering 142–143; sexuality, psychoanalytic understanding through art 130–133, 134–135; "synthetism," artistic 137
substitute formation 56
Swoboda, Herman 56–57, 62nn28–29

Tábory, Elemér *see The Caliph Stork (A gólyakalifa)* (Babits)
Takács, J. 71
Tardieu, Ambroise 78
Teige, Karel 138–139, 146n3
text–spoken word relationship 12–15, 35–36, 59n2
A Thousand Plateaus (Deleuze, Guattari) 19
Three Essays on the Theory of Sexuality (Freud) 55, 73, 78, 164–165, 191
Totem and Taboo (Freud) 3, 144
trauma: castration 140–141; *The Discovery of the Self* (Severn) 115, 229–231; dreams and 115–117; modernity 117; neurosis 112–113, 115–116; theory (Ferenczi, Severn) 207, 222–230
The Trauma of Birth (Rank) 147n8, 176
Twilight of the Idols (Nietzsche) 184
two-person psychology 53, 207, 223; *see also* mutual analysis

Uranians, Uranism 73, 82, 84, 88n11

Vay, Sándor (Sarolta) 77–78, 79, 164
Vienna: fin-de-siècle Vienna, characteristics 3–4; psychoanalysis, development 3
Vienna Psychoanalytic Society 7, 11, 123
Viennese modernism 3–4
Vojvodík, Josef 122, 130, 137–138, 139, 140

Was muss das Volk vom dritten Geschlecht wissen! (*What People Should Know about the Third Sex*, Hirschfeld) 81–82
Weininger, Otto 56–57, 62nn28–29, 83–84, 152

Weltlein, Thomas 185–186, 238
Wilde, Oscar 97, 98
Will, Herbert 211
Williams, Bernard 201n13
Windholz, Emanuel 123
Wittels, Fritz 7, 11, 35
Włast, Piotr Odmieniec (Maria Komornicka), transgenderism 150–170; biographical background 150; *The Devils* as literary self-reflection 158–159, 162, 169n8; epistolographic self-reflection 154; *Forpoczty* (Vanguards) 150; gender transgression and institutional response 151–155; hermaphroditism (Freud vs Oszacki) 158–167; infantilism 160, 161–163, 165, 167; "Materials on the Life and Work of Maria Komornicka" (Pigoń) 151, 156–157; as modernist writer 150, 159–161; naming 155; Oszacki's psychographic essay 158–167; psycho-medical images of 156–157; self-articulation, medical narrative 152; self-articulation, violation and spiritual experience 152–155, 158–159, 162
Wolff, Larry 229
writer's block 193, 216–219

Yearning for Pure Love (Pór) 76
"The Young Ones" (Die Jungen) 2

Zarathustra (Nietzsche) 186
Zweigeschlechtlichkeit 54–55; *see also* bisexuality

For Product Safety Concerns and Information please contact our EU
representative GPSR@taylorandfrancis.com
Taylor & Francis Verlag GmbH, Kaufingerstraße 24, 80331 München, Germany

www.ingramcontent.com/pod-product-compliance
Ingram Content Group UK Ltd.
Pitfield, Milton Keynes, MK11 3LW, UK
UKHW021606250926
R4271200001B/R42712PG475702UKX00001B/1
9781032579757